Evidence Report/Technology Assessment
Number 70

Criteria for Determining Disability in Infants and Children: Low Birth Weight

Volume 2. Evidence Tables

Prepared for:
Agency for Healthcare Research and Quality
U.S. Department of Health and Human Services
2101 East Jefferson Street
Rockville, MD 20852
www.ahrq.gov

Contract No. 290-97-0019

Prepared by:
Tufts New England Medical Center EPC, Boston, MA

Principal Investigator
Cynthia Cole, MD, MPH

Investigators
Geoffrey Binney, MD, MPH
Patricia Casey, RNC, MS, NNP
John Fiascone, MD
James Hagadorn, MD
Chiwan Kim, MD

EPC Staff
Joseph Lau, MD, Director
Chenchen Wang, MD, MSc., Project Leader
Deirdre DeVine, M Litt, Project Manager
Kimberly Miller, BA, Research Assistant

AHRQ Publication No. 03-E010
December 2002

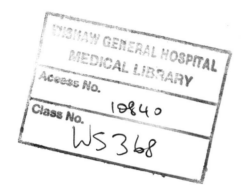

Contents

Evidence Tables

Criteria for Determining Disability in Infants and Children: Low Birth Weight

Evidence Tables

Evidence Table 1. Studies Evaluating Association of LBW and Multiple Outcomes: CNS, Eye, Lung, Growth, etc.

Part I

Author, Year UI#	Demographics	Inclusion Criteria	Exclusion Criteria	Disease/Condition Type (N)	Study Design (Duration)
Akerman 1992 93255928	Location: Sweden Years of Birth: ND Median GA (range), wk: 7 pairs < 37 wks Median BW (range), g: 37 < 2500 g (23 of these > 37 wks) Male: 46% Race: ND Enrolled: 35 parents who were expecting twins Evaluated: 68 (34 twin pairs) Number of sites: 1	ND (35 parents who were expecting twins)	ND (One child in a twin pair was stillborn)	Low born twins (68, or 34 pairs)	Prospective longitudinal cohort (at 9, 18 months, and 4 years)
Thompson 1993 93234177	Location: South African Years of Birth: 1988 to 1989 Mean GA (range), wk: 32±2.5 (26.8-40) Mean BW (range), g: 1044±149 (600-1250) Male: 50% Race: ND Enrolled: 143 Evaluated: 143 Number of sites: 1	BW <1250 g ventilated infants Survived to hospital discharge	Infants <900g and <28week are not routinely ventilated	VLBW ventilated infants (143)	Prospective cohort (2 years)
Rademaker 1994 95003452	Location: Netherlands Years of Birth: 9/1989-9/1992 Mean GA (range), wk: 25-32 Mean BW (range), g: 820-2200 Male: 70% Race: ND Enrolled: 20 Evaluated: 20 Number of sites: 1	GA ≤ 32 weeks Unilateral parenchymal involvement on cranial ultrasound associated with GLH Germinal layer hemorrhage or IVH	ND	Preterm infants (GA 32 weeks or less) with diagnosis of unilateral parenchymal involvement (20)	Prospective cohort

3

Evidence Table 1. Studies Evaluating Association of LBW and Multiple Outcomes: CNS, Eye, Lung, Growth, etc.
Part I

Author, Year UI#	Demographics	Inclusion Criteria	Exclusion Criteria	Disease/Condition Type (N)	Study Design (Duration)
Vonderveid 1994 94297368	Location: Italy Years of Birth: 1987-1988 Mean GA: ND Mean BW : ND (only range: 500-1499 g) Male: ND Race: ND Enrolled: 634 Evaluated: 390 (alive at 2 yrs) Number of sites: 8	All newborns with BW: 500-1500 g BW Admitted in one of the 8 participating NICUs Born between 1/1987-12/1988	ND	Sample 1: VLBW (500-1000 g): (191) Sample 2: LBW (1000-1499f): (443)	Prospective cohort study (24 mo CA)

4

Evidence Table 1. Studies Evaluating Association of LBW and Multiple Outcomes: CNS, Eye, Lung, Growth, etc.
Part I

Author, Year UI#	Demographics	Inclusion Criteria	Exclusion Criteria	Disease/Condition Type (N)	Study Design (Duration)

Kraybill 1995 95264242	Location: USA
	Years of Birth: 1986-1989
	Sample with F/up at 1 year
	Mean GA:
	Sample 1: 28.2 ±1.9
	Sample 2: 28.1 ±2.0
	Mean BW:
	Sample 1: 1022 ±177
	Sample 2: 1028 ±184
	Male:
	Sample 1: 51% Sample 2: 52%
	Race:
	Sample 1: White: 21%, Black: 53%, Hispanic: 23%, Other: 4%
	Sample 2: White: 34%, Black: 42%, Hispanic: 22%, Other: 2%
	Enrolled: 323 (survivors at 1 yr)
	Evaluated: 258 (at 1 yr f/up)
	Sample with F/up at 2 years
	Mean GA: Sample 1: 28.3 ±1.8
	                   Sample 2: 28.1 ±1.8
	Mean BW: Sample 1: 1043 ±165
	               Sample 2: 1005 ±184
	Male:
	Sample 1: 49% Sample 2: 43%
	Race:
	Sample 1: White: 35%, Black: 60%, Other:5%
	Sample 2: White: 43%, Black: 54%, Other: 3%
	Enrolled: 136 (survivors at 2 yrs)
	Evaluated: 118
	Number of sites: 2
		Premature VLBW:
		700-1350 g
		(Detailed description available in another article)
			ND	At 1 yr f/up
				Sample 1:
				Synthetic Surfactant at
				Birth via ET tube: 5 ml/kg (136)
				
				Sample 2:
				Air placebo via ET tube at birth (122)
				
				At 2 yr F/up
				Sample 1:
				Synthetic surfactant at birth (57)
				
				Sample 2:
				Air placebo (61)
					Randomized placebo-controlled double blind trial
					(at 1 year and at 2 years CA)

5

Evidence Table 1. Studies Evaluating Association of LBW and Multiple Outcomes: CNS, Eye, Lung, Growth, etc. Part I

Author, Year UI#	Demographics	Inclusion Criteria	Exclusion Criteria	Disease/Condition Type (N)	Study Design (Duration)

Speechley 1995 96356544	Location: Canada
	Years of Birth: 1978-1980
	Mean GA:
	  Sample 1: 37 (28-43)
	  Sample 2: 40 (37-44)
	Mean BW:
	  Sample 1: 2790 (850-4550)
	  Sample 2: 3503 (2660-5170)
	Male:
	  Sample 1: 56%
	  Sample 2: 50%
	Race:
	  Sample 1: whites : 90%
	  Sample 2: whites: 90%
	(Original study: was a randomized interventional study of having a family volunteer visit the home on a regular base for 6 months)
	Eligible (for the original study): 828
	Enrolled (for the original RCT): 312
	Evaluated (at 12 yrs): 253
	Number of sites: 1
		All infants born at a tertiary care hospital in Ontario
		Born between 1978-1980
		Transferred to NICU or Normal Neonatal Nursery (NNN)
			Family residence more than 120 Km from hospital
			Newborn's survival was in question
			Language barrier
			Refused to participate to the original RCT.
				Sample 1:
				Former NICU graduates: [116]
				
				Sample 2:
				Former NNN graduates [137]
					Prospective, longitudinal, comparative, observational study
					(12 yrs)

6

Evidence Table 1. Studies Evaluating Association of LBW and Multiple Outcomes: CNS, Eye, Lung, Growth, etc.
Part I

Author, Year UI#	Demographics	Inclusion Criteria	Exclusion Criteria	Disease/Condition Type (N)	Study Design (Duration)
Hack 1996 97060805	Location: US Years of Birth: 1/1977 to 12/1979 Mean GA (range), wk: 30±2 Mean BW (range), g: 1177±218 Male: ND Race: Mother black race 56% Enrolled: 249 Evaluated: 249 (363 controls) Number of sites: 1	VLBW infants, BW <1500gm, survived to 2 years of age NBW: randomly selected NBW children (the selection method was described in the prior papers)	ND	VLBW infants (249) Sample 1: AGA (199) Sample 2: SGA (50) NBW infants: (363)	Prospective cohort (8 years)

Hack 1996 97066007	Location: US
	Years of Birth: 7/1982-6/1988, 1/1990-12/1992
	Mean GA (range), wk:
	  Sample 1: 25.9±2 (22-31)
	  Sample 2: 25.7±2 (22-31)
	Mean BW (range), g:
	  Sample 1: 688.6±73 (560-740)
	  Sample 2: 670.6±56 (502-742)
	Male:
	  Sample 1: 28%
	  Sample 2: 29%
	Race: White
	  Sample 1: 31%
	  Sample 2: 37%
	Enrolled: 280
	Evaluated: 280
	Number of sites: 1
		BW 500-759 g
		Survived to 20 months corrected Age
			ND	Sample 1: VLBW survived infants born in 1990-1992 (surfactant/dex era) (114)
				Sample 2: VLBW survived infants born in 1982-1988 (surfactant and less dex. era) (166)
					Prospective cohort (followed to 20 months corrected age)

7

Evidence Table 1. Studies Evaluating Association of LBW and Multiple Outcomes: CNS, Eye, Lung, Growth, etc.
Part I

Author, Year UI#	Demographics	Inclusion Criteria	Exclusion Criteria	Disease/Condition Type (N)	Study Design (Duration)
Northern Neonatal Nursing Initiative Trial Group 1996 96304894	Location: UK Years of Birth: 1990-1992 Mean GA (range), wk: 29 (27-31) Mean BW (range), g: 1253 (965-1543) Male: 39% Race: ND Enrolled: 776 Evaluated: 776 Number of sites: 16	GA <32 weeks; resident in northern UK	ND	Experiment 1: fresh frozen plasma treatment (257) Experiment 2: gelatin plasma substitute (261) Glucose controls (258)	Randomized controlled trial (2 years)
Sethi 1996 96334245	Location: UK Years of Birth: 1989-1992 Mean GA (range), wk: ND Mean BW (range), g: ND Male: ND Race: ND SES: ND Enrolled: 93 Evaluated: 92 Number of sites: 1	Liveborn infants BW <1501 g Survived until discharged	ND	VLBW infants 92	Prospective cohort (2 years)
Wilkinson 1996 97087405	Location: Australia Years of Birth: 1/1989-12/1991 Mean GA (range), wk: 27.7 (23-34) Mean BW (range), g: 1144 (700-1725) Male: 50% Race: ND Enrolled: 12 Evaluated: 10 Number of sites: 1	All NICU admissions <35 weeks GA or BW<1500g who had cranial US with cystic PVL	ND	VLBW preterm infants (10)	Retrospective cohort

8

Evidence Table 1. Studies Evaluating Association of LBW and Multiple Outcomes: CNS, Eye, Lung, Growth, etc.

Part I

Author, Year UI#	Demographics	Inclusion Criteria	Exclusion Criteria	Disease/Condition Type (N)	Study Design (Duration)

DeReginer 1997 98041177	Location: US
	Years of Birth: 1987-1991
	Mean GA (range), wk:
	  Sample 1: 28.0±1.5
	  Sample 2: 27.1±1.2
	  Sample 3: 27.5±1.7
	Mean BW (range), g:
	  Sample 1: 1030±140
	  Sample 2: 1007±122
	  Sample 3: 1007±140
	Male: ND
	Race: ND
	Enrolled: 174
	Evaluated: 164
	Number of sites: 2
		BW ≤1500 g survived until
		Discharged
		Able to match to a patient in other
		  two respiratory groups
			Presence of LBW independent of chronic lung disease known to adversely affect neurodevelopment, sensory, or growth, i.e. severe intracranial abnormalities, congenital anomalies or viral infections, etc.
			Unable to match to a patient in other groups
			Died after discharged (6)
			Lost to follow-up (4)
				Sample 1:
				No chronic lung disease (58)
				
				Sample 2:
				Mild chronic lung disease (58)
				
				Sample 3:
				Severe chronic lung disease (58)
					Retrospective chart review with marched subject group
					(1 year of adjusted age)

Dezoete 1997 97359687	Location: New Zealand Years of Birth: 1990-1992 Mean GA (range), wk: 26.7±1.9 Mean BW (range), g: 834.6±120.0 Male: 51% Race: European 63%, Maori 20%, Other 22% SGA: 32% Enrolled: 110 Evaluated: 105 Number of sites: 1	BW<1000g and survived to hospital discharge.	Died after discharge Congenital malformations Lost to follow-up	VLBW infants (105)	Prospective cohort (18 months)

9

Evidence Table 1. Studies Evaluating Association of LBW and Multiple Outcomes: CNS, Eye, Lung, Growth, etc.
Part I

Author, Year UI#	Demographics	Inclusion Criteria	Exclusion Criteria	Disease/Condition Type (N)	Study Design (Duration)
O'Shea 1997 98049056 *overlapped sample with 98190123	Location: US Years of Birth: 1979-1994 Mean GA (range), wk: Sample 1: 25 (22-31) Sample 2: 25 (22-30) Sample 3: 25 (22-29) Mean BW (range), g: Sample 1: 673 (522-790) Sample 2: 670 (527-800) Sample 3: 688 (520-793) Male: Sample 1: 49% Sample 2: 51% Sample 3: 48% Race: White Sample 1: 61% Sample 2: 60% Sample 3: 56% Enrolled: 513 Evaluated: 513 → 216 (1 year of age) Number of sites: 2	BW 501-800g Born to mother's residing in 17 countries in NW N.Carolina Survived to 1 year of age	ND	Sample 1: VLBW infants born between 7/1/1979 and 6/30/1984 (120 → 24) Sample 2: VLBW infants born between 7/1/1984 and 6/30/1989 (175 → 63) Sample 3: VLBW infants born between 7/1/1984 and 6/30/1994 (218 → 129)	Retrospective cohort (1 year corrected age)

Evidence Table 1. Studies Evaluating Association of LBW and Multiple Outcomes: CNS, Eye, Lung, Growth, etc.

Part I

Author, Year UI#	Demographics	Inclusion Criteria	Exclusion Criteria	Disease/Condition Type (N)	Study Design (Duration)
Piecuch 1997 97456215	Location: US Years of Birth: 1979-1991 Median GA (range), wk: Sample 1: 25.9±1.5 (24-29) Sample 2: 25.8±1.6 (24-32) Sample 3: 26.3±1.5 (24-32) Sample 4: 27.1±1.4 (24-34) Sample 5: 27.8±1.7 (25-35) Mean BW (range), g: Sample 1: 560±28 Sample 2: 653±28 Sample 3: 747±29 Sample 4: 850±29 Sample 5: 942±30 Male: Sample 1: 25% Sample 2: 24% Sample 3: 48% Sample 4: 47% Sample 5: 48% Race: ND Enrolled: 518 Evaluated: 445 Number of sites: 2	BW<1000g Discharged from Mt. Zion Hospital + M.C. & UCSF	Genetic diagnosis {Died after discharge (14) Lost to follow-up (58) Late genetic diagnosis (1)}	Sample 1: BW 500-599 (15) Sample 2: BW 600-699 (38) Sample 3: BW 700-799 (92) Sample 4: BW 800-899 (135) Sample 5: BW 900-999 (165)	Prospective cohort (1 year)

11

Evidence Table 1. Studies Evaluating Association of LBW and Multiple Outcomes: CNS, Eye, Lung, Growth, etc.
Part I

Author, Year UI#	Demographics	Inclusion Criteria	Exclusion Criteria	Disease/Condition Type (N)	Study Design (Duration)
Piecuch 1997 98012134	Location: US Years of Birth: 1990-1994 Mean GA (range), wk: Sample 1: 24 Sample 2: 25 Sample 3: 26 Mean BW (range), g: Sample 1: 668±91 (450-850) Sample 2: 790±115 (550-1000) Sample 3: 842±158 (505-1260) Male: Sample 1: 50% Sample 2: 73% Sample 3: 50% Race: ND SES: high social risk Sample 1: 89% Sample 2: 43% Sample 3: 68% Enrolled: 94 Evaluated: 86 Number of sites: 1	24, 25 or 26 week GA Non-anomalous Born at University of California, San Francisco	ND (Died after discharge (2) Accidental severe central nervous system insult after discharge (1) Lost to follow-up (5)}	Sample 1: GA 24 weeks (18) Sample 2: GA 25 weeks (30) Sample 3: GA 26 weeks (38)	Prospective cohort (at 12months, 18 months, 2 ½ years, 4 ½ years. 7-8 years)

Evidence Table 1. Studies Evaluating Association of LBW and Multiple Outcomes: CNS, Eye, Lung, Growth, etc.

Part I

Author, Year UI#	Demographics	Inclusion Criteria	Exclusion Criteria	Disease/Condition Type (N)	Study Design (Duration)

Singer 1997 98049057
 	
Singer 2001 21163669
	Location: US
	Years of Birth: 1989-1991
	Mean GA (range), wk:
	  Sample 1: 27±2
	  Sample 2: 30±2
	  Controls: 40±2
	Mean BW (range), g:
	  Sample 1: 956±248
	  Sample 2: 1252±178
	  Controls: 3451±526
	Male:
	  Sample 1: 52%
	  Sample 2: 43%
	  Controls: 50%
	Race: White
	  Sample 1: 55%
	  Sample 2: 48%
	  Controls: 51%
	SES: Hollingshed classification:
	  Sample 1: 3.5±1
	  Sample 2: 3.6±1
	  Controls: 3.6±1
	Enrolled: 464
	Evaluated: 206 (123 controls)
	Number of sites: 3
		Cases (sample 1&2): premature infants, BW < 1500g
		Controls: term infants with no diagnosed medical illness or abnormalities at birth, >36 weeks, GW>2500g
			Major congenital abnormality
			Drug exposure
			Maternal illness
			HIV
			Maternal mental retardation
			>2 hours driving time from hospital
				Sample 1: VLBW infants with BPD infants (122)
				Sample 2: VLBW without BPD (84)
				Sample 3: Full term infants (123)
					Prospective cohort (followed to 3 years corrected age)

13

Evidence Table 1. Studies Evaluating Association of LBW and Multiple Outcomes: CNS, Eye, Lung, Growth, etc.
Part I

Author, Year UI#	Demographics	Inclusion Criteria	Exclusion Criteria	Disease/Condition Type (N)	Study Design (Duration)
Victorian Infant Collaborative study Group, 1997 98026322 *This study is also in CNS table	Location: Australia Years of Birth: 1979-80, 1985-87, 1991-92 Mean GA (range), wk: ND Mean BW (range), g: ND Male: ND Race: ND Enrolled: 453 (242 controls) Evaluated: 448 (242) Number of sites: 3	ELBW infant (Sample 1-3ts, BW 500-999 g born in Victoria, Australia survived to age of 2 years Controls: Normal birth weight (>2499 g) infants born in 1991-1992	Excluded infants born in 1979-1980 for current review	ELBW infants (448): Sample 1: born in 1985-1987 (212) Sample 2: born in 1991-1992 (241) Controls: Normal BW (>2499 g) infants (242)	Retrospective cohort (2 years)
Victorian Infant Collaborative study Group, 1997 97466059	Location: Australia Years of Birth: 1979-80, 1985-87, 1991-92 Mean GA (range), wk: ND Mean BW (range), g: ND Male: ND Race: ND Enrolled: 36 Evaluated: 35 Number of sites: 3	ELBW infants, BW 500-999 g born outside the level III perinatal centers in Victoria, Australia survived to age of 2 years	Excluded infants born in 1979-1980 for current review	ELBW infants (36): Sample 1: born in 1985-1987 (19) Sample 2: born in 1991-1992 (16)	Retrospective cohort (2 years)
Cheung 1998 99059896	Location: Canada Years of Birth: 12/93-10/97 Mean GA (range), wk: 25 (24-30) Median BW (range), g: 860 (340-1460) Male: 67% Race: ND Enrolled: 24 Evaluated: 10 Number of sites: 1	VLBW survivors, BW < 1500 g, Requiring inhaled nitrous oxide (INO) (continues to be hypoxenic) at >90% O_2 and MAP 15 ± 2)	Mosaic trisomy 18 Potter's syndrome Survived to 1 year of chronological age	VLBW infants treated with INO (10)	Prospective cohort

14

Evidence Table 1. Studies Evaluating Association of LBW and Multiple Outcomes: CNS, Eye, Lung, Growth, etc.

Part I

Author, Year UI#	Demographics	Inclusion Criteria	Exclusion Criteria	Disease/Condition Type (N)	Study Design (Duration)
Finnström 1998 99041345	Location: Sweden Years of Birth: 1990-1992 Mean GA (range), wk: ND Mean BW (range), g: 798±144 Male: ND Race: ND Enrolled: 370 Evaluated: 362 Number of sites: ND	BW ≤ 1000 g and GA ≥ 23 weeks Survived to the age of 1 year	ND	Preterm infants (362)	Prospective cohort of a previously published study (followed to the median corrected age of 36 months)
Gregoire 1998 98232532	Location: Canada Years of Birth: 1987-1992 Mean GA (range), wk: Sample 1: 27.3±1.1 Sample 2: 26.8±1.3 Comparison: 27.9±0.8 Mean BW (range), g: Sample 1: 997±195 Sample 2: 930±178 Comparison: 1129±181 Male: Sample 1: 45% Sample 2: 56% Comparison: 45% Race: ND Enrolled: 217 Evaluated: 217 Number of sites: 1	Inborn infants GA 24-28 weeks, Admitted to NICU Survival to 18 months CA	ND	Sample 1: BPD-1 group – preterm infants who received O_2 at 28 days but not at 396 weeks' GA (48) Sample 2: BPD-2 group – preterm infants with oxygen dependency at 36 weeks' GA (93) Comparison: preterm infants who were not oxygen-dependent at 28 days of age (76)	Prospective cohort (18.5±1.1 months)

Evidence Table 1. Studies Evaluating Association of LBW and Multiple Outcomes: CNS, Eye, Lung, Growth, etc.
Part I

Author, Year UI#	Demographics	Inclusion Criteria	Exclusion Criteria	Disease/Condition Type (N)	Study Design (Duration)

Kurkinen-Raty 1998 98387235
 	
(All+Lung)
 	
*sample from the same big population as 20284814
	Location: Finland
	Years of Birth: 1990-1996
	Mean GA (range), wk:
	  Cases: 28.2 (23.8- 37.2)
	  Controls: 28.4 (22.9-36.9)
	Mean BW (range), g:
	  Cases: 1138.3±434
	  Controls: 1272.4±547.2
	Male: ND
	Race: ND
	Enrolled: 78 (78 controls)
	Evaluated: 78 (78)
	Number of sites: 1
		Preterm PROM between 17-30 weeks gestation; singleton; delivered > 2 hr after rupture
		Controls: preterm no PROM; spontaneous preterm delivery matched for GA and year of delivery.
			Rupture unconfirmed or transient	Sample 2: Preterm rupture (78)
				Sample 2: Preterm delivery no rupture (78)
					Retrospective cohort

16

Evidence Table 1. Studies Evaluating Association of LBW and Multiple Outcomes: CNS, Eye, Lung, Growth, etc.

Part I

Author, Year UI#	Demographics	Inclusion Criteria	Exclusion Criteria	Disease/Condition Type (N)	Study Design (Duration)
Lee 1998 98442293	Location: Canada Years of Birth: 1990-1995 Mean GA: ND Mean BW: Sample 1: 763 ±157 Sample 2: 807±176 Male: ND Race: ND Enrolled: ND (total N not given, data only for enrolled cases with candidemia: N= 29) Evaluated: 50 Assessed for outcome: 35 (14 cases and 21 controls) Number of sites: 2	For cases: Prematures with BW<1250 g Admitted in the NICU s of UAH and RAH from 1990-1995 Diagnosis of candidemia: by at least one positive blood culture Diagnosis of candidal meningitis: By isolation of candida in the CSF or >45x10 ^{6} WBCs in the CSF and candidemia. For controls: Prematures with BW <1250 g Admitted to the same NICUs during the same period without candidal infection	Neonates with major congenital anomalies	Sample 1: Premature infants <1250 with candidemia and/ or candida meningitis (25) Sample 2: Premature neonates with BW <1250 matched with cases for BW, GA, sex and admission dates, without candidal infection (25)	Retrospective longitudinal comparative study with case control design and cases defined based on exposure to candidemia and matched controls (f/up between 37 and 70 mo CA) Average age at assessment: for cases :31 ±19 mo, and for controls: 28 ±20 mo
Lefebvre 1998 98387703	Location: Canada Years of Birth: 1987-1992 Mean GA (range), wk: 27.0±1.2 Mean BW (range), g: 961±179 (585-1450) Male: 52% Race: ND Enrolled: 139 Evaluated: 121 Number of sites: 1	GA<28 weeks 3 or more cranial ultrasounds Survival to discharge	ND	Preterm infants (121): Low risk (50) Moderate risk (37) High risk (34)	Prospective cohort (CA 18.6±1.2 [17-19] months)

17

Evidence Table 1. Studies Evaluating Association of LBW and Multiple Outcomes: CNS, Eye, Lung, Growth, etc.
Part I

Author, Year UI#	Demographics	Inclusion Criteria	Exclusion Criteria	Disease/Condition Type (N)	Study Design (Duration)
Millet 1998 98212544	Location: France Years of Birth: ND Mean GA (range), wk: 31±3 (25-36) Mean BW (range), g: 1243±400 Male: 75% Race: ND Enrolled: 60 Evaluated: 40 (20 controls) Number of sites: 1	Neonates considered at risk of neurologic impairment	Severe neurologic abnormalities (HIE, PVL, brain malformations and congruental infections)	Premature infants (40) Term infants (20)	Prospective cohort (3-6 months correlated age)

Evidence Table 1. Studies Evaluating Association of LBW and Multiple Outcomes: CNS, Eye, Lung, Growth, etc.

Part I

Author, Year UI#	Demographics	Inclusion Criteria	Exclusion Criteria	Disease/Condition Type (N)	Study Design (Duration)

Piecuch 1998 98446413	Location: USA
	Years of Birth:
	  Sample 1: 1989-1991
	  Sample 2: 1984-1986
	  Sample 3: 1979-1981
	Mean GA:
	  Sample 1: 29 ±2
	  Sample 2: 30 ±2
	  Sample 3: 30 ±2
	Mean BW:
	  Sample 1: 1221 ±142
	  Sample 2: 1235 ±140
	  Sample 3: 1246 ±146
	Male:
	  Sample 1: 56%
	  Sample 2: 50%
	  Sample 3: 46%
	Race: ND
	Enrolled: 563
	Evaluated: 450
	Number of sites: 4
		Prematurity
		BW: 1000-1499 g
		Discharged from NICUs of 5 Hospitals
		Born in one of the three time periods:
		1989-1991 (Recent)
		1984-1986 (Middle)
		1979-1981 (Early)
			Congenital anomalies	Comparison of the outcome of infants 1000-1499 g born in three time periods:
				Most recently born
				Born at a middle period
				Born at an early period
				
				Sample 1:
				Born most recently, between 1989-1991 (186)
				
				Sample 2:
				Born in a middle period, between: 1984-1986 (155)
				
				Sample 3:
				Born in an early period, between 1979-1981 (109)
					(Not clearly stated)
					Retrospective longitudinal comparative cohort study
					
					Age for outcome assessment was not specified. It could be done up to 7.5-8 yrs of age
					
					(Mean ages of f/up were: 24, 54, 75 mo for the 3 periods)

19

Evidence Table 1. Studies Evaluating Association of LBW and Multiple Outcomes: CNS, Eye, Lung, Growth, etc.

Part I

Author, Year UI#	Demographics	Inclusion Criteria	Exclusion Criteria	Disease/Condition Type (N)	Study Design (Duration)

Sajaniemi 1998 99041674	Location: Finland
	Years of Birth: 1989-1991
	Mean GA:
	  Sample 1: 28.9 (23-35)
	  Sample 2: 39.4 (36-43)
	Mean BW:
	  Sample 1: 1205 (560-2360)
	  Sample 2: 3461 (2510-5360)
	Male: ND
	Race: ND
	Enrolled: ND
	Evaluated : 160
	Number of sites: 1
		For Preterm Group (sample 1):
		GA: 23-34 wks
		Mother being referred to University Central Hospital of Helsinki for threatened preterm delivery
		Born between 1989-1991
		
		For Full term group (Sample 2):
		Born in Metropolitan Helsinki
		Visiting pediatric services in Helsinki for acute infectious diseases
			For Preterm group
			If mothers had chorioamnionitis
			If mother had insulin dependent diabetes
			Children with congenital anomalies, by U/S
			
			For Full term group
			Chronic diseases
			Developmental delay
				Sample 1:
				Preterm infants (80)
				
				Sample 2
				Full term enrolled at: 20-28 mo of age (80)
					Retrospective comparative study (24 mo CA)

Scherjon 1998 98429216	Location: Netherlands Years of Birth: 1989 Mean GA: ND [median and range given: 30.4 (26.1-32.8)] Mean BW: ND (median and range given: 1295 (605-2295)] Male: ND Race: ND Enrolled: 106 Evaluated: 96 (at 3 yrs) Number of sites: 1	Pregnant mother admitted to Obstetric Department of Amsterdam university with threatened preterm delivery GA < 33 wks. Admitted during a 10 month period in 1989	Pregnancies with known congenital or chromosomal anomalies	Infants born prematurely between 26-33 wks (96)	Prospective observational cohort study (3 yrs CA)

20

Evidence Table 1. Studies Evaluating Association of LBW and Multiple Outcomes: CNS, Eye, Lung, Growth, etc.

Part I

Author, Year UI#	Demographics	Inclusion Criteria	Exclusion Criteria	Disease/Condition Type (N)	Study Design (Duration)
Cheung 1999 99146391	Location: Canada Years of Birth: 1990-1993 Mean GA (range), wk: Sample 1: 25 (22-29) Sample 2: 26 (24-30) Sample 3: 28 (23-32) Mean BW (range), g: Sample 1: 660±56 Sample 2: 873±73 Sample 3: 1127±71 Male: total 57% Race: ND Enrolled: 187 Evaluated: 164 Number of sites: 2	BW<1250 gm GA < 32 weeks Mild or no significant respiratory disease (O_2 < 30%, RR < 70)	Major congenital abnormalities, syndromes Infants with neurologic insult after discharge from NICU.	Sample 1: BW 500-749 g (26) Sample 2: BW 750-999 g (63) Sample 3: BW 1000-1249 g (75)	Prospective cohort (followed to 24 months adjusted age)
Duvanel 1999 99207097	Location: Switzerland Years of Birth: 1982-1990 Mean GA: Sample 1: 31.9 ±2.1 Sample 2: 31.9 ±1.7 Mean BW (range) Sample 1:1142 ±285 Sample 2: 1186 ±229 Male: Sample 1: 47% Sample 2: 57% Race: ND Enrolled: : ND Evaluated: 85 Number of sites: 1	Prematurity (< 34 weeks GA) SGA (BW < 10% percentile) Cases: hypoglycemia: glucose level < 47 mg/dl Controls-matched: (not specified for which parameters): blood glucose > 47 mg/dl	Major malformations Metabolic diseases Periventricular leukomalacia Grade IV cerebral hemorrhage Psychiatric illness detected in follow up study Very low socioeconomic status	Sample 1 Hypoglycemic (62) Sample 2: Euglycemic (23)	Retrospective longitudinal cohort study with case control design. Cases defined based on exposure. Control group matched with cases (not specified for which parameters)

21

Evidence Table 1. Studies Evaluating Association of LBW and Multiple Outcomes: CNS, Eye, Lung, Growth, etc. Part I

Author, Year UI#	Demographics	Inclusion Criteria	Exclusion Criteria	Disease/Condition Type (N)	Study Design (Duration)
Pennefather, 1999 20002011 Pennefather, 2000 20217908 * This study is also in eye table	Location: UK Years of Birth: 1/1/90-12/31/91 Mean GA (range), wk: ND Mean BW (range), g: ND Male: ND Race: ND Enrolled: 566 Evaluated: 558 Number of sites: ND	All surviving children <32wk GA born in geographically deprived region in Northern UK Survived to 2 years old	No examined at age 2 years old	Preterm infants (558)	Prospective cohort and retrospective review of patient records (2-3 years)
Ambalavanan 2000 21031370	Location: US Years of Birth: 1/1990 to 12/1994 Mean GA (range), wk: 26±2 Mean BW (range), g: 829±123 Male: 45% Race: African-American 66% Enrolled: 218 Evaluated: 218 Number of sites: 1	ELBW infants, BW <1000 g	ND	ELBW infants (218)	Retrospective cohort (followed to 18 months of age)
Cioni 2000 20150341	Location: Italy Years of Birth: 1/1989 to 2/1994 Mean GA (range), wk: 31±2.8 (24-36) Median BW (range), g: ND Male: ND Race: ND Enrolled: 29 Evaluated: 29 Number of sites: 1	All premature newborns with brain lesions on HUS who have abnormal neurological exam at term who are enrolled in neonatal follow-up study	Severe ROP (≥ stage 3), major refraction problems, and optic nerve atrophy, and infants with "congenital diseases"	All premature newborns with brain lesions who have abnormal neuro-logical exam at term (29)	Prospective cohort (1 yr [8-16 months] and 3 years [30-47 months])

Evidence Table 1. Studies Evaluating Association of LBW and Multiple Outcomes: CNS, Eye, Lung, Growth, etc.
Part I

Author, Year UI#	Demographics	Inclusion Criteria	Exclusion Criteria	Disease/Condition Type (N)	Study Design (Duration)
Hack 2000 20358826	Location: US Years of Birth:: 1/1/1992-2/31/1995 Mean GA (range), wk: 26.4±1.8 Mean BW (range), g: 813±125 Male: 43% Race: ND Enrolled: 333 Evaluated: 221 Number of sites: 1	BW<1000g	Major congenital malformations	VLBW infants (221)	Prospective cohort
Jankov 2000 20188680	Location: Canada Years of Birth: 1990-1996 Mean GA (range), wk: Sample 1: 23 (20-28) Sample 2: 25 (23-33) Mean BW (range), g: Sample 1: 669 (400-750) Sample 2: 515 (255-745) Male: Sample 1: 51% Sample 2: 46% Race: ND Enrolled: 281 Evaluated: 269 Number of sites: 1	Infants ≤ 750 g and GA ≥ 20 weeks who received CPR in the delivery room	Charts were not available for review (5) Major congenital abnormalities (4) Those infants not intubated in the delivery room (3)	Sample 1: Resuscitated (198) Sample 2: Non-resuscitated (71)	Retrospective cohort

23

Evidence Table 1. Studies Evaluating Association of LBW and Multiple Outcomes: CNS, Eye, Lung, Growth, etc. Part I

Author, Year UI#	Demographics	Inclusion Criteria	Exclusion Criteria	Disease/Condition Type (N)	Study Design (Duration)
Kurkinen-Raty, 2000 20284814 ***sample from the same big population as 98197235**	Location: Finland Years of Birth: 1990-1997 Mean GA (range), wk: Cases: 30.5±2.1 Controls: 30.4±2.1 Mean BW (range), g: Cases: 1294±469 Controls: 1605±427 Male: ND Race: ND Enrolled: 103 (103 controls) Evaluated: 103 (103) Number of sites: 1	Cesarean delivered singleton, GA 24-33 weeks Controls: spontaneous delivered singleton after regular contractions and/or preterm rupture of the membranes no more than 24 hrs before. The mothers were matched one-to-one by gestational age at delivery plu7s or mines 1 week.	ND	Sample 1: Indicated preterm (i.e., preterm birth 'indicated' for maternal/fetal reasons)(103) Sample 2: Spontaneous preterm delivery due to preterm labor (103)	Retrospective cohort

24

Evidence Table 1. Studies Evaluating Association of LBW and Multiple Outcomes: CNS, Eye, Lung, Growth, etc.
Part I

Author, Year UI#	Demographics	Inclusion Criteria	Exclusion Criteria	Disease/Condition Type (N)	Study Design (Duration)
Marlow 2000 20150342	Location: UK Years of Birth: 1990-1994 Mean GA: ND (Median and Range) Sample 1: 28 (26-31) Sample 2: 28 (26-31) Mean BW: ND (Median and range) Sample 1: 960 (600-2914) Sample 2: 1026 (410-2814) Male: ND Race: ND Enrolled: 27 Evaluated: 15 Number of sites: 1	For sensorineural hearing loss (SNHL) group GA: <33 wks Family resident of Greater Bristol area Records at Hearing Assessment Center of Royal Hospital for Sick children. Born during 1990-1994 Diagnosis of SNHL of 50 dB For control group: Matched controls 2:1 to cases Admitted to the same NICUs as cases Matched for sex and GA and next and preceding matching children in the admission books of St Michael's and Sothmead hospitals	ND	Sample 1: SNHL group [15] Sample 2: Control group [30] Matched with cases for sex, GA, admission dates in NICU	Retrospective case control study with a longitudinal component (unclear if retrospective or prospective) (12 mo CA)

Evidence Table 1. Studies Evaluating Association of LBW and Multiple Outcomes: CNS, Eye, Lung, Growth, etc. Part I

Author, Year UI#	Demographics	Inclusion Criteria	Exclusion Criteria	Disease/Condition Type (N)	Study Design (Duration)
Victorian Infant Collaborative study Group, 2000 20307288 *some subjects overlapped with Doyle, 2001	Location: Australia Years of Birth: 1991-92 Mean GA (range), wk: Sample 1: 25.5±1.3 Sample 2: 27.3±1.9 Mean BW (range), g: Sample 1: 797±147 Sample 2: 932±149 Male: Sample 1: 61.2% Sample 2: 39.5% Race: ND Enrolled: 346 Evaluated: 346 Number of sites: 4	BW<1000 or GA<28 consecutive births, survived to 5 years of age	ND	Preterm infants (120): Sample 1: infants treated with corticosteroids Sample 2: infants not treated with corticosteroids (226)	Non-randomized comparison trial (5 years)
Wood 2000 20373840	Location: UK and Ireland Years of Birth: 1995-1996 Mean GA (range), wk: 22-25 Mean BW (range), g: ND Male: ND Race: ND Enrolled: 314 Evaluated: 283 Number of sites: 276	GA 20-25 weeks survivors	ND	Preterm infants (283)	Prospective cohort (30 [28-40] months)

26

Evidence Table 1. Studies Evaluating Association of LBW and Multiple Outcomes: CNS, Eye, Lung, Growth, etc. Part I

Author, Year UI#	Demographics	Inclusion Criteria	Exclusion Criteria	Disease/Condition Type (N)	Study Design (Duration)
Doyle 2001 21326609 Victorian Infant Collaborative study Group, 1997 97290716 J Paediatr Child Health ***some subjects were overlapped with 20307288 (stated in text)** ***possibly overlapped with 98026322**	Location: Australia Years of Birth: 1991-92 Mean GA (range), wk: 23-27 Mean BW (range), g: ND Male: ND Race: ND Enrolled: 225 Evaluated: 225 (265 controls) Number of sites: 1	Cases: GA 23-27 weeks, survived to 2 and 5 years of age Controls: randomly selected contemporaneous normal birth weight controls (BW > 2499 g)	ND	Sample 1: Preterm survivors (N= 401) Controls: Randomly selected contemporaneous normal birth weight controls (BW>2499 grams) (N=265)	Prospective cohort (Doyle - 5 years; Victorian – 2 years)

27

Evidence Table 1. Studies Evaluating Association of LBW and Multiple Outcomes: CNS, Eye, Lung, Growth, etc.
Part I

Author, Year UI#	Demographics	Inclusion Criteria	Exclusion Criteria	Disease/Condition Type (N)	Study Design (Duration)
Gaillard 2001 21221175	Location: UK Years of Birth:1994-1996 Mean GA: ND (only median and range given) Sample 1: 26 (23-34) Sample 2: 26 (23-33) Mean BW: ND (only median and range given) Sample 1: 852 (520-2710) Sample 2: 745 (580-1620) Male: Sample 1: 57% Sample 2: 50% Race: ND Enrolled: 100 Evaluated: 84 Number of sites: 1	Retrospective cohort : All infants born from 1/1/1994 to 12/31/1996 Born at Liverpool Women's Hospital Ventilated beyond 27 postnatal days	If transferred from another hospital after first postnatal week (mostly surgical referrals) If ventilated after 27 postnatal days after a surgical procedure requiring anesthesia	Sample 1 : Ventilated beyond 27 (but not 50) postnatal ds (56) Sample 2: Ventilated beyond 49ds (28)	First component: Retrospective longitudinal cohort with case-control design and cases defined based on exposure (length of ventilation). Unmatched. (3 years) Second component: Retrospective longitudinal cohort study With two historical control groups (3 years)
Roth 2001 21262686	Location: UK Years of Birth: 1979-1988 Mean GA (range), wk: Sample 1: 29 (24-32) Sample 2: 29 (24-32) Mean BW (range), g: Sample 1: 1350 (600-2500) Sample 2: 1324 (535-2390) Male: Sample 1: 49% Sample 2: 53% Race: ND Enrolled: 854 Evaluated: 782 Number of sites: 1	GA < 33 weeks During 1980, for logistic reasons, only infants who were either less than 1250 g or mechanically ventilated were enrolled	ND	Sample 1: children had been studied by linear array US scanning (205) Sample 2: children had been studied by mechanical sector scanning (577)	Retrospective cohort (followed to age of 7 years and 2 months, and 10 years and 6 months)

Evidence Table 1. Studies Evaluating Association of LBW and Multiple Outcomes: CNS, Eye, Lung, Growth, etc.
Part I

Author, Year UI#	Demographics	Inclusion Criteria	Exclusion Criteria	Disease/Condition Type (N)	Study Design (Duration)

Saigal 2001 21376729
 	
 * **Important paper**
	Location: Canada
	 Years of Birth: 1977-1982
	 Mean GA (range), wk:
	   Cases: 27±2
	   Controls: "Term"
	 Mean BW (range), g:
	   Cases: 835±124
	   Controls: 3401±481
	 Male:
	   Cases: 31%
	   Controls: 36%
	 Race: ND
	 SES: middle class
	   Cases: 30%
	   Controls: 30%
	 Enrolled: 179 (145 controls)
	 Evaluated: 154 (125)
	 Number of sites: 1
		ELBW survivors, BW= 501-1000g
		 Controls: term infants recruited at 8 years of age from a random list obtained through the directors of 2 school boards and matched for gender, age, and SES to each case
			ND
			
			 (Died after discharge (10)
			 Lost to follow-up (8)
			 Refusal (5)
			 Unable to be reached (2)
			 Controls:
			 Lost to follow-up (10)
			 Refusal (8)
			 Unable to be reached (2))
				Cases: ELBW infants (154)
				 Controls: Term infants (125)
					Prospective cohort (followed to 12-16 years age)

29

Evidence Table 1. Studies Evaluating Association of LBW and Multiple Outcomes: CNS, Eye, Lung, Growth, etc.
Part I

Author, Year UI#	Demographics	Inclusion Criteria	Exclusion Criteria	Disease/Condition Type (N)	Study Design (Duration)
Schmidt 2001 21298249	Location: Canada, USA, Australia, New Zealand, Hong Kong Years of Birth: 1996-1998 Mean GA: Sample 1: 25.9 ±1.8 Sample 2: 26 ±1.9 Mean BW: Sample 1: 782 ±131 Sample 2: 783 ± 130 Male: 51% Race: Sample 1:White: 69%, black: 13%, Asian: 5%, other: 12% Sample 2: White: 67%, black: 14%, asian: 7%, other: 12% Enrolled: 2756 Evaluated: 1202 Number of sites: 32	BW: 500-999g 2 hrs old Born in 1 of the 32 participating centers in Canada, USA or Australia. Born during 1/1996-3/1998	Excluded total 981 (not eligible) Unable to administer study drug within 6 hrs of birth , n=469 Structural heart disease Renal disease or both, or strongly Suspected (n=24) Dysmorphic feature or congenital abnormalities likely to affect life expectancy or neurologic development or to be associated with structural heart disease or renal disease (n=49) Maternal tocolytic therapy with indomethacin or another prostaglandin inhibitor within 72hr before delivery (n=245) Overt clinical bleeding at more than one site (n=8) Platelet count <50.000 (n=25) Hydrops (n=9) Not considered viable (n=171) Unlikely to be available for f/up (n=31)	Sample 1: Indomethacin group [574] Sample 2: Placebo group [569]	Randomized, multicenter, placebo/controlled, double-blind trial (18 mo CA)

Evidence Table 1. Studies Evaluating Association of LBW and Multiple Outcomes: CNS, Eye, Lung, Growth, etc.

Part II

Author, Year	Predictors	Predictor Measures	Outcomes	Outcome Measures
Akerman 1992 93255928	General: BW, GA, Twinning Other: Mother's negative or ambivalent expectations concerning the twin pregnancy	Interviews with mother prior to delivery	**CNS:** Motor delay Cognitive delay Behavioral disorders **Ophthalmology:** Visual Impairment **Audiology:** Deafness Speech	Griffith's Mental Development Scales: including locomotor, personal-social, hearing and speech, hand and eye coordination, performance, and practical reasoning scores
Thompson 1993 93234177	Birth weight GA	ND	**CNS:** Motor delay CP Cognitive delay Mental retardation **Ophthalmology:** Visual impairment **Audiology:** Hearing disorders	Griffith's scale
Rademaker 1994 95003452	CNS: 1) Intracranial / Intraventricular hemorrhage 2) White Matter Disorder 3) Periventricular leukomalacia	US grading GLH-IVH	**CNS:** Cognitive delay Mental retardation Post Hemorrhagic Hydrocephalus (PHH) **Ophthalmology:** Visual impairment **Audiology:** Hearing disorders	Griffith's mental development scale Amiel-Tison, Greniers and Touwen scores IQ

Evidence Table 1. Studies Evaluating Association of LBW and Multiple Outcomes: CNS, Eye, Lung, Growth, etc. Part II

Author, Year	Predictors	Predictor Measures	Outcomes	Outcome Measures
Vonderveid 1994 94297368	**General:** 1) BW (in 100 g intervals) 2) GA (in wks) 3) Gender 4) SGA(<10% vs > 10%) 5) Type of pregnancy 6) Fetal presentation 7) Antenatal steroid 8) Place of birth 9) Apgar score 1 min 10) Apgar score 5 min 11) Transport 12) On admission to NICU: Spontaneous respirations (present or absent); Body temperature (<35 vs >35); PH (<7.00 vs 7.00-7.09 vs > 7.09); PCO2: 80 vs 60-79 vs 40-59 vs <40 **Pulmonary:** 1) RDS 2) Maximum FIO2 required **CNS:** 1) Peri-intra-ventricular hemorrhage 2) PVL **Others:** 1) Sepsis 2) Maximum bilirubin level 3) Hypoglycemia (< 25 mg/dl) 4) Hyperglycemia (>175 mg/dl) 5) Acidosis (pH<7.20)	ND	**CNS--Audiology-Ophthalmology:** 1) Neuromotor disorders: > impairment > disability > handicap > (including CP, Blindness, Deafness) 2) Developmental quotients	1) Each limb was evaluated separately: > 0= nl function > 1= impairment with no loss of function > 2= mild motor disability > 3= severe motor disability > 4= complete loss of function 2) Cerebral palsy: Monoplegia, diplegia, paraplegia, hemiplegia, quadriplegia) 3) Developmental quotients: Brunet-Lezine test (24 mo CA)

32

Evidence Table 1. Studies Evaluating Association of LBW and Multiple Outcomes: CNS, Eye, Lung, Growth, etc.
Part II

Author, Year	Predictors	Predictor Measures	Outcomes	Outcome Measures
Kraybill 1995 95264242	**General:** 1) Surfactant (single dose 5 ml/kg given via ET tube at birth)	Infants were treated, as soon as after birth, either with 5 ml/kg of surfactant or air placebo, via ET tube.	**1 yr assessment (NCMH and HCHD cohort):** **General:** Overall survival **Pulmonary:** Need for O2 via Nasal canula Need for O2 via CPAP CLD **2 yr assessment (NCMH cohort only)** **General:** Overall survival Hospitalization for respiratory illness **Pulmonary:** Bronchodilator regular use Tracheostomy **1 and 2 yr assessment:** **Growth:** Height for age Weight for age HC for age Mean MDI score MDI scores < 2 SDs Mean PSI score PDI scores < 2 SDs Severity of impairments Types of Impairments Any surgery Assessment between 28 ds-12mo: **Ophthalmology:** ROP Tx for ROP ROP presence at latest exam Severe ROP	No further specifications given, except for the followings: Oxygen via Nasal canula : providing alveolar O2 concentrations of : 26%-40%, based on NC flow and NC O2 concentration **General:** Overall survival Bayley Scale of Infant Development: 1) MDI= Mental Development Index Score 2) PDI: Psychomotor Development Index Score ROP : (no further definitions) 1) No ROP, 2) Mild/moderate 3) Severe CP (no further definitions) 1) Mild 2) Moderate/Severe Severity of impairments: 1) Severe 2) Mild/Moderate Types of impairments: 1) MDI<69 2) MDI: 69-84 3) Moderate/severe CP 4) Mild CP 5) Bilateral sensorineural deafness 6) Deafness not requiring amplification 7) Bilateral blindness 8) Visual defect (1 yr and 2 yr CA)

Evidence Table 1. Studies Evaluating Association of LBW and Multiple Outcomes: CNS, Eye, Lung, Growth, etc.
Part II

Author, Year	Predictors	Predictor Measures	Outcomes	Outcome Measures
Speechley 1995 96356544	General: 1) Former NICU graduate (of any BW) 2) Gender	Not further specified	Physical health outcome at 12 yrs 1) Chronic physical health (mother's report) 2) Lifetime hospitalizations (mother's report) 3) Physical impairments (mother's report) 4) Perception of child's heath (child's report) 5) Perception of child's health (mother's report) Emotional and social wellbeing at 12 yrs: 1) Internalizing problems (child's report) 2) Externalizing problems (child's report) 3) Social competence (child's report) 4) Social support (child's report) 5) Self esteem (child's report) 6) School performance (mother's report)	Based on responses on an interviewer administered and self-report questionnaire. Physical health outcome at 12 yrs 1) Chronic physical health (mother's report): Precoded 25 chronic illnesses 2) Lifetime hospitalizations (mother's report) 3) Physical impairments (mother's report):response to a question asking whether their child had any physical impairments 4) Perception of child's heath (child's report): 4-item scale 5) Perception of child's health (mother's report): 4-item scale Emotional and social well being at 12 yrs: 1) Internalizing problems (child's report) 3-item scale 2) Externalizing problems (child's report) 3-item scale 3) Social competence (child's report) 36-item scale 4) Social support (child's report) 24-item scale 5) Self-esteem (child's report) 10-item scale 6) School performance (mother's report) 5-item scale

34

Evidence Table 1. Studies Evaluating Association of LBW and Multiple Outcomes: CNS, Eye, Lung, Growth, etc.
Part II

Author, Year	Predictors	Predictor Measures	Outcomes	Outcome Measures
Hack 1996 97060805	General : 1) VLBW vs. NBW 2) GA 3) SGA/IUGR 4) Sex CNS: Neurosensory Development IA+II, I Other: Maternal Factors, race, education, height, martial	VLBW<1500gm (AGA+SGA) to compare growth with FT NBW infants	**CNS:** Major neurosensory abnormal. **Growth:** Weight Height Head Circumference	ND
Hack 1996 97066007	General: Birth Weight	500-750 gm	**CNS:** Cerebral palsy Motor and cognitive delay **Ophthalmology:** Blindness **Audiology:** Deafness	Neurosensory status BSID: MDI, PDI

Evidence Table 1. Studies Evaluating Association of LBW and Multiple Outcomes: CNS, Eye, Lung, Growth, etc.
Part II

Author, Year	Predictors	Predictor Measures	Outcomes	Outcome Measures
Northern Neonatal Nursing Initiative Trial Group 1996 96304894	Cardiovascular or Pulmonary Predictors: use of FFP or plasma substitute to expand vascular volume prophylactically	ND	**CNS Outcomes:** Motor delay Cerebral palsy Seizure disorder Post hemorrhagic hydrocephalus **Ophthalmology:** Visual impairment Blindness **Audiology Outcomes:** Hearing disorders Speech **Other outcomes:** a. blind, deaf, or unable to walk – combined outcome b. no severe disability – combined outcome c. overall developmental quotient – Griffith's	Motor delay: Griffith's gross motor quotient >350 below mean Griffith's quotient for speech + hearing >350 below mean
Sethi 1996 96334245	General Predictors: 1) Birth weight	1) 2) <1000g 3) 1000g – 1500 g	**CNS Outcomes:** Cerebral palsy Cognitive delay Seizure disorder **Ophthalmology outcomes:** Blindness ROP - eye exam **Audiology outcomes:** Deafness **Other outcomes:** Survival	"abnormal neurodevelopmental outcome" - not defined "major impairment" - any CP blindness, deafness, "significant" developmental delay or hydrocephalus requiring a shunt deafness OAE testing before discharge and at 7 months "minor impairment" - squint, refractive error, mild auditory impairment (< 50 dB loss), stable epilepsy, or needing speech therapy assessment

36

Evidence Table 1. Studies Evaluating Association of LBW and Multiple Outcomes: CNS, Eye, Lung, Growth, etc.
Part II

Author, Year	Predictors	Predictor Measures	Outcomes	Outcome Measures
Wilkinson 1996 97087405	CNS predictors: Periventricular leukomalacia (severe cystic PVL)	Changes not seen on first scan Multiple cysts must be present (excludes cases with flare only) The cysts are bilateral The cysts are distributed in the periventricular area involving the region of the trigones and variable involvement anterior to the trigones	**CNS outcomes:** Motor delay Cerebral palsy Cognitive delay Mental retardation **Ophthalmology outcomes:** Visual impairment Blindness **Audiology outcomes:** Hearing disorders	Not specifically defined. Spastic quadriparesis, cortical blindness, seizures presumably self-evident.
DeReginer 1997 98041177	Cardiovascular/ Pulmonary: Chronic lung disease	Classification based on the duration of supplemental oxygen requirements. "No CLD" – breathing room air at 28 days "Mild CLD" – requiring supplemental oxygen at 28 days but not at 36 weeks PMA Sever CLD" – requiring oxygen at 28 days and 36 weeks PMA	**General:** Motor and cognitive delay Cerebral palsy **Opthalmology:** Visual impairment Blindness **Audiology:** Hearing loss Deafness **Growth:** Weight Z score Length Z score Head circumference Z score **Other:** any adverse outcome	Bayley PDI & MDI

37

Evidence Table 1. Studies Evaluating Association of LBW and Multiple Outcomes: CNS, Eye, Lung, Growth, etc.
Part II

Author, Year	Predictors	Predictor Measures	Outcomes	Outcome Measures
Dezoete 1997 97359687	**General:** 1) Birth weight 2) GA 3) SGA/IUGR **CNS:** Intracranial/Intraventricular Hemorrhage **Cardiovascular/** **Pulmonary:** Chronic Lung disease	Clinical measures	**CNS:** Motor delay Cerebral palsy Cognitive delay **Ophthalmology:** Visual impairment Blindness **Audiology:** Deafness	Stratify outcome into 4 categories base on severity of disability. "Severe disability" / Category I – ≥1 of the following: (1) Sensorineural deafness (requiring hearing aids). (2) Bilateral blindness. (3) Severe cerebral palsy. (4) Developmental delay (adjusted Bayley mental scores 2 or more SD below mean). Category II – – ≥1 of the following: (1) Adjusted Bayley mental scores between 1 and 2 SD below mean. (2) Mild-moderate CP w/o developmental cognitive delay. (3) Impaired vision requiring spectacles. Category III – Presence of tone disorder or motor delay (adjusted Bayley motor score more than one SD below mean but adjusted mental score within average rage.) Category IV / "apparently normal" – (1) No apparent tone disorder, and (2) No apparent developmental delay when mental and motor scores adjusted for GA.

Evidence Table 1. Studies Evaluating Association of LBW and Multiple Outcomes: CNS, Eye, Lung, Growth, etc.
Part II

Author, Year	Predictors	Predictor Measures	Outcomes	Outcome Measures
O'Shea 1997 98049056 *overlapped sample with 98190123	General: BW, GA, Yr of birth CNS: 1) Intracranial/ Intraventricular hemorrhage 2) White matter disorder 3) Periventricular leuko-malacia	Hemorrhage disease diagnosed by cranial US finding, classified by Stewart's method	**CNS:** Cerebral palsy Cognitive delay Major neurosensory impairments **Ophthalmology:** Blindness **Growth:** Head Circumference<10th percentile at 1 yr Weight<10% Length<10% **Other:** Rehospitalization	CP – presence of definitely abnormal position and posture attributable to impaired neuromotor function Bayley scales – MDI, PDI
Piecuch 1997 97456215	General: 1) Birth weight 2) GA 3) SGA/IUGR 4) Social Risk CNS: Intracranial/Intraventricular Hemorrhage, Periventricular leukomalacia Cardiovascular/Pulmonary: Chronic lung disease Other: 1) Inborn-Outborn 2) Year of birth 3)Sex	Well defined in text	**CNS:** Motor delay Cerebral palsy Cognitive delay **Ophthalmology:** Visual Impairment **Audiology:** Hearing Disorder	Neuromotor problems, OP Neurosensory-blindness/hearing loss Cognitive outcome-abnormal if <2 SD below mean testing

39

Evidence Table 1. Studies Evaluating Association of LBW and Multiple Outcomes: CNS, Eye, Lung, Growth, etc.
Part II

Author, Year	Predictors	Predictor Measures	Outcomes	Outcome Measures
Piecuch 1997 98012134	*General predictors:* 1) GA *CNS predictors:* 1) intracranial/ intraventricular hemorrhage 2) periventricular leukomalacia *Cardiovascular or pulmonary predictors:* 1) chronic lung disease *Other predictors:* 1) social risk: economic 2) social risk: substance abuse	CLD - at 36 weeks PCA, requirement for supplemental O$_2$ IVH grade 3 or 4 & PVL, according to sonogram Social risk economic - maternal education <12 grade; complete unemployment in household; or government assistance for health insurance Social risk substance abuse - positive toxicology screens or confirmed history of drug or alcohol abuse	**CNS outcomes:** cerebral palsy cognitive delay **Ophthalmology outcomes:** visual impairment **Audiology outcomes:** hearing disorders	`Visual – Near point tests or Snellen eye charts Audiologic - behavioral testing followed by BAER or pure tone audiometry. Cognitive outcome - Bayley scales at 12 and 18 months; Stanford-Binet at 2.5-4 years; McCarthy scales at 4-6 years. Abnormal neurological outcome - CP, quadriplegia, dysplegia, hemiplegia Suspicious neurological outcome – clumsiness, tremors Severe neurosensory abnormalities – Bilateral hearing loss, blindness Mild neurosensory abnormalities - high frequency hearing loss without hearing aids, visual deficit without glasses
Singer 1997 98049057	Cardiovascular or pulmonary predictors: 1) Bronchopulmonary dysplasia General : BW, Neurologic risk Other: Race, Socioeconomic status	BPD: preterm, <1500g BW, oxygen for >28 days with radiographic evidence of CLD	**CNS outcomes:** Cerebral palsy Cognitive delay Mental retardation **Ophthalmology outcomes:** Visual impairment **Audiology outcomes:** Hearing disorders Speech Language Communication disorder	Bayley Scales of Infant Development
Singer 2001 21163669				Language (speech/communication) measured by Battelle Developmental Communication Subscale Domain→ receptive, expressive and total communication scores converted to DQ mean 100 and SD 15.

40

Evidence Table 1. Studies Evaluating Association of LBW and Multiple Outcomes: CNS, Eye, Lung, Growth, etc.
Part II

Author, Year	Predictors	Predictor Measures	Outcomes	Outcome Measures
Victorian Infant Collaborative study Group, 1997 98026322 *This study is also in CNS table	General: BW Other: period of time when born	Each sample were subdivided into BW=500-749 g and BW=750-999 g 1985-1987 vs. 1991-1992	**CNS:** Cerebral palsy Neurodevelopmental: Cognitive and motor delay Disability **Ophthalmology:** Blindness **Audiology:** Deafness or hearing aid	CP was not defined Bayley Scales of Infant Development DQ, using the published mean and SD Disability: "Severe" – bilateral blindness, cerebral palsy with the child unlikely ever to walk, or a DQ score <-3SD; "Moderate" – bilateral sensorineural deafness requiring hearing aids, cerebral palsy in children not walking at 2 but expected to walk, or a DQ score from –3SD to <-2 SD; "Mild" – cerebral palsy but walking at 2 , or a DQ score form –2 SD to <-1 SD.
Victorian Infant Collaborative study Group, 1997 97466059	Other: time period of birth	ND	**CNS:** Cerebral Palsy Cognitive delay Post Hemorrhagic Hydrocephalus (PHH) Ophthalmology: Blindness **Audiology:** Deafness **Other:** Sensorineural disability: severe, mental, moderate, none.	CP neurologic exam Bayley MDI, PDI scores Blindness-not stated Deafness-not stated Degrees of sensorineural delay are defined as an aggregate measure and are approximated.

41

Evidence Table 1. Studies Evaluating Association of LBW and Multiple Outcomes: CNS, Eye, Lung, Growth, etc. Part II

Author, Year	Predictors	Predictor Measures	Outcomes	Outcome Measures
Cheung 1998 99059896	Cardiovascular or Pulmonary Predictors: Inhaled nitric oxide (INO)	ND	**CNS Outcomes:** Post Hemorrhagic Hydrocephalus (PHH) "Neurodevelopmental outcomes" Intraventricular hemorrhage **Audiology Outcomes:** Deafness **Pulmonary Outcomes:** BPD or CLD (with or without meds) Aspiration pneumonia **Growth Outcomes:** Wt, HC, length (height)	PDI + MDI of Bayley Scales of Infant Developmental Index were used. "Neurodevelopmental" outcomes: Disability: one of more of: 1. CP (all types or severity) 2. Legal blindness (corrected visual acuity of the better eye <20/200 3. Hearing loss (sensorineural hearing loss of >30 dB in the better ear) 4. Severe mental retardation (MDI >3 SD below the mean) Delay: does not have disability and either MDI or PDI was >2 SD below the mean. Normal: free of disability or delay and MDI and PDI were within 2 SD of the mean.

42

Evidence Table 1. Studies Evaluating Association of LBW and Multiple Outcomes: CNS, Eye, Lung, Growth, etc.

Part II

Author, Year	Predictors	Predictor Measures	Outcomes	Outcome Measures
Finnström 1998 99041345	General Predicators 1) GA 2) SGA/IUGR 3) Apgar score 4) Other: gender CNS Predicators 1) Intracranial/Intraventricular hemorrhage 2) Periventricular leukomalacia Ophthalmology Predicators 1) Retinopathy of Prematurity (ROP) Cardiovascular or Pulmonary Predictors 1) Chronic Lung Disease 2) Other: Mechanical ventilation Other Predicators 1) Other: PDA	Self-explanatory	**CNS Outcome:** Cerebral palsy **Ophthalmology:** Visual impairment **Audiology:** Deafness **Growth:** Height Weight Head circumference	CP: spastic diplegia, spastic hemiplegia, spastic hemiplegia Scheffzek's categories of functional disabilities are not defined in this article. They refer to a previous article which is written in German. "Major Handicaps" (category 3-4) CP, severe visual impairment, CP+ severe visual impairment, mental retardation and cardiomyopathy, hearing less
Gregoire 1998 98232532	Cardiovascular/Pulmonary: 1) Chronic Lung Disease 2) Bronchopulmonary dysplasia Compared O_2 dependence at 28 days with O_2 dependence at 36 wk	ND	**CNS:** Cerebral palsy Motor and cognitive delay **Audiology:** Hearing Disorders→ Free field audiograms **Pulmonary:** Respiratory readmissions PICU admissions **Growth:** Weight, height, head circumference **Other:** Health Outcomes	Giffith's Mental Development Scales Neurologic examinations

Evidence Table 1. Studies Evaluating Association of LBW and Multiple Outcomes: CNS, Eye, Lung, Growth, etc.
Part II

Author, Year	Predictors	Predictor Measures	Outcomes	Outcome Measures
Kurkinen-Raty 1998 98387235 (All+Lung) *sample from the same big population as 20284814	General : PROM	Diagnose was through clinical assessment or with the use of a PROM-test, which detects insulin growth factor binding protein-1 in the cervico-vaginal secretions, or with the use of a nitrazine test.	**CNS:** Motor delay Cerebral delay **Ophthalmology:** Visual Blindness **Audiology:** Hearing disorders **Pulmonary:** Chronic lung disease **Growth:** weight percent **Other:** Days of re-hospitalization Steroid therapy at followed up	Neurologic exams Diagnosis of CLD was made if infants required oxygen, continuous bronchodilator, or steroid tx because of respiratory signs and symptoms. Diagnoses of RDS were made based on need for respiratory support, radiologic findings, and clinical assessments

Evidence Table 1. Studies Evaluating Association of LBW and Multiple Outcomes: CNS, Eye, Lung, Growth, etc.

Part II

Author, Year	Predictors	Predictor Measures	Outcomes	Outcome Measures
Lee 1998 98442293	**General:** 1) Candidemia and/or Candidal meningitis	Diagnosis of Candidemia: by at least one positive Blood Culture Diagnosis of Candidal meningitis: by isolation of Candida in the CSF or >45x10 ^{6} WBCs in the CSF and candidemia.	**CNS:** Neurodevelopmental disabilities (NDDs) Cognitive delay Cerebral palsy **Ophthalmology:** Legal blindness **Audiology:** Hearing loss **Growth:** Growth retardation	1) Bayley Scales of Infant development; MDI, PDI for ages < 24 mo. 2) Stanford-Binet Intelligence Scale and Peabody Development Motor Scales for ages > 24 mo 3) Scores obtained by psychologists, psychometricians, pediatricians specialized. Neurodevelopmental Disabilities: 1) Cerebral palsy (all types and severity) 2) Legal blindness (corrected VA of the better eye<20/200) 3) Hearing loss (neurosensory hearing loss in the better ear > 30 dB) (done by certified audiologist 4) And/or cognitive delay (MDI>3 SDs below the mean) Growth retardation: Weight, Height, HC > 2 SDs below the mean (Between 3-6 yrs CA)

Evidence Table 1. Studies Evaluating Association of LBW and Multiple Outcomes: CNS, Eye, Lung, Growth, etc.
Part II

Author, Year	Predictors	Predictor Measures	Outcomes	Outcome Measures
Lefebvre 1998 98387703	Other: Neurobiologic risk score (NBRS)	Items in NBRS: ventilation, PH, surgeries, IVH< PVL, infection, hypoglycemia-items scored zero or greater in progression	**CNS:** Cerebral palsy Cognitive delay Other neurodevelopmental impairment **Ophthalmology:** Blindness **Audiology:** hearing disorders-free fetal audiogram	Neurologic exam Griffith's mental development scale Mental retardation-Griffith's mental development scale 1) Global developmental quotient (DA) 2) Mild/moderate: DA 80-89 or CP 3) Severe: DA<80, severe CP unilateral blindness or severe hearing defect 4) Normal: more of the above Areas of Griffith's Developmental Scales: - Locomotor - Personal-social - Hearing and speech - Eye and hand coordination - Performance Control mean DA=110+or- in literature
Millet 1998 98212544	CNS: MRI findings at 3-6 months	ND	**CNS:** Motor delay Cerebral palsy Cognitive delay Behavioral disorders **Ophthalmology:** Visual impairment **Audiology:** Hearing loss **GI:** Dysphagia	Neurodevelopmental outcome poorly defined

46

Evidence Table 1. Studies Evaluating Association of LBW and Multiple Outcomes: CNS, Eye, Lung, Growth, etc.

Part II

Author, Year	Predictors	Predictor Measures	Outcomes	Outcome Measures
Piecuch 1998 98446413	**General:** 1) Birth in a recent period vs early period vs midpoint period (the authors wanted to assess whether changes in neonatology for the care of VLBW infants have changed the outcome of LBW infants: 1000-1500g) 2) Birth weight 3) GA 4) Gender 5) Place of birth (inborn vs outborn) 6) Weight for age (AGA vs SGA) **CNS:** 1) Intracranial hemorrhage (ICH) **Pulmonary:** 1) Duration of mechanical ventilation 2) Duration of O2 requirements (CLD)	Birth in a recent period: 1989-1991 Birth in an early period : 1979-1981 Birth in a midpoint period:1984-1986	**CNS:** 1) Neurologic: normal, suspect, abnormal 2) Cognitive: Average or above, Mild delays, Moderate/severe delays **Ophthalmology-Audiology:** Significant visual and/ or auditory deficits (B/L blindness or need for hearing aids)	Neurologic: 1) Normal 2) Suspect: (clumsiness, tremors, mild tone and reflexes changes, but without fixed impairment) 3) Abnormal: moderate/ severe: fixed impairments such as CP, diplegias, hemiplegias Sensory 1) Visual acuity screening 2) Behavioral screening assessment Cognitive: < 24 mo: Bayley Scale >24 mo: Stanford-Binet scale Carthy Scale 7-8 yrs: Wechsler Intelligence Scale for Children Revised 1) Average or above 2) Mild delays: 1-2 SDs below mean 3) Moderate/severe delays: > 2 SDs below mean Time of outcome assessment not specified: It could be done up to age 7.5-8 yrs (Mean age at assessment in the cohort was: 24 mo)

47

Evidence Table 1. Studies Evaluating Association of LBW and Multiple Outcomes: CNS, Eye, Lung, Growth, etc.

Part II

Author, Year	Predictors	Predictor Measures	Outcomes	Outcome Measures
Sajaniemi 1998 99041674	**General:** 1) Prematurity per se 2) Premature with BW< 1000 g vs premature with BW > 1000 g 3) Pre-eclampsia 4) SGA 5) Duration of NICU stay **CNS:** 1) PVL 2) IVH **Pulmonary:** 1) Duration of ventilation	Not further specified	**CNS:** Neurologic outcome Developmental outcome Temperament profile Behavioral profile	Neurologic outcome: 1) Cerebral palsy 2) Free of major disabilities Developmental outcome: 1) Bayley Scales of Infant Development 2) Mental Development Index (MDI) Temperament: Toddler Temperament questionnaire (TTQ) (contains 97 statements) 9 temperament dimensions: 1) Activity 2) Rhythmicity 3) Approach 4) Adaptability 5) Intensity 6) Mood Persistence 7) Distractability 8) Threshold Behavior: Infant Behavior Record: 1) Social responsiveness 2) Attention 3) Affect 4) Energy level 5) Goal directedness during the test (24 mo CA)

Evidence Table 1. Studies Evaluating Association of LBW and Multiple Outcomes: CNS, Eye, Lung, Growth, etc.

Part II

Author, Year	Predictors	Predictor Measures	Outcomes	Outcome Measures
Scherjon 1998 98429216	**CNS:** 1) U/C ratio: Doppler finding of umbilical/cerebral artery pulsatility index (U/C ratio: raised vs normal) 2) Neonatal Cranial Ultrasound findings **General:** 1) Fetal growth ratio 2) GA	1) U/C ratio: The ratio between umbilical artery and cerebral artery pulsatility index (used as a marker of fetal blood redistribution to the brain, and indirect marker of placental insufficiency) 2) Neonatal cranial Ultrasound: Normal: No intracranial or subependymal bleeding, Echodensities less bright than choroid plexus Moderate: IVH (< 50% of lumen filled) some echodensity brighter than choroid plexus, lasting less than 3 days. Abnormal: IVH (>50% of lumen filled) Intraparenchymal bleeding Some echodensities brighter than choroid plexus and lasting longer than 3 days 3) Fetal growth ratio (observed birth weight divided by expected mean BW for GA)	**Growth:** Growth (Weight, Height, HC) **CNS:** Neurodevelopmental outcome Behavioral outcome	Hempel outcome: 1) Specific for toddlers 2) Observed children while playing in a standardized situation 3) 89 items Motor aspects of Hempel examination: Classification of infants: 1) Normal 2) Mildly abnormal (e.g., slight asymmetry, or mild hypo-, hyper-tonia which does not lead to handicapping condition) 3) Abnormal (e.g., CP, which leads to handicap in daily life) Behavioral aspects of Hempel examination: 1) Information based on parental questionnaire on child's cognitive function and 2) language skills (level of activity, nocturnal enuresis, eating, sleeping disturbances, language development, comprehensibility, passive understanding, number of words used in sentences) Hempel outcome assessment was done by a person blind to prior medical history of child. (3 yrs CA)

49

Evidence Table 1. Studies Evaluating Association of LBW and Multiple Outcomes: CNS, Eye, Lung, Growth, etc.

Part II

Author, Year	Predictors	Predictor Measures	Outcomes	Outcome Measures
Cheung 1999 99146391	*General predictors:* 1) BW 2) GA 3) Apgar score *CNS predictors:* 1) intracranial/ intraventricular hemorrhage *Cardiovascular or pulmonary predictors:* 1) days of ventilation 2) days of O_2 use *Other predictors:* 1) frequency of apnea 2) mean desaturation of apnea 3) mean frequency of apnea 4) Blisten index (socioeconomic status)	ND	**CNS outcomes:** Motor delay Cerebral palsy Cognitive delay Mental retardation Seizure disorder Neurodevelopmental disability **Ophthalmology outcomes:** Blindness **Audiology outcomes:** Hearing disorders **Growth outcomes:** Weight > 2 SD below the mean Height > 2 SD below the mean HC > 2 SD below the mean	Bayley scores Stanford-Binet Intelligence Scale Peabody Developmental Motor Scale Neurodevelopmental disability: "children with 1 or more of a) cerebral palsy b) legal blindness c) hearing loss d) convulsive disorder e) cognitive delay
Duvanel 1999 99207097	**General:** 1) Hypoglycemia: 2) Severity of hypoglycemia (0-11 mg/dl, 11-29 mg/dl, 29-47 mg/dl), and 3) Frequencies of hypoglycemic episodes	Blood glucose level in the first 24 hours of less than 47 mg/dl by reagents sticks, or confirmed by glucose analyzer for stick measurements less than 36mg/dl. About the frequency of episodes: no Precise information on the frequency Of performance of glucose measurements.	**CNS:** Scores in psychometric tests done for neurodevelopmental assessment at: 6 moths 12 moths 18 months 3.5 yrs 5 yrs. **Growth:** Head circumference at 6, 12, 18 months, 3.5 yrs, 5 yrs Growth rates for weight, length, and HC for time intervals: 6-18 months 6-3.5 yrs 6-5 yrs	Griffith's test (6 items): at 6, 12, 18 mo McCarthy test (6 items) : 3.5 yrs, 5 yrs

50

Evidence Table 1. Studies Evaluating Association of LBW and Multiple Outcomes: CNS, Eye, Lung, Growth, etc.
Part II

Author, Year	Predictors	Predictor Measures	Outcomes	Outcome Measures
Pennefather, 1999 20002011	*Genera Predictor:* GA	ND	**CNS:** Cerebral palsy	Retrospective review of patient records
Pennefather, 2000 20217908 * **This study is also in eye table**	**CNS:** 1) IVH 2) Periventricular leukomalacia 3) Ventriculomegaly/Ventricular Dilation Ophthalmology: 1) ROP 2) Refractive error Other: Family Hxg strabismus, Developmental disability, CP		**Ophthalmology:** Visual impairment (cortical)(CVI) Cicatricial ROP Strabismus	Visual acuity, Visual fields
Ambalavanan 2000 21031370	General: BW, GA, Antenatal steroids, Apgar score Other: Race, Gender Multiple gestation, Maternal education, Maternal age CNS: Intracranial hemorrhage Periventricular/Ventricular Dilation Bronchopulmonary dysplasia GI: Necrotizing "entrocolitis" Interinal perforation, Chorioamnionitis Multiple gestation Maternal education Maternal age	Extensive list of the 21 predictor variables	**CNS:** Motor delay Cerebral palsy Cognitive delay Mental retardation PHH Neurologic exam Major handicap **Ophthalmology:** Visual impairment Blindness **Audiology:** Hearing disorders Deafness	Bayley Scales of Infant Development Major handicap-presence of one or any poor outcome (i.e. CP, deadness, blindness). Mental retardation (MDI or PDI <70), PHH requiring sheet

Evidence Table 1. Studies Evaluating Association of LBW and Multiple Outcomes: CNS, Eye, Lung, Growth, etc.
Part II

Author, Year	Predictors	Predictor Measures	Outcomes	Outcome Measures
Cioni 2000 20150341	CNS intracranial hemorrhages, white matter disorder, Ventriculomegaly	MRI findings Total MRI score (the higher the worse, range 7-21) made by summation of subscores of following categories: Size of Lateral ventricles, white matter abnormal signal intensity, white matter reduction, cysts, size of subarachnoid space, corpus callosum, cortical gray matter; MRI score of visual cortex and optic radiations	**CNS:** CP **Ophthalmology:** Visual assessment Developmental	**Neurological examination:** Normal Mildly abnormal (mild retardation and/or mild abnormal neurological signs, but not CP. CP with relatively normal head and trunk control. CP without head and trunk control. **Visual assessment:** Grating acuity: assessed with binocular Teller acuity card procedure (cycles per second) Visual Field (kinetic perimetry) Horizontal optokinetic nystagmus (OKN) Oculomotor behaviour (following and fixation) and strabismus. **Developmental Assessment:** Griffith's developmental scales (global and each subscale: locomotor, personal-social, hearing-speech, hand-eye co-ordination, and performance) Scores $\geq$85 = normal Borderline 84-71 Abnormal $\leq$70

Evidence Table 1. Studies Evaluating Association of LBW and Multiple Outcomes: CNS, Eye, Lung, Growth, etc.

Part II

Author, Year	Predictors	Predictor Measures	Outcomes	Outcome Measures
Hack 2000 20358826	General: 1) Birth weight 2) GA 3) SGA/IUGR 4) Antenatal steroids 5) Jaundice CNS: 1) Intracranial/Intraventricular Hemorrhage 2) Periventricular leukomalacia 3) Ventriculomegaly/ ventricular dilation Cardiovascular/Pulmonary: Chronic lung disease Gastrointestinal: Necrotizing "entroclitis" Other: 1) Infectious Disease 2) Dexamethasone 3) Perinatal factors (chorioamnionitis) 4) Multiple birth 5) C-section 6) Social risk 7) Male sex	ND	**CNS:** Cerebral palsy Motor delay Cognitive delay MDI score<70 Post hemorrhagic Hydrocephalus **Ophthalmology:** Blindness **Audiology:** Deafness	Neurologic abnormality- includes: CP, hypotonia, hypertonia Shunt-dependent hydrocephalus
Jankov 2000 20188680	Cardiovascular predictors: 1) CPR Other predictors: 1) Apgar scores	1) 2) Use of CPR in delivery room 3) Assignment of Apgar scores in the delivery room	**CNS outcomes:** Cerebral palsy Cognitive delay Mental retardation Adverse outcome **Ophthalmology outcome:** Blindness **Audiology outcome:** Hearing disorders	Adverse outcome defined as: 1) CP causing non-ambulation beyond 2 years or spastic quadriparesis 2) Intellectual delay = below 2 SD 3) Hearing loss requiring aids 4) Legal blindness (<20/200)

Evidence Table 1. Studies Evaluating Association of LBW and Multiple Outcomes: CNS, Eye, Lung, Growth, etc.
Part II

Author, Year	Predictors	Predictor Measures	Outcomes	Outcome Measures
Kurkinen-Raty, 2000 20284814 *sample from the same big population as 98197235	General predictors: Birth weight GA Antenatal steroids Cord pH Bronchopulmonary dysphasia (BPD) Other predictors: Indicated preterm delivery Spontaneous preterm delivery	BPD diagnoses were based on radiologic finding	**CNS:** Motor delay Cerebral palsy **Ophthalmology** Visual impairment **Audiology** Hearing disorder **Pulmonary** Chronic lung disease (CLD) at 1 year **Growth:** Wt, Ht, HC	Motor delay = abnormalities of tone or reflexes but functionally normal or borderline CP = spastic diplegia or hemiplegia or spastictetraplegia Diagnosis of CLD was made if infants required oxygen, continuous bronchodilator, or steroid tx because of respiratory signs and symptoms.

Evidence Table 1. Studies Evaluating Association of LBW and Multiple Outcomes: CNS, Eye, Lung, Growth, etc.
Part II

Author, Year	Predictors	Predictor Measures	Outcomes	Outcome Measures
Marlow 2000 20150342	**General:** 1) Birth weight 2) Apgar score 3) CRIB scores **CNS:** 1) Maximum bilirubin level 2) Abnormal cerebral US scan **Audiology:** 1) Sensorineural hearing loss **Cardiovascular/Pulomonary:** 1) Duration of intubation, respiratory support, oxygen, pH<7.2, base excess 2) Dopamine excess 3) Furosemide 4) Indomethacin use **Other:** 3) Netilmicin 6) Vancomycin 7) Positive blood cultures 8) Bilirubin >200 Ꝓmol/l 9) Bilirubin>GA x 10 10) Creatinine >60 mmol/l 11) Netilmicin 12) Vancomycin Combination of the above: 1) Bili 200 + acidosis 2) Bili> 200 + sepsis 3) Bili >200+ netilmicin 4) Bili> 200+ vancomycin 5) Bili>200+ furosemide 6) Peak bili+ acidosis 7) Peak bili+ sepsis 8) Peak bili+ netilmicin 9) Peak bili+ furosemide 10) Creatinine>60+ netilmicin or vancomycin or furosemide 11) Netilmicin+furosemide 12) Vancomycin+ furosemide	Not further specified	In case control component: **Audiology:** Sensorineural hearing loss (SNHL) of 50 dB within 9 months from birth In Longitudinal component: **CNS:** Cerebral palsy at 12 months of age in the 2 groups (SNHL and control group)	Cases of SNHL were identified if the hearing loss had been identified within 3 months of discharge home, (within 9 mo from birth); after excluding cases with conductive hearing loss, possible congenital cause, or had neonatal bacterial meningitis

Evidence Table 1. Studies Evaluating Association of LBW and Multiple Outcomes: CNS, Eye, Lung, Growth, etc.
Part II

Author, Year	Predictors	Predictor Measures	Outcomes	Outcome Measures
Victorian Infant Collaborative study Group, 2000 20307288 *some subjects were overlapped with Doyle, 2001	Other: Dexamethasone- Postnatal	ND	**CNS:** Cerebral palsy Cognitive delay **Ophthalmology:** Blindness **Audiology:** Deafness	Wechsler PPSI-R
Wood 2000 20373840	*General:* 1) GA 2) Gender Other: Perinatal Factors → Multiple gestation	ND	**CNS:** Motor delay Cognitive delay Seizure disorder Overall development **Ophthalmology:** Visual impairment Blindness **Audiology:** Hearing disorders Deafness Speech Communication disorder **Other:** Severely disabled Other disability No disability Disability of hearing, vision, or communication	Bayley scales Severe disability = need of physical assistance to perform daily activities. If disability did not fit into this category = "other disability"

Evidence Table 1. Studies Evaluating Association of LBW and Multiple Outcomes: CNS, Eye, Lung, Growth, etc.

Part II

Author, Year	Predictors	Predictor Measures	Outcomes	Outcome Measures

Doyle 2001 21326609
 	
Victorian Infant Collaborative study Group, 1997 97290716
 	
*some subjects were overlapped with 20307288 (stated in text)
*possibly overlapped with 98026322
	General predictors:
	1) GA
	2) SGA/IUGR
	3) antenatal steroids
	4) gender (female)
	5) postnatal age
	CNS predictors:
	1) intracranial/ intraventricular hemorrhage
	2) periventricular leukomalacia
	Cardiovascular or pulmonary predictors:
	1) bronchopulmonary dysplasia
	Other predictors:
	1) dexamethasone
	2) perinatal factors
	  a) multiple birth
	  b) cesarian section
	3) socioeconomic variables
	  i) Asian mother
	  ii) higher SEC
	  iii) no English-speaking at home
	4) surgery in primary hospital
	5) patient with no adverse events
		1) SGA/IUGR - BW ratio <0.8
		2) intracranial/ intraventricular hemorrhage - Papille system
		3) periventricular leukomalacia - cystic lesions in PVWM dx < discharge
		4) bronchopulmonary dysplasia - ROS + O_2 Rx after 28 days age
		5) dexamethasone - postnatal steroid use
			CNS:
			Motor delay
			Cerebral palsy
			Cognitive delay
			Mental retardation
			
			Ophthalmology outcomes:
			Blindness
			
			Audiology outcomes:
			Hearing disorders
			Deafness
			
			Other outcomes:
			Survival without major disability at 5 years age
			Survival with major neurosensory disability at 5 years age
				1) motor delay, cognitive delay - WPPSI-R and alternative IQ tests
				2) cerebral palsy - not walking or walking with difficulty
				3) mental retardation - IQ < 2 SD below mean for NBW group

Evidence Table 1. Studies Evaluating Association of LBW and Multiple Outcomes: CNS, Eye, Lung, Growth, etc.
Part II

Author, Year	Predictors	Predictor Measures	Outcomes	Outcome Measures
Gaillard 2001 21221175	In retrospective case-control component: **General:** 1) shorter length of ventilation beyond 27 (but not 50) postnatal ds vs more prolonged ventilation beyond 49 ds 2) Number of days "off" ventilator in the groups of 27-49 postnatal ds ventilation and the group of >49ds ventilation In retrospective cohort with historical control group component: **General:** 1) Birth in a period where Antenatal steroids and Surfactant were more routinely used vs birth in pre-surfactant pre-antenatal steroid period	Not further specified	**CNS:** Neurodevelopmental outcome: 1) Normal 2) Mild disability 3) Moderate disability 4) Severe disability	Normal neurodevelopmentally: no clinically apparent neurodevelopmental abnormality causing functional disability Mild disability: e.g. myopia, language delay, mild hearing loss, hyperactivity or motor clumsiness. Moderate disability: for example: spastic diplegia, hemiplegia or moderate learning disability (Developmental Quotient: 50-69) Severe disability: e.g. spastic quadriplegia, blindness, deafness (loss of 70 decibel or more), uncontrolled epilepsy, or severe learning disability (developmental quotient <50). Infants with multiple disabilities. (3 yrs CA)

Evidence Table 1. Studies Evaluating Association of LBW and Multiple Outcomes: CNS, Eye, Lung, Growth, etc.
Part II

Author, Year	Predictors	Predictor Measures	Outcomes	Outcome Measures
Roth 2001 21262686	**CNS:** 1) intracranial/Intraventricular hemorrhage 2) white matter disorder 3) Periventricular leukomalacia 4) Ventriculomegaly/ventricular dilation 5) Ultrasound methodology: linear array vs mechanical sector	ND	**CNS:** Motor delay Cerebral palsy Cognitive delay Mental retardation School problems Learning disabilities **Ophthalmology:** Visual impairment Blindness **Audiology:** Hearing disorder Deafness	Outcome categories: 1) No neurodevelopmental impairment 2) Detectable impairment with disability (included neuromotor impairment with functional conse-quences, high tore hearing loss with need for aid, IQ 70-79, informal "help" in mainstream school) 3) Impairment leading to disability (included neuromotor impairment leading to disability sensory neural hearing loss, requiring aids, blindness or registered partial sight, IQ<70 or requirement for formal extra educational provision
Saigal 2001 21376729 * **Important paper**	Birth weight GA	ELBW=500-1000 g	**CNS:** Motor delay Cognitive delay Other: neurosensory impairment **Ophthalmology:** Visual impairment **Growth:** 1) height 2) weight 3) head circumferences 4) BMI (wt/ht2) **Other:** 1) Health status and problems ; current and past 2) Extra health care expenses 3) Utilization and health care resources	Reported previously in the authors' other paper Growth reference population was using the age- and gender- specific reference data provided by the NCHS growth chart

59

Evidence Table 1. Studies Evaluating Association of LBW and Multiple Outcomes: CNS, Eye, Lung, Growth, etc.

Part II

Author, Year	Predictors	Predictor Measures	Outcomes	Outcome Measures
Schmidt 2001 21298249	1) Prophylactic indomethacin administration : 0.1 mg/kg Q24 hrs X 3 days (vs NS placebo) in VLBW infants, during first 6 hrs of life	Nor further specified	Primary outcomes at 18 months of age: 1) Composite outcome: death or impairment 2) Death before 18 mo corrected age 3) Cerebral palsy 4) Cognitive delay (MDI<70) 5) Hearing loss requiring amplification 6) Bilateral blindness Secondary long term outcomes outcomes: 1) Hydrocephalus, necessitating the placement of shunt 2) Seizure disorders 3) Microcephaly (HC<3 d %)	1) Death before a corrected age of 18 months or documentation in survivors of one of the following: CP, Cognitive delay, Hearing loss requiring amplification, B/L blindness 2) Cerebral palsy diagnosed if had nonprogressive motor impairment with abnormal muscle tone and decreased range or control of movements. 3) Cognitive delay: as MDI less than 70 (2SD below the mean of 100) on the Bayley scale between 85-114: classified as normal, Scores below 70: marked cognitive delay. 4) Documentation of composite primary outcome: required documentation that the infant had died or had survived with one of the 4 types of impairment. A single missing component of the f/up assessment would result in designation of missing for primary outcome. A priori criteria for definitions of presence or absence of component of the primary outcome. 5) In cases it was difficult to obtain Audiologic test results, deafness requiring amplification was assumed to be absent if no such indication was present during the Bayley test. (n=27) 6) Blindness: a corrected visual Acuity of less than 20/200. F/up evaluation around 18 mo: allowed range 18-21 mo. (Home visits were permitted when necessary)

60

Evidence Table 1. Studies Evaluating Association of LBW and Multiple Outcomes: CNS, Eye, Lung, Growth, etc.

Part III

Author, Year	Associations found	Potential Biases	Comments
Akerman 1992 93255928	Physical and Emotional Problems at 4yrs: Psychomotor retardation----------11.8% Impaired hearing----------2.9% Impaired vision----------2.9% Delay in speech/language----------11.8% Emotional Problems----------2.9% No physical or psychological problems----------67.7% All except 3 infants with physical and emotional problems were either premature or weighed less than 2500 gms at birth. Of the 22 infants with physical or psychomotor impairment, 17 were males	No infant weighed less than 1250 g Population homogeneous middle class with access to medical care	No data on funding source
Thompson 1993 93234177	Two years CA neurodevelopmental outcome and Griffith's scores for a cohort of South African infants with BW < 1250 g, n = 96. Mechanical ventilation not routinely used when BW < 900g. Percent with outcome Normal 75% CP 6% DQ < 70 and CP 3% DQ < 70, no CP 1% DQ 70-79 and CP 0 DQ 70-79, no CP 15% Hyperactive 3% "Squint" 0 Developmental delay 0 Scores on Griffith's scales for most items fell significantly (P < 0.001) between one and two years of CA. Overall major handicap rate rose between years 1 and 2 CA from 14% to 22%	(None)	Study was private funded

Evidence Table 1. Studies Evaluating Association of LBW and Multiple Outcomes: CNS, Eye, Lung, Growth, etc.
Part III

Author, Year	Associations found	Potential Biases	Comments
Rademaker 1994 95003452	3.6% of the Preemie population (≤ 32 weeks) have unilateral intracranial parenchymal lesion. Not all unilateral parenchymal lesions are the same. Size of the lesion, location of the lesion, and whether the lesion communicates with the ventricle at any time all have important role in prediction of neurodevelopmental outcome. For example, if the initial lesion is triangular/fan-shaped and does not communicate with the ventricle at any time and is located in the fronto-parietal area, overall prognosis is favorable. But if the lesion is globular-shaped, continuous with the ventricle and extends beyond the trigone into the occipital periventricular white matter, risk for death and developing moderate to severe hemiplegia is significantly increased.	Small sample size	No data on funding source Cases series

Evidence Table 1. Studies Evaluating Association of LBW and Multiple Outcomes: CNS, Eye, Lung, Growth, etc.
Part III

Author, Year	Associations found	Potential Biases	Comments
Vonderveid 1994 94297368	Of all these 22 predictors/variables evaluated for **CNS** outcomes : • PVL was associated with more than 5-fold increase in the risk of **CP** (OR: 5.8; 95% CI: 3.8-8.8) • Acidosis during hospitalization was associated with more than 1.5-fold increase in the risk of CP (OR: 1.6; 95% CI: 1.1-2.4) Overall in this NICU cohort: there were: 443/634 (70%) LBW and 191/634 (30%) were VLBW Overall **CNS outcomes** at 2 yrs: 1) Functionally normal were: • 52% of all prematures • 25% of VLBWs • 63% of LBWs 2) 62/634 (10%) children had one or more disabilities • 46/62 (74%) had CP of severity score 2-4 • 2 had peripheral motor disability • 9 had DQ< 80 (without motor or sensory disability) **Ophthalmology outcome:** 1) 8 were blind due to ROP (3 also had CP) **Audiology outcome:** 1) 1 was deaf (was also blind and had CP) A definite handicap was considered for: • 21/62 (34%) disabled children • (21/634=3%) (according to WHO definitions)	• Cannot exclude Diagnosis bias as no information is given on blinding of personnel doing the outcome assessment on PMHx of the child. • Cannot exclude false Association found due to high number of predictors analyzed for the number of CP events (22 predictors for 46 CP cases)	

Evidence Table 1. Studies Evaluating Association of LBW and Multiple Outcomes: CNS, Eye, Lung, Growth, etc.
Part III

Author, Year	Associations found	Potential Biases	Comments
Kraybill 1995 95264242	Predictor evaluation for **Pulmonary, Growth and Neurodevelopmental outcomes at 1 yr.** Single dose Surfactant tx at birth was not associated with the pulmonary, growth, neurodevelopmental and neurosensory status of VLBW premature infants at 1 yr of corrected age *Placebo group vs Surfactant group, at 1 yr of age:* 1) Overall survival at 1 yr: 160/193 (83%) vs 163/192 (85%) **Pulmonary:** 1) Oxygen via NC: 4/122 (3%) vs 2/136 (1.5%) 2) Oxygen via CPAP: 0/122 vs 1/136 3) CLD: 8/122 (6.5%) vs 10/136 (7%) **Growth:** 1) Distribution of pts in both groups across different percentiles: Ht/age, Weight/age and HC/age: were not s/s different across the two groups. **CNS:** 1) Mean MDI score: 85 ± 20 vs 88 ±22 (not ss)) 2) MDI scores< 2SDs : 11/118 vs 23/133 3) Mean PDI score: 89±22 vs 91 ±23 (not ss) 4) PDI scores < 2 SDs: 11/118 vs 8/133 5) No impairment: 69/119 (58%) vs 78/134 (58%) 6) Impairment present (total): 50/119 (42%) vs 56/134 (42%) 7) Severe impairment: 29/119 (24%) vs 37/ 134 (28%) 8) Mild/Moderate impairment: 21/119 (18%) vs 19/134 (14%) 9) Types of impairment: MDI<69: 21/119 (18%) vs 27/134 (20%) MDI: 69-84: 19/119 (16%) vs 20/134 (15%) Moderate/severe CP: 10/119 (8%) vs 9/134 (7%) Mild CP: 10/119 (8%) vs 12/ 134 (9%) **Audiology:** 1) Bilateral sensorineural deafness: 0% vs 0% 2) Deafness not requiring amplification 1/119 (1%) vs 2/134 (1%) **Ophthalmology:** 1) Bilateral blindness: 4/119 (3%) vs 2/134 (1%) 2) Visual defect: 9/119 (8%) vs 9/134 (7%) Assessment from 28ds-12 mo:		

Evidence Table 1. Studies Evaluating Association of LBW and Multiple Outcomes: CNS, Eye, Lung, Growth, etc.

Part III

Author, Year	Associations found	Potential Biases	Comments

Kraybill
1995
95264242
(continued)

- No ROP: 50/132 (38%) vs 57/143 (40%)
- Present ROP overall: 82/132 (62%) vs 86/143 (60%)
- Mild/Moderate ROP: 79/132 (60%) vs 84/143 (59%)
- Severe ROP: 3/132 (5%) vs 2/143 (2%)
- Treatment for ROP overall:7/132 (5%) vs 10/ 143 (7%)
  Surgery: 4/132 (3%) vs 3/143 (2%)
  Cryotherapy: 4/132 (3%) vs 8/143 (6%)

In the NCMH cohort there was no difference in impairments (present or absent), the severity of impairments and the types of impairments at the 1yr of age assessment of this cohort)

Predictor evaluation for Pulmonary, Growth and Neurodevelopmental outcomes at 2 yr.

Single dose of Surfactant tx at birth was not associated with the pulmonary, growth, neurodevelopmental and neurosensory status of VLBW premature infants at 2 yrs of corrected age24/52 (46%)

Placebo group vs Surfactant group, at 2 yr of age:

- Overall survival at NCMH only at 2 yrs: 68/60 (13%) vs 67/83 (81%)

Pulmonary:
1) Hospitalized for respiratory illness: 9/84 (82%) vs 9/52 (17%)
2) Bronchodilator regular use: 10/61 (16%) vs 6/57 (11%)
3) Tracheostomy: 2/61 (3%) vs 0/57

Growth:
1) Distribution of pts in both groups across different percentiles: Ht/age, Weight/age and HC/age were: not s/s different across the two groups

CNS:
1) Mean MDI score: 89 ±21 vs 90 ±19
2) MDI scores< 2SDs: 5/58 (9%) vs 2/48 (4%) (NS)
3) Mean PDI score: 89 ±18 vs 88 ±16
4) PDI scores < 2 SDs: 4/58 (8%) vs 3/48 (7%)
5) No impairment: 32/60 (53%) vs 24/52 (46%)
6) Impairment present (total): 28/60 (47%) vs 28/52 (54%) (NS)
7) Severe impairment: 11/60 (18%) vs 7/52 (13%)
8) Mild/Moderate impairment: 17/60 (28%) vs 21/52 (40%)

Evidence Table 1. Studies Evaluating Association of LBW and Multiple Outcomes: CNS, Eye, Lung, Growth, etc.
Part III

Author, Year	Associations found	Potential Biases	Comments
Kraybill 1995 95264242 Continued	9) Types of impairment: MDI<69: 8/60 (13%) vs 2/52 (4%) MDI: 69-84: 14/60 (23%) vs 18/52 (35%) (NS) Moderate/severe CP: 6/60 (10%) vs 5/52 (10%) (NS) Mild CP: 2/60 (3%) vs 3/52 (6%) (NS) **Audiology:** 1) Bilateral sensorineural deafness: 0 vs 0 2) Deafness not requiring amplification: 0 vs 0 **Ophthalmology:** 1) Bilateral blindness: 0 vs 3/52 (6%) 2) Visual defect: 8/60 (13%) vs 2/52 (4%) (not ss) **Others:** 1) Any surgery (between 1-2 yrs): 10% vs 9 % Administration of single dose surfactant at birth in premature VLBW infants, with BW: 700-1350 g, results in improved survival rates up to 28 ds, without BPD and is not associated with adverse physical or neurodevelopmental outcomes at 1 yr or 2 yr corrected age.		

66

Evidence Table 1. Studies Evaluating Association of LBW and Multiple Outcomes: CNS, Eye, Lung, Growth, etc.
Part III

Author, Year	Associations found	Potential Biases	Comments
Speechley 1995 96356544	**General Health outcome:** Among boys around 12 yrs of age: NICU graduates as opposed to normal boys: 1) Are living with more chronic health problems 2) Are more likely to have a physical impairment 3) And have been hospitalized more often. Among girls around 12 yrs of age: NICU graduates as compared to normal girls: No statistically significant differences in their physical health outcome. Among NICU graduates, boys were not different from girls in their long-term physical health outcomes. **Emotional and Social well being outcomes:** Among girls around 12 yrs of age: NICU graduates as opposed to normal girls: 1) Had significantly lower social competence 2) Lower social support 3) And Lower self-esteem. Among boys around 12 yrs of age: NICU graduates as compared to normal boys: 1) They had no difference in their emotional or social well being. There was no interaction between family's socioeconomic status and long term outcomes among NICU graduates. Analytically: The **physical health outcomes** at 12 yrs were (**Boys NICU** grads vs Boys NNN grads/ **Girls NICU** grads vs Girls NNN grads) • Chronic physical health (mother's report): 2.8 vs 1.8 (p<0.005)/ 2.4 vs 1.3 • Lifetime hospitalizations (mother's report): 2.5 vs 1.6 (p<0.005)/ 1.7 vs 0.4 • Physical impairments (mother's report): 0.29 vs 0.10 (p<0.005)/ 0.22 vs 0.06 • Perception of child's heath (child's report): 21.6 vs 22.2/ 21.1 vs 21.9 • Perception of child's health (mother's report): 16.9 vs 17.7/ 16.8vs 18.0 **Emotional and social well being at 12 yrs:** (Boys NICU grads vs Boys NNN grads, Girls NICU grads vs Girls NNN grads) • Internalizing problems (child's report):15.3 vs 15.5/ 18.2 vs 14.8 • Externalizing problems (child's report): 15.9 vs 16.0 / 14.3 vs 13.5 • Social competence (child's report): 109.1 vs 113.9 / 101.7 vs 115.7 (p<0.005 • Social support (child's report): 81.6 vs 83.2/ 79.9 vs 86.1 (p<0.005) • Self esteem (child's report): 31.9 vs 32.4/ 29.8 vs 32.5 (p<0.005) • School performance (mother's report): 4.5 vs 4.6/ 4.8 vs 5.3	1) There is an inconsistency in mother's appreciation of their child's physical health: mothers of NICU graduate boys reported that their children had more physical impairments than NNN boy graduates; however, their overall perception of their child's health status was not any different from NNN boys graduates. 2) Some of the outcomes collected are prone to recollection bias (e.g., frequency of lifetime hospitalizations).	1) In this NICU cohort, only 36% of infants had BW<2500 g and only 5% had BW < 1500 gs, reflecting more NICU populations in the 1970s and early 1980s than the current ones. 2) It is unclear whether statistically significant differences in psychometric scales, with 10-36 items each, reflect clinically significant differences in the emotional and social well wellbeing of these children. 3) Conversely, given the fact of many negative findings, post hoc power analyses demonstrated that the study had an 80% power to detect a 40% difference between the 2 groups. (considering 20% as small effect and 50% as medium effect) 4) The fact that girl NICU graduates had a more substantial psychological effect than boys may reflect that girls are further into adolescence than the boys, experiencing the sequelae earlier. Thus in order to determine whether the differences observed are a temporary effect/related to adolescence, this cohort had to be followed further into their teenage years

Evidence Table 1. Studies Evaluating Association of LBW and Multiple Outcomes: CNS, Eye, Lung, Growth, etc. Part III

Author, Year	Associations found	Potential Biases	Comments
Hack 1996 97060805	At 8 year age, 10% of VLBW (24/249) had major neurosensory abnormality vs. 0% of Normal Birth Weight. At 8 years age, VLBW vs. Normal Birth weight were significantly less for each of the growth outcomes: weight, height, and head circumference (p<0.001) Significantly greater % of former VLBW infants with (22%) vs. without (7%) major neurosensory abnormal had significantly greater subnormal growth at 8 yr (OR 3.91, 95% CI 1.18-12.88). VLBW with major neurosensory abnormal had no catch-up growth after 20 months age. VLBW +SGA had increased odds of subnormal growth at 8 years (OR 3.89, 95%CI 1.35-11.23)	(None)	No data on funding source ELBW: Lost to follow-up (22), families refused (17), families moved out of state (20)
Hack 1996 97066007	MR (MDI<84) CP Blind Deaf Major Neurosensory abnormal +MDI<80 1982-1988 52% 10% 10% - 49% 1990-1992 34% 10% 2% 6% 35% 20-month Neurodevelopmental outcomes did not change appreciably between the 2 eras. 20% of infants had subnormal cognitive function (MDI<70) and 10% had CP during 1990-1992 period. One third of infants with BW 500-750 gram had major neurosensory abnormalities and / or MDI<80.	(None)	No data on funding source
Northern Neonatal Nursing Initative Trial Group 1996 96304894	No significant differences by Griffith's Developmental quotients, incidence of CP, seizures, hearing disorders. Initial demographics available in an earlier study.	(None)	Study was government and privately funded

68

Evidence Table 1. Studies Evaluating Association of LBW and Multiple Outcomes: CNS, Eye, Lung, Growth, etc.
Part III

Author, Year	Associations found	Potential Biases	Comments
Sethi 1996 96334245	Single evaluation at 2 years age. Follow-up information available for 99% of cohort. Normal 70% Major impairment 11% Minor impairment 19% Cerebral palsy 8.7% Blindness 2%	Results are from a single district general hospital No accounting for confounders: IVH, antenatal steroids, etc. Very little information provided to characterize groups BW distribution, degree of illness, IVH, BPD, etc. Inadequate information about population and about determination of cognitive function	No data on funding source 93 infants; follow-up available for 92; 20 infants had follow-up data from local medical care center rather than clinic visits
Wilkinson 1996 97087405	Among 10 surviving infants GA<35 wk/ BW<1500 gm who had severe cystic PVL, all (100%) had severe neurodevelopmental outcome (CNS [spastic quadriplegia, abnl neuro exam, seizures], impaired vision and hearing) at mean 27.3 mo age.	10/12 examined (8 by single neurologist/ 2 by pediatrician and neurologist) 9/10 eye examined in NICU 7/10 followed as outpatients Not a complete population sample of all GA<35 weeks or BW<1500 g with complete scanning data Small sample size	No data on funding source

69

Evidence Table 1. Studies Evaluating Association of LBW and Multiple Outcomes: CNS, Eye, Lung, Growth, etc.
Part III

Author, Year	Associations found	Potential Biases	Comments
DeReginer 1997 98041177	**Chronic lung disease** Any adverse outcome: 2/54 12/54　　P<0.001 18/56 Sensorineural hearing loss: 0/54 0/54　　P<0.05 3/56 Low MDI<2 SD from mean: 0/54 4/54　　P<0.05 5/56 Low PDI<2 SD from mean: 1/54 4/54　　P<0.05 7/56 Weight Z-score: No numbers given　　<0.05 Chronic lung disease and cerebral palsy, unilateral blindness, length Z-score, head circumference Z-score are not significant.	Matching scheme used is likely to be ineffective Large proportion of study population excluded by their matching strategy: subjects excluded were: 329/387=85% with no chronic lung disease; 53/111=47.7% with mild chronic lung disease; 122/180=68% with severe chronic lung disease	No data on funding source
Dezoete 1997 97359687	Outcome of category I & II: SGA: No difference between SGA and AGA infants IVA gr. III, IV: signify more cat I & II outcome with gr III-IV IVA vs I+II　　P= 0.01 Category IV: CLD: Children with CLD more likely to be normal (category IV)　　P<0.01	Entry criteria of infants that admitted to NICU; don't know standards of resuscitation in all 276 centers and it expertise of resuscitators creates a different kind of population.	No data on funding source

70

Evidence Table 1. Studies Evaluating Association of LBW and Multiple Outcomes: CNS, Eye, Lung, Growth, etc.
Part III

Author, Year	Associations found	Potential Biases	Comments
O'Shea 1997 98049056 *overlapped sample with 98190123	*Major neurosensory impairment:* Grade 3 LVH or PVE: 6.21(2.56, 15.101) *CP:* Total: (N=216) 14% (17/129 survivors) *Blindness:* Total: (N=126) 4% (5/129 survivors) *MDI<68* Total: (N=216) 14% (17/129 survivors)	(None)	Study was government funded
Piecuch 1997 97456215	Neurologic abnormal, neurosensory abnormal, cognitive abnormal BW No association Neurologic: GA Negative association Neurologic/neurosensory: ICH/PVL Significant association with abnormal outcome Cognitive: CLD Significant association with poor outcome Social risk Strong association No association was found between outcome and birth weight.	(None)	No data on funding source

Piecuch 1997 98012134	Mean age at follow-up was 32 months. Bayley exams were done at 18 months. Neurologic abnormalities and CP did not differ significantly across the gestational ages of 24 to 26 weeks. Between 67% and 89% were normal in each gestational age group. Significant differences (P = 0.036) related to gestational age were found in 18 month Bayley exam scores when group as normal borderline or deficient
	
	        Normal Deficient
	24 wk 28% 39%
	25 wk 47% 30%
	26 wk 71% 11%
	Significant differences (P = 0.008) related to gestational age were found in the combined end point of CP or an abnormal Bayley exam score:
	       Neither One Both
	24 wk 28% 39% 33%
	25 wk 47% 23% 30%
	26 wk 63% 34% 3%
		All inborn infants	No data on funding source

Evidence Table 1. Studies Evaluating Association of LBW and Multiple Outcomes: CNS, Eye, Lung, Growth, etc.
Part III

Author, Year	Associations found	Potential Biases	Comments
Singer 1997 98049057	Evaluation at 36 months corrected age. VLBW, VLBW with BPD, full term (FT). **Bayley MDI** **% with MDI below 70** VLBW 90 ± 16 (38-126) 11% VLBW w/ BPD 84 ± 24 (10-116) 21% FT 96 ± 12 (57-127) 4% P = 0.001 for VLBW vs. VLBW w/ BPD	Single region, but at least it is a region Unclear if examiners were blinded to group status	Study was government funded
Singer 2001 21163669	**Bayley PDI** **% with PDI below 70** VLBW 98 ± 20 (33-122) 9% VLBW w/ BPD 84 ± 29 (8-127) 9% FT 103 ± 15 (58-128) 1% P = 0.001 for VLBW vs. VLBW w/ BPD At 3 years BPD predicted poorer motor outcome but not poorer mental outcome. **Receptive DQ:** BPD < VLBW < Term, p < .05 **Receptive DQ < 85:** BPD 49%, VLBW 34%, Term 30%, BPD < VLBW + Term p < .05 **Expressive DQ:** BPD < VLBW + Term, p < .05 **Expressive DQ<85:** BPD 44%, VLBW 25%, Term 25% BPD < VLBW + Term p < .05 **Communication DQ:** BPD < VLBW + Term, p < .05 **Communication DQ < 85:** BPD 43%, VLBW 31%, Term 28%, NS Rank order listing of risk factors in order of magnitude of effect and the number of communication DQ lowered by the risk factor: PDA lowered DQ by 13 points, Minority race by 6 points, lower socioeconomic status by 5 points, and higher neurologic risk by 5 points. p .001 **Bayley Scales MDI:** BPD 83.7 ± 24, VLBW 90 ±16, Term 96.4 ± 12, BPD < VLBW < Term, p< 0.05 **Bayley Scales PDI:** BPD 84.1 28, VLBW 97.4 19, Term 102.8 14 BPD < VLBW + Term, p< .05 **ROP:** BPD 43%, VLBW 4%, p= .001 **Seizures:** BPD 7%, **Neurologic score:** BPD 1.3 ± 2, VLBW 58 ± 1, p < .001		

Evidence Table 1. Studies Evaluating Association of LBW and Multiple Outcomes: CNS, Eye, Lung, Growth, etc.
Part III

Author, Year	Associations found	Potential Biases	Comments
Victorian Infant Collaborative study Group, 1997 98026322	Birth weight < 1000g; assessed at 2 years corrected age.	Incomplete reporting of demographic data, methods and results.	Study was government funded
	Cohort n DQ <-3 SD DQ -3 to -2 SD DQ -2 to -1 SD DQ> -1 SD		
	'91-'92 237 5.9% 6.3% 13.9% 73.4%		
	'85-'87 211 6.2% 4.3% 14.2% 75.4%		
*This study is also in CNS table	Cohort n Mild CP Mod. CP Severe CP Any CP Blindness Deaf		
	'91-'92 237 3.8% 1.7% 3.8% 9.3% 2.1% 0.8%		
	'85-'87 211 NS NS NS 6.6% 4.3% 0.5%		
	Cohort No disability Mild Disability Moderate disability Severe disability		
	'91-92 71.3% 14.8% 7.2% 6.8%		
	n = 237		
	'85-'87 71.6% 15.6% 6.2% 6.6%		
	n = 211		
Victorian Infant Collaborative study Group, 1997 97466059 Arch Dis Child	All children born outside the level III perinatal centers. Assessment at 2 years corrected age.	Incomplete reporting of demographic data, methods and results.	Study was government funded
	1985-1987 1991-1992		
	n 19 16		
	Cerebral Palsy 19.1% 12.5%		
	Cognitive delay 19.1% 18.8%		
	Blind 5.6% 6.2%		
	Deaf 0 0		
	Sensorineural disability		
	Mild 15.8% 6.2%		
	Moderate 0 0		
	Severe 5.3% 12.5%		

73

Evidence Table 1. Studies Evaluating Association of LBW and Multiple Outcomes: CNS, Eye, Lung, Growth, etc. Part III

Author, Year	Associations found	Potential Biases	Comments
Cheung 1998 99059896	Mean MDI 81 ± 21, PDI 64 ± 22 Normal development 31% Neurodevelopmental delay 20% Disabled 50% Severe mental retardation 10% Spastic diplegic CP 30% Hemiplegic CP 10% <3rd %ile for weight 20% <3rd%ile for height 40% <3rd%ile HC 30% BPD 80% Need bronchodilators for CLD 10% Recurrent wheezing but did not need meds 40% Grade 4 IVH 20% Grade 3 IVH 20% VP shunt 30% PVL 10% Sensorineural hearing loss 10%	Very small sample size Descriptive study with no control group for comparison	No data on funding source
Finnström 1998 99041345	**CP** in 23-24 wks: 14%, in 25-26 wks 10%, ≥27 wks 3%, p<0.02 CP 25-26 wks AGA: 8%, SGA 24% **Major handicap by GA:** 23-24 wks: 14% 25-26 wks: 9% ≥27 wks: 3% **Major handicap by predictors:** Grade ≥ 3 IVH and/or PVL: 29%, OR 5.6 (95%CI 2.4-12.9) Stage ≥ 3 ROP 19%, OR 2.8 (1.1-7.6) Oxygen-dependent at 36 wks: 11%, OR 2 (0.9-4.1) PDA requiring treatment: 10%, OR 1.2 (0.5-2.8) Apgar score 0-3 at 1 min: 15%, OR 1.7 (0.7-4.0) Mechanical ventilation: 7%, OR 1.3 (0.4-4.5) After adjusting for GA, significant increased risk of handicap in infants with Grade ≥ 3 IVH/PVL and Stage ≥ 3 ROP **The mean height, weight and head circumferences were** significantly lower than reference values.	Exams done by infants' own pediatrician who is not blinded. Also they were not specifically trained in the evaluation so that results may be inconsistent. No control group. Scheffzek's categories not well defined. Infants were in the era of limited use of antenatal steroids and surfactant so that they may have been much sicker. How GA was determined not reported.	No data on funding source Possible that because of national recommendation that mothers should not be treated actively on fetal indications before completion of 25 weeks that only the fittest survive and this may underestimate Incidence of CP in this study. {Died by the follow-up exam (1) Left the country (6) Incomplete identification Number (1)}

74

Evidence Table 1. Studies Evaluating Association of LBW and Multiple Outcomes: CNS, Eye, Lung, Growth, etc. Part III

Author, Year	Associations found				Potential Biases	Comments
Gregoire 1998 98232532	Neurodevelopmental Outcome at 18 Months				Exam of SGA infants in BPD-2 group	Study was private and hospital funded
		Control	BPD-1	BPD-2	Higher receipts of postnatal steroids in BPD-2 groups	
	N	76	48	93	Higher rate of severe IVH in BPD-2 groups	
	Developmental quotient (DQ)	97.4 (15.6)	97.9 (11.6)	90.7 *(19.3)		
	DQ when no grade 4 IVH or PVL	97.4 (15.6)	99.9 (9.1)	93.0 *(19.3)		
	Percent w/ DQ ≤ 93	25%	29%	46%*		
	Percent w/ DQ ≤ 82	13%	13%	24%		
	Total CP	14%	17%	17%		
	Severe CP	13%	13%	17%		
	Total disabilities	29%	31%	50%**		
	BPD-1: supplemental O2 at 28 days but not at 36 weeks PCA. BPD-2: supplemental O2 at 36 weeks PCA. *P < 0.05 for comparison between BPD-1 vs. BPD-2. ** P < 0.05 for control group vs. BPD-2 and for BPD-1 vs. BPD-2.					
Kurkinen-Raty 1998 98387235 (All+Lung) *sample from the same big population as 20284814	Retrospective controlled cohort study of early PROM between 17 and 30 weeks of gestation. Assessments at one year corrected age. N = 55 for early PROM and 56 for control.				(None)	No data on funding source
	Outcome	Early PROM 18%	Control 16%	OR (CI) 1.2 (0.4, 3.1)		
	Cerebral palsy Delayed motor					
	Development	9%	16%	0.5 (0.2, 1.7)		
	Visual disability	4%	4%	1.0 (0.1, 7.5)		
	Hearing loss	7%	9%	0.8 (0.2, 3.2)		
	Good nuerosensory development	67%	61%	1.2 (0.6, 2.2)		
	Early PROM seems to be a major obstetric and neonatal problem with pulmonary ramifications extending beyond the neonatal period. However, most of these infants can be saved.					

Evidence Table 1. Studies Evaluating Association of LBW and Multiple Outcomes: CNS, Eye, Lung, Growth, etc.
Part III

Author, Year	Associations found			Potential Biases	Comments
		Cases	Controls		
Lee 1998 98442293	**Growth, CNS and Audiology, and ophthalmology outcomes** for prematures<1250 g with candidemia/candida meningitis			1) Cannot exclude missed association due to the small number of patients analyzed n both groups	
	Growth:				
	1) No difference in Growth retardation:	7/14 survivors(50%)	11/21 survivors (50%)		
	CNS:				
	1) No difference in MDIs of survivors	83 ±20	90 ±20 (p>0.05)		
	2) Lower PDIs in survivors	71 ±21	87±18 (p<0.05)		
	3) No difference in overall Neurodevelopmental disabilities (NDDs)	4/14 (29%)	3/21 (14%) (p>0.05)		
	4) Cerebral palsy	4/14 (29%)	3/21 (14%)		
	Ophthalmology:	2/14 (14%)	1/21 (5%)		
	1) Vision loss				
	Audiology:	2/14 (14%)	1/21 (5%)		
	1) Hearing loss (All the children with NDDs had Cerebral palsy with or without visual or hearing deficit)				
	Prematures<1250 g with candidemia/candida meningitis had: Higher Combined mortality and NDDs	60% (OR=3.9; 1.2-12.6)	28% (p< 0.05)		

Evidence Table 1. Studies Evaluating Association of LBW and Multiple Outcomes: CNS, Eye, Lung, Growth, etc.

Part III

Author, Year	Associations found	Potential Biases	Comments
Lefebvre 1998 98387703	Assessed at 18 months corrected age. Divided into low, moderate and high-risk group based on Neurobiologic risk score (NBRS). Tested with Griffith's Developmental Scales.	(None)	Study was privately funded
	Griffith's Developmental Score Category		
		Severe impairment, <80	All < 80		
	Risk Group n			
	Low 50	0%	12%		
	Moderate 37	22%	24%		
	High 34	50%	71%		
	Significance: for severe or any delay the NBRS was predictive, P < 0.0001		
		Severe CP (+)	Any CP		
	Risk Group n			
	Low 50	0%	4%		
	Moderate 37	13%	19%		
	High 34	26%	41%		
	Significance: NBRS predictive of CP, severe CP, P < 0.0009, any CP P < 0.0001		
Millet 1998 98212544	*Motor deficits:* Diffuse brain damage (N=26); 14	This paper has serious flaws	No data on funding source
	Moderate CP: Diffuse brain damage (N=26); 6	There is little demographic information and sparse reporting of CNS outcome. No statistical testing is report	
	Visual impairment: Diffuse brain damage (N=26); 12		
	Sensorineural hearing loss: Diffuse brain damage (N=26); 2		
	Cognitive impairment: Diffuse brain damage (N=26); 16		
	Epilepsy(in..? spasm) : Diffuse brain damage (N=26); 2		

Evidence Table 1. Studies Evaluating Association of LBW and Multiple Outcomes: CNS, Eye, Lung, Growth, etc.
Part III

Author, Year	Associations found	Potential Biases	Comments
Piecuch 1998 98446413	**Neural/Neurosensory outcome** 1) Neurologic and cognitive outcomes were relatively stable over the 3 time periods (1989-1991, 1984-1986, 1979-1981) for infants of 1000-1499 g BW. 2) > 90% of the infants born in each time period were neurologically normal. 3) There was a non-statistically significant trend towards an increased number of infants with neurologic abnormalities in the more recent period. 4) The incidence of CP was stable over the 3 time periods. Born in a recent period vs Born in a midpoint period vs Born in an Early period • Normal: 168/186 (90%) vs 143/155 (92%) vs 102/109 (94%) • Suspect: 10/186 (5%) vs 3/155 (2%) vs 1/109 (1%) • Abnormal: 8/186 (4%) vs 9/155 (6%) vs 6/109 (5%) More than 80% of infants in each group had normal cognitive outcome. Cognitive outcome: • Average/Above average: 152/182 (83%) vs 122/150 (81%) vs 86/102 (84%) • 1-2 SD< mean: 23/182 (13%) vs 19/150 (13%) vs 12/102 (12%) • > 2 SDs< mean: 7/182 (4%) vs 9/150 (6%) vs 4/102 (4%) 5) MDI scores declined slightly over time. But, mean PDI scores and MDI scores were not "clinically" significant across the 3 periods. More recent periods the infants born were smaller, younger, and had longer CLD Mean PDI: 96.6 vs 98.5 vs 96.9; Mean MDI: 101.0 vs 103.4 vs 106.9 In all the infants from the 3 time periods: General Predictors evaluation: Univariate analyses of predictors showed different relationships between outcome depending on inborn or outborn, with inborn having better neurologic and cognitive outcome. Predictors associated with poor neurologic/neurosensory (suspect and abnormal) or poor cognitive outcome (p< 0.02) were: Place of birth (outborns vs inborns); GA; male gender; ICH; CLD. When infants of suspect or abnormal neurologic outcome and infants of abnormal neurosensory outcome were grouped together and compared with infants of normal neurologic/neurosensory outcome (multivariate): For inborns: ICH, GA were predictors of poor outcome; For outborns:ICH, CLD were predictors of poor outcome. When infants of mild and moderate to severe cognitive deficits were grouped together and compared with infants of normal cognitive outcome (multivariate): For inborns: males had poorer outcome; For outborns: CLD was associated with poorer outcome	Concern about generalizability of findings in other populations with higher socieconomic status and higher maternal education. (For 50% of infants families were on public assistance and had maternal education of <12 yrs) Predictors were assessed for their association with the outcomes; but the outcomes were measured with different scales for the different age groups (Bayley, Stanford-Binet, McCarthy, Wechler Intelligence scale) and the mean age at assessment were different in the 3 periods	Severe cognitive delay may be apparent at 26 mo CA (the mean age of assessment of the youngest group in the study). However, subtle or late appearing cognitive problems may not have yet been diagnosed. Thus, the study had a limitation in detecting borderline cognitive or academic problems.

Evidence Table 1. Studies Evaluating Association of LBW and Multiple Outcomes: CNS, Eye, Lung, Growth, etc. Part III

Author, Year	Associations found	Potential Biases	Comments
Sajaniemi 1998 99041674	The neurological outcome of preterm infants was: For Cerebral palsy: Free from major disabilities MDI 1) All prematures: 17.5% 82.5% 103 2) Prematures < 1000 gs: 23.5% 23.5% 98 3) Prematures >1000 gs: 13.5% 85.6% 107 The developmental outcome: Preterm infants had significantly lower MDI scores when compared to full terms (Full terms 124) When temperament was considered: the premature children were significantly less active; more adaptive; less intensive; more positive in mood and had lower sensory threshold than the healthy control term children. When behavior was assessed (Infant's Behavior Records): the preterms were significantly less goal directed; less attentive and; had lower in endurance than the controls. When Bayley neurodevelopmental was assessed: 1) The preterms performed significantly less well than the controls. 2) Low Bayley scores correlated with temperament scores of high rythmicity, positive mood, low persistence and high threshold 3) Low Bayley scores correlated with IBR scores 4) No strong relationship between temperament characteristics and cognitive performance. Preterm infants had significantly lower MDI compared to full terms: • Preterm infants were different in 5/9 items of temperament profile compared to full terms: less active (p<0.008), more adaptive (p<0.02), less intense (p<0.01), more positive in mood (p<0.0004), lower in threshold to respond (p<0.0003) • Preterm infants were different in 3/5 items in IBR profile, when compared to full terms: less goal directed, less attentive, lower in endurance Predictors evaluation: • From the perinatal risk factors: pre-eclampsia, SGA, PVL and IVH were not associated with developmental outcome or temperament profiles. • PVL, IVH were associated with shorter attention span (1/5 items in IBR profile); when preterms compared to full terms. • Duration of NICU stay was not associated with Bayley score • Duration of ventilation was not associated with Bayley score • Duration of ventilation and days in NICU were associated with the 5 items of IBR profile; Duration of ventilation was associated with 1/9 items of temperament profile	• Post hoc multiple comparisons were done between preterms and full terms for the multiple individual items of the tests used. • Cannot exclude selection bias • No matching between groups cannot exclude the presence of confounders. • Interactions between predictors may have masked some real associations; possible interactions were not formally tested • Cannot exclude diagnosis bias, as no information is given on the blinding of the personnel doing the outcome evaluation of the child's PMHx.	

79

Evidence Table 1. Studies Evaluating Association of LBW and Multiple Outcomes: CNS, Eye, Lung, Growth, etc.
Part III

Author, Year	Associations found	Potential Biases	Comments
Scherjon 1998 9842916	**Predictors for Neurodevelopmental outcomes** (Univariate analysis) Adverse neurodevelopmental outcome at 3 years, measured with the Hempel test, was related to: 1) neonatal cranial ultrasound abnormalities of neonatal periventricular echodensities- as a sign of cerebral ischemia or intracranial haemorrhages (p< 0.0001) 2) low head circumference at 3 years. (when compared to normal and moderate abnormal findings) (p< 0.0001) Hempel test was not related to the umbilical/cerebral artery pulsatility index (raised vs normal) (p=0.23) Fetal growth retardation (IUGR) or gestational age was not related to behavioral aspects, language and speech skills using a parental questionnaire. Abnormal neurosonographic findings had an influence on Hempel outcome, only if these findings occurred in combination with a normal U/C ratio. However, abnormal neurosonographic findings with raised U/C ratio were not associated with a poor Hempel outcome. (Raised U/C ratio reflects a more favorable adaptation to prematurity related risks, preventing the infant from having severe intracranial pathology) **Predictors for Growth outcomes** at 3 yrs (Univariate model) In preterm infants born 26-33 wks, lower median HC at 3 yrs was associated with 1) fetal Doppler findings of raised Umbilical/cerebral artery pulsatility index (U./C ratio) (vs Normal U/C ratio) (p=0.01) Weight or height at 3 yrs was not associated with this predictor. **Predictors for Growth and Neurodevelopmental outcome** (multivariate) 1) Cranial U/S findings of IVH and ED were associated a) with Hempel outcome (p<0.001), and b) with HC at 3 yrs. (p=0.01) (it is not clear if it refers to moderate or abnormal U/S classification, or both) 2) U/C ratio, fetal growth ratio and GA were not associated with Hempel outcome	Cannot exclude possible confounders between compared groups.	The methods used for evaluation of qualitative behavioral and language differences at the age of 3 years between infants with and without placental insufficiency, possibly was not sensitive enough. There was blinding for the Hempel outcome assessment on the patients PMH or cranial U/S findings. The focus of this study was on motor development and quality of motor function. However, as there is weak association between neurodevelopmental outcome at 3 yrs and at school age yrs, it remains to reevaluate these children for their cognitive function at school age.

Evidence Table 1. Studies Evaluating Association of LBW and Multiple Outcomes: CNS, Eye, Lung, Growth, etc.
Part III

Author, Year	Associations found	Potential Biases	Comments
Cheung 1999 99146391	*Mental score:* Days of ventilation: (N=64) <0.0001 *Motor Score:* Days of ventilation: (N=164) <0.004 *Mental Score:* Grade of IVH: (N=164) 0.003 *Motor Score:* Grade of IVH: (N=164) <0.0001 *Mental Score:* Infants <1250g with gr. 3 or 4 IVH: (N=50) <0.001 *Motor Score:* Infants <1250g with gr. 3 or 4 IVH: (N=50) <0.001	(None)	No data on funding source

Evidence Table 1. Studies Evaluating Association of LBW and Multiple Outcomes: CNS, Eye, Lung, Growth, etc.
Part III

Author, Year	Associations found	Potential Biases	Comments

Duvanel 1999 99207097	There was no association of hypoglycemia with scores in Griffith's test at 6, 12, 18 months and in the McCarthy's test at 5 years.
	
	There was association of hypoglycemia with significantly lower scores in 2 items of the McCarthy's test (the perceptive index and the motricity index score) at 3.5 years
	
	Repeated episodes of hypoglycemia were associated with significantly decreased scores for 2/6 items in the McCarthy's test (perceptive performance and motricity scale index) only at 3.5 years. ($p< 0.05$)
	
	          Hypoglycemic Euglycemic group
	One episode of hypoglycemia:
	Mean MDI perception score at 3.5 yrs: 44.00 50.33 ($p<0.01$)
	>6 episodes of hypoglycemia
	MDI perception score at 3.5 yrs 44.89 50.33 ($p<0.05$)
	
	>7 episodes of hypoglycemia:
	• MDI perception score at 3.5 yrs 42.64 50.33
	  ($P<0.01$)
	• Motricity index score at 3.5 yrs 43.00 52.53
	  ($p<0.05$)
	
	Moderate hypoglycemia (11-29 mg/dl) was associated with significantly lower score in 2/6 items (perceptive performance and motricity scale index) in the McCarthy's test only at 3.5 years. ($p< 0.005$)
	No data on the association between the severity of hypoglycemia and the outcomes at 6, 12, 18 months and 5 years. (No complete data reporting)
	Infants with recurrent mild hypoglycemia had lower neurodevelopmental scores than the group with 1 unique severe episode of hypoglycemia. (Multiple subgroup comparisons, between subgroups of the independent variable and subgroups of the dependent variable)
	Hypoglycemia was not associated with growth rates for Weight, length, and HC at intervals 6-18 months, 6 mo-3.5 yrs, or 6mo -5 yrs.
	Hypoglycemia was associated with significantly reduced HC at 12, 18 mo and 5 yrs. ($p<0.05$)
		1) Selection bias
		2) Information bias (in the measurement of the independent variable/glucose levels)
		3) Confounders between the 2 groups
		4) Multiple subgroup comparisons. Hypothesis generating analyses.
			Selected Population/Potential Selection bias:
			Apparently a high-risk population was studied as the frequency of hypoglycemia identified was much higher than usually anticipated.
			
			Methods:
			Not clear for which parameters the matching between the 2 groups was done. Did not describe the flow of patients (Enrolled, excluded, lost to follow up, eligible for the analysis)
			
			Statistical analysis:
			No predefined in the Method section of primary and secondary outcomes to be studied. Many exploratory, hypothesis generating, subgroup analyses, which were not predefined in the Method sections.
			
			Information bias:
			Not consistent measurement of the predictor (glucose level) across different categories of hypoglycemia. Dextrosticks if glucose> 36mg/dl vs glucose analyzer if glucose<36 mg/dl)

Evidence Table 1. Studies Evaluating Association of LBW and Multiple Outcomes: CNS, Eye, Lung, Growth, etc.
Part III

Author, Year	Associations found	Potential Biases	Comments
Pennefather, 1999 20002011	Strabismus in 70/558 (12.5%) infants GA<32 week. **The incidence of strabismus increased with decreasing GA (p=0.0004),** increasing severity of ROP (p=0.0001), and decreasing general developmental quotient (GMDS) (p<0.0001).	Prospective evaluation but retrospective collection of neonatal data; therefore, probable incomplete collection of variable reason for present and absent data	No data on funding source
Pennefather, 2000 20217908	Stabismus present in 28 (52%) of patients with CP (P< 0.001) **OR (95% CI) of Strabismus if following predictor was present:** Cicatricial ROP: 4.94 (1.1-22.12), p0.037 Fam Hx of Strabismus: 4.15 (2.19-7.88), p<0.00005	No demographic data was report (the cohort was described elsewhere)	
* This study is also in eye table	Refractive Error: 2.71 (1.3-5.66), p=0.008 GMDS 78-100: 3.34 (1.46-7.64), p =0.004 GMDS <77: 46.2 (17.1-125), p<0.00005 This study confirms findings of other studies that strabismus is increasing in premature infants with decreasing GA and is increased with increasing severity of ROP and CP. Independent factors related to strabismus are cicatricial ROP, refractive error, family hx of strabismus, and developmental delay (especially delayed hand-eye coordination)		

Evidence Table 1. Studies Evaluating Association of LBW and Multiple Outcomes: CNS, Eye, Lung, Growth, etc. Part III

Author, Year	Associations found	Potential Biases	Comments
Ambalavanan 2000 21031370	ELBW: MDI<68 : 12% PDI<68: 20% Major handicap: 28% CP:28% MR 16% Post-hemorrhagic hydrocephalus: 5% Deaf 1.4% Blindness 1% Predictors of major handicap (Low MDI and/or PDI): Grade of IVH, PVL, absence of chorio (in this population, not in most others), NEC>II; race; multiple gestation, BPD, maternal education For ELBW infants without IVH, the prevalence of major handicap, low MDI, and Low PDI was 25%, 17%, 16%, respectively. For ELBW infants with grade III IVH, the prevalence of major handicap, low MDI, and Low PDI was 33%, 29%, 24% respectively. For ELBW infants with grade IV IVH, the prevalence of major handicap, low MDI, and Low PDI was 69%, 44%, 63% respectively. This study identifies major determinants of adverse neurodevelopmental outcome (i.e. major handicaps, low MDI, low PDI) of ELBW (<1 kg) infants born 1990-1994. Grade of IVH is strong predictor of adverse outcome. But note large % of ELBW without IVH who had major handicap, low MDI, and Low PDI. **BPD** was a significant determinant of low MDI and PDI. Mat education level was significant determinant of neurodevelopmental outcome. NEC, race, multiple gestation, PVL independently contributed to poor outcome in ELBW infant. Lower BW predicted low PDI.	Retrospective, relatively small samples size (218).	No data on funding source

Evidence Table 1. Studies Evaluating Association of LBW and Multiple Outcomes: CNS, Eye, Lung, Growth, etc.
Part III

Author, Year	Associations found	Potential Biases	Comments
Cioni 2000 20150341	Multivariate analysis found that periventricular leukomalacia in premature infants is highly, significantly correlated with visual impairment and abnormal neurodevelopment at 1 and 3 years age. The degree of visual impairment correlated well with degree of neurodevelopmental abnormality at 1 and 3 years age. Strong association between visual impairment and involvement of optic radiation on MRI. 28 of 29 infants had abnormal neurological examination at follow-up (6 mild abnormal; 22 had CP). 23/29 premature infants with PVL abnormality on MRI had at least one abnormality of visual function, and 50% had multiple visual function abnormalities. 8/29 severe 'fixation and following' disorders 19/29 had strabismus abnormal grating visual acuity 13/29 reduced visual field 9/29 OKN abnormalities 17/29	(None)	Study was government funded Visual function plays a strong role in early global development. But the presence of exceptions to these results also illustrate the complex, multifactorial nature of neurodevelopmental outcome. This study also illustrates the importance of a comprehensive assessment that includes various aspects of visual function. No single visual assessment will detect all visual abnormalities.

85

Evidence Table 1. Studies Evaluating Association of LBW and Multiple Outcomes: CNS, Eye, Lung, Growth, etc.
Part III

Author, Year	Associations found	Potential Biases	Comments

Hack 2000 20358826	MDI Score < 70:
	CLD: 55% (49/89); 2.18 (1.20-3.94)
	MDI Score<70 (multi stepwise logistic regression)
	Male sex: 2.73 (1.52-4.92)
	Social risk: 1.48 (1.09-2.00)
	CLD: 2.18 (1.20-3.94)
	OR adjusted for sex, social risk & BW:
	
	Gr III-IV IVH:
	   50% (16/32); 8.55 (3.52-20.76)
	   50% (8/16); 4.45 (1.54-12.84)
	   50% (17/34); 5.48 (2.41-12.47)
	CLD: 30% (27/89); 3.09 (1.51-6.35)
	Sepsis: 14% (13/93); 3.47 (1.16-10.36)
	Jaundice: 26% (6/23); 5.15 (1.63-16.22)
	Mult. Stepwise Logistic regression:
	Male sex: 2.79 (1.02-7.62)
	Sepsis: 3.15 (1.05-9.48)
	Jaundice: 4.80 (1.46-15.73)
	Predictors of neurologic abnormality were a severely abnormal finding on cerebral ultrasound (OR, 8,09; 95% CI 3.69-17.71) and chronic lung disease (OR 2.46; 95% CI 1.12-5.40); predictors of deafness were male sex (OR 2.79 95% CI 1.02-7.62), sepsis (OR 3.15 95 % CI 1.05-9.48), and jaundice (maximal bilirubin level >171)
			The authors concluded that there is an urgent need for research into the etiology and prevention of neonatal morbidity.

Evidence Table 1. Studies Evaluating Association of LBW and Multiple Outcomes: CNS, Eye, Lung, Growth, etc.
Part III

Author, Year	Associations found	Potential Biases	Comments
Jankov 2000 20188680	Infants CPR in delivery room -9 survived to discharge 8/9 were free of severe neurologic disability 1/9 was legally blind DR resuscitation beyond PPVin <750 gms was associated with high mortality but without unnecessary prolongation of life Persistent Apgar score <5 and delayed onset of respirations beyond 5 mins in CPR recipients were associated with death or severe disability. Did not find a high rate of severe neurodevelopmental disability in CPR recipients	Incomplete disclosure of data as it relates to the subgroups Small sample size Opposite results to other studies might be explained by decisions in many cases not to resuscitate infants that are extremely high risk which would be resuscitated in other centers	No data on funding source

87

Evidence Table 1. Studies Evaluating Association of LBW and Multiple Outcomes: CNS, Eye, Lung, Growth, etc. Part III

Author, Year	Associations found	Potential Biases	Comments
Kurkinen-Raty, 2000 20284814 *sample from the same big population as 98197235	**CLD at 1 year age:** Indicated PT delivery: (81) 12/81 (15%) Spontaneous PT delivery: (94) 3/94 (3%) RR 4.6 (1.4, 1.6) **Growth:** Indicated PT delivery: (81) Spontaneous PT delivery: (94) Weight RR =0.03 (-5.3, 0.3) L RR = 0.002 HC RR = 0.03 **CP:** Indicated PT delivery: (81) 5/81 (6%) Spontaneous PT delivery: (94) 10/94 (11%) RR=0.6 (0.25-1.6) **Delayed motor:** Indicated PT delivery: (81) 8/81 (6%) Spontaneous PT delivery: (94) 8/94 (9%) RR 1.2 (0.5-3.0) **Visual disability:** Indicated PT delivery: (81) Spontaneous PT delivery: (94) RR =1.9 (0.5, 7.8) **Hearing loss:** Indicated PT delivery: (81) Spontaneous PT delivery: (94) RR =1.9 (0.5, 7.8) This study demonstrated that premature infants who were born due to 'indicated maternal/fetal reasons' vs. spontaneous preterm delivered infants had worse pulmonary outcome a 1 yr age. More infants in 'indicated' group were SGA and were significantly smaller than control group at 1 yr in Wt, HT, and HC. There was no difference between groups in neurosensory outcomes.	Outcome not well defined Difficult to know if lack of difference between groups is due to sample size or event rate.	No data on funding source

Evidence Table 1. Studies Evaluating Association of LBW and Multiple Outcomes: CNS, Eye, Lung, Growth, etc.
Part III

Author, Year	Associations found	Potential Biases	Comments
Marlow 2000 20150342	**Pulmonary and Other predictors evaluation for Audiology outcome.** Children with sensorineural hearing loss [15] as compared to control group[30] had longer periods of: 1) Intubation, (14 ds vs 2 ds) 2) Ventilation (34 ds vs 6 ds) 3) Oxygen therapy (57 ds vs 10 ds) 4) Acidosis (12 ds vs 0.5 ds), and 5) More treatments with dopamine (33% vs 7%)or 6) Furosemide (87% vs 53%) 7) Neither P/T of aminoglycosides 8) nor duration of jaundice 9) or level of bilirubin varied between the 2 groups. SNHL was more likely when : 1) netilmicin use coexisted with the peak of bilirubin (87% vs 14%) 2) when acidosis occurred when bilirubin was over 200 μmol/l, (31% vs 4%) 3) when furosemide was used in the face of high creatinine levels (64% vs 27%) 4) when furosemide was used with netilmicin (67% vs 37%) **CNS outcome at 12 mo:** At 12 months of age evidence of cerebral palsy was present in 7/15 (47%) of children with SNHL vs 2/30 (7%) of children without SNHL.(p=0.022)	1) Very small sample size (cases with SNHL only 15) 2) Analyzed too many predictors and combination thereof, for very few outcomes. Very wide confidence intervals; and even those predictors found to be associated with the SNHL this may have been due to chance. 3) The association found between SNHL and cerebral palsy was <u>not</u> based on an adjusted analyses for possible confounders; 4) The 2 groups were different in many factors that were associated with both SNHL and CP	Not reported source of funding

Evidence Table 1. Studies Evaluating Association of LBW and Multiple Outcomes: CNS, Eye, Lung, Growth, etc. Part III

Author, Year	Associations found				Potential Biases	Comments
		Cortocosteroids	No Cortocosteroids	P-value	(None)	No data on funding source
Victorian Infant Collaborative study Group, 2000 20307288				Cerebral		
	n	98	195			
	Palsy	22.7%	3.6%	<0.0001		
	Blindness	5.2%	0.5%	<0.02		
	Deafness	1%	1.5%	ns.		
*some subjects were overlapped with Doyle, 2001	IQ scores			<0.0001		
	≥-1SD	46.4%	68.2%			
	-2 SD to <-1 SD	27.8%	24.1%			
	-3 SD to <-2 SD	13.4%	4.6%			
	<-3 SD	12.4	3.1			
	Sensorineural disability			<0.0001		
	Mild	26.8%	23.6%			
	Moderate	18.6%	6.7%			
	Severe	13.4%	3.6%			

Subgroup case-control study: cases (subjects with cortocosteroids treatment) and controls (subjects w/o with cortocosteroids treatment) were well matched in most perinatal variable

	Cortocosteroids	No Cortocosteroids	P-value
			Cerebral
n	60	60	
Palsy	21.7%	5.0%	<0.002
Blindness	1.7%	1.7%	ns.
Deafness	1.7%	3.3%	ns.
IQ scores, SDS	-1.26	-0.86	<0.05
Sensorineural disability			
Mild	26.7%	26.7%	
Moderate	21.7%	6.7%	
Severe	10%	8.3%	

Evidence Table 1. Studies Evaluating Association of LBW and Multiple Outcomes: CNS, Eye, Lung, Growth, etc.
Part III

Author, Year	Associations found	Potential Biases	Comments
Wood 2000 20373840	Infants 22-25 weeks GA developmentally assessed at median 30 months	(None)	Severe disability common children born extremely premature
	• 138/283 had disability 49% (64 met criteria for severe disability)		
	• 49% no disability		
	• 53/283 severely delayed 19% (Bayley below 3 SD)		
	• 32/283 2-3 below SD 11%		
	• 28 severe neuromotor disability 10%		
	• 7 blind or perceived light only 2%		
	• 8 hearing loss that was uncorrectable or required hearing aids 3%		
	Survived without overall disability		
	22 wks----------0.7 %		
	23 wks----------5%		
	24 wks----------12%		
	25 wks----------23%		
	Severe disability at 30 months		
	22 ------------0.7%		
	23 ------------3%		
	24 ------------6%		
	25 ------------9%		
	• no relation between morbidity pattern and either gestational age &multiple birth		
	• boys were likely to be disabled than girls		

Evidence Table 1. Studies Evaluating Association of LBW and Multiple Outcomes: CNS, Eye, Lung, Growth, etc. Part III

Author, Year	Associations found	Potential Biases	Comments

Doyle 2001 21326609
 	
Victorian Infant Collaborative study Group, 1997 97290716 J Paediatr Child Health
 	
*some subjects were overlapped with 20307288 (stated in text)
 	
*possibly overlapped with 98026322
	Evaluation at 5 years corrected age:
	CP : 23-27 wk survivors (11.3%) 25/221 Blindness : 23-27 wk (1.8%) 4/221
	   FT controls (0%) FT control 0%
	  Deafness : 23-27 wk (0.9%) 2/221
	FT control 0%
	IQ <-2 SD: 23-27 wk (15.4%) 34/221
	Major neurosensory disability
	23 –27 wk (19.6%) 44/225 FT control (4.1%) 10/245
	Major disability among survivors
	23 wk GA: 2/5 (40%) 24 wk GA: 7/21 (33%)
	25 wk GA: 13/51 (25%) 26 wk GA: 17/71 (24%)
	27 wk GA: 5/79 (6%) Overall 23-27 wk: 19%
	OR for survival with major disability at 5 years:
	OR each 1 wk increase in GA = 0.59 (95% CI 0.43, 0.8)
	Prognostic factors with major disability at 5 years: IVH, cystic PVL, surgery during primary hospitalization, postnatal steroid treatment.
	Rates of survival free of major disability for surviving PT infants:
	None 96/103 =93% One 59/71 =83 %
	Two 23/43 =53 % Three 3/9 =33%
	Four 0/1 = 0
	Evaluation at 2 years corrected age. Data shown are for births in 1991-1992.
	Gestational age Sensorineural disability (% of survivors)
	
		Gestational age	n	Severe	Moderate	Mild	None

---	---	---	---	---	---
23 weeks	5	29%	20%	40%	20%
24 weeks	21	14.3%	19%	33.3%	33.3%
25 weeks	51	5.9%	21.6%	25%	47%
26 weeks	68	8.8%	11.8%	20.6%	58.8%
27 weeks	74	1.4%	10.8%	23%	64.9%

Overall	219	6.4%	14.6%	24.2%	54.8% |
					
					Decrease in disability with increase in gestational age was significant, p = 0.014.
					Also showed significant fall in severe disability with increase in gestational age,
					   Odds ratio = 0.58 (0.36-0.94)
					Comparison of cohorts born in 1985-1987 vs. 1991: 1992 did not demonstrate
					   any difference between cohorts.
						Perinatal data lacking on some infants,
						Especially outborn (in level II or I)
						Different methods of testing IQ
						Different times of assessing Neurodevelopmental outcome
						Some children not evaluated at 5 years
						(evaluated at 2 years)
						210/401 preterm infants were assessed at
						both 2 and 5 years
						The classification of disability or no disability
						was the same at both 2 and 5 years (90.5% agreement; k=0.691)
						Inadequate discussion of study population,
						Demographic
						Also various surrogate data
							Study was government funded

92

Evidence Table 1. Studies Evaluating Association of LBW and Multiple Outcomes: CNS, Eye, Lung, Growth, etc. Part III

Author, Year	Associations found	Potential Biases	Comments
Gaillard 2001 21221175	**Predictors for Neurodevelopmental outcome:** 1) Shorter length of ventilation (beyond 27(but not 50) postnatal days) was associated with better neurodevelopmental outcome : 59% (33/56) neurodevelopmentally normal or only mildly disabled survivors vs 25% (7/28) with more prolonged ventilation(> 49 ds) *Ventilated beyond 27 (but not 50)ds vs Ventilated beyond 49 ds* Total: 56 vs 28 Survived: 48/56 (86%) vs 14/28 (50% Normal neurodevelopmentally: 26/48 (54%) vs 5/14 (36%) Mild disability: 7/48 (15%) vs 2/14 (14%) Moderate disability: 11/48 (23%) vs 4/14 (29%) Severe disability: 4/48 (8%) 3/14 (21%) 2) Number of days "off"" ventilator was not associated with the neurodevelopmental outcome at 3 yrs neither in the groups of 27-49 postnatal ds ventilation nor in the group of >49ds ventilation (but had only 1,4 and 9 survivors in the 3 subgroups respectively) *Ventilated beyond 27 (but not 50)ds and O ds "off" ventilator vs 1-7 ds "off" ventilator vs > 7 ds off ventilator* Total: 18 vs 17 vs 21 Survived: 13 (72%) vs 15 (88%) vs 20 (95%) Neurodevelopmentally normal: 8 (44%) vs 7 (41%) vs 11 (52%) Mild disability: 2 (11%) vs 2 (12%) vs 3 (14%) Moderate disability: 3 (17%) vs 4 (24%) vs 4 (19%) Severe disability: 0 vs 2 (12%) vs 2 (10%) (In the second component: comparison of the retrospective cohort with the historical control) 3) Birth in a period where antenatal steroids and exogenous surfactant was more routinely used was associated with better neurodevelopmental outcome (69% vs 40% and 45% respectively in the 2 historical control cohorts)	In First component: Retrospective cases control design: 1) the 2 groups were unmatched for possible confounders, thus cannot exclude false associations 2) Cannot exclude selection Bias as only 62 survivors were analyzed from the 84 initially included in the 2 groups In the Second component: 3) Problems of confounders due to historical control group could be even greater	ND

93

Evidence Table 1. Studies Evaluating Association of LBW and Multiple Outcomes: CNS, Eye, Lung, Growth, etc.
Part III

Author, Year	Associations found	Potential Biases	Comments
Roth 2001 21262686	Neurodevelopment Impairment: Liner array- all impairments 58 (28%) Disabling impairment 24 (12%) Mech sector all impairments 207 (36%) Disabling impairment 80 (14%)	Groups outcome into large categories of Disability unable to specify motor vs cognitive Vs hearing vs vision	

Evidence Table 1. Studies Evaluating Association of LBW and Multiple Outcomes: CNS, Eye, Lung, Growth, etc.
Part III

Author, Year	Associations found	Potential Biases	Comments

Saigal 2001 21376729
 	
* Important paper
	Neurosensory Impairment:: ELBW 28%, FT Controls 2%, p= 0.001
	Growth: Weight: diff. between ELBW and FT (mean z scores) –5.78 (p<0.0001)
	Visual Problems: ELBW 57%, FT Controls 21%, p=<0.001 (OR 5.1, CI 2.89-9.05)
	
	Current Health Problems (multiple/patient: ≥3 Health Problems: ELBW 35%, FT Controls 7%, p<0.0001
	Past Health Problems:
	  Seizures: ELBW 11%, FT Controls 2%, p<0.005
	  Asthma: ELBW 25%, FT Controls 14%, p=0.05
	  Recurrent bronchiolitis/pneumonia: ELBW 14%, FT Controls 3%, p=0.005
	Current (at 12-16 yr age) Functional Limitation (Table 4 page 411) (multiple/patient)
	  Visual difficulty: ELBW 57%, FT Controls 21%, p<0.001
	  Hearing Difficulty: ELBW 7%, FT Controls 5%, ns.
	  Emotional problems: ELBW 4%, FT Controls 1%, ns
	  Mental problems: ELBW 4%, FT Controls 1%, ns.
	  Clumsiness: ELBW 25%, FT Controls 1%, p<0.001
	  Developmental Delay: ELBW 26%, FT Controls 1%, p<0.001
	  Learning Disability: ELBW 34%, FT Controls 10%, p<0.001
	  Hyperactivity: ELBW 9%, FT Controls 2%, p=0.04
	  Reduced self-abilities: ELBW 5%, FT Controls 0%, p=0.02
	Limitation in school or in normal activity: ELBW 31%, FT Controls 9%, **p<0.002**
	Any functional limitation: **ELBW 81%, FT Controls 42%, p<0.001**
	Functional limitation/child [Mean (SD)]: **ELBW 2.0 (1.8) FT Controls 0.6 (0.8), p<0.001**
	Utilization of Health Care Resources:
	  Pediatrician: **ELBW 34%, FT Controls 14%, p<0.0002**
	  Ophthalmologist: **ELBW 62%, FT Controls 34%, p<0.0001**
	  Ear/nose/throat: **ELBW 14%, FT Controls 6%, p<0.05**
	  Occupational therapist: **ELBW 7%, FT Controls 1%, p=0.002**
	  Speech therapist: **ELBW 8%, FT Controls 0%, p<0.002**
	  Special Education: **ELBW 48%, FT Controls 10%, p<0.0001**
	  Prescription Glasses: **ELBW 36%, FT Controls 10%, p<0.001**
		Didn't specify exclusion criteria but these are implied based on clear industry criteria
		
		Limits to generalizability:
		1) different era of natural care
		2) white race
		3) access to universal health care in Canada
			Study was private funded

Evidence Table 1. Studies Evaluating Association of LBW and Multiple Outcomes: CNS, Eye, Lung, Growth, etc.
Part III

Author, Year	Associations found	Potential Biases	Comments
Schmidt 2001 21298249	1) There was no difference in primary outcomes between the 2 groups at 18 months of age. 2) Among the 574 infants who were assigned to prophylaxis with indomethacin, 271 (47%) died or survived with impairment as compared with 261 of 569 infants (46%) assigned to placebo (OR: 1.1; 95% Confidence intervals; 0.8-1.4) 3) In VLBW infants, prophylaxis with indomethacine does not improve the rate of survival without neurosensory impairments at 18 months of age 4) There was no difference in any of the secondary outcomes between the 2 groups , at 18 months of age. **Primary: Composite / CNS Outcomes:** **Indomethacin vs. Placebo** • Death or impairment 271/574(47%) vs. 261/569 (46%) • Death before 18 mo 121/595 (21%) vs 111/594 (19%) • Cerbral palsy 58/467 (12%) vs 55/477 (12%) • Cognitive delay (MDI<70 by Bayley scale 118 /444 (27%) vs 117/457 (26%) **Audiology outcome:** • Hearing loss requiring amplification 10/456 (2%) vs 10/466 (2%) **Ophthalmology outcome:** • Bilateral blindness 9/456 (2%) vs 7/472 (1%) (Odds ratios adjusted for BW stratum and Center) **Secondary CNS outcomes** were not affected by indomethacin administration: • Hydrocephalus requiring shunt 15/470 (3%) vs 9/480 (2%) • Seizure disorder 8/470 (2%) vs 7/483 (1%) • Microcephaly 49/461 (11%) vs 54/475 (11%) Kaplan Meier estimates of survival in the 2 groups: • 0 months n=601 vs 601 • 6 months n=479 (80%) vs 490 (82%) • 12 months n=473 (79%) vs 487 (81%) • 18 months n=470 (78%) vs 483 (80%)		1) By using the Bayley test at 18 mo the authors found that more than one quarter of all surviving infants had moderate to severe cognitive delays, defined by MDIs< 70. The validity of the MDI score at this age as a predictor of later intellectual functioning remains to be determined. 2) At a post hoc calculation the study had a 90% power to detect a 20% reduction in risk, had it existed 3) Authors report that the outcome assessments were done blindly by investigators unaware of treatment groups assignments. 4) Authors report that they had almost complete ascertainment for the primary outcome at 2 yrs of age.

Evidence Table 2. Randomized Controlled Trials for LBW Infants and Multiple Outcomes: CNS, Eye, Lung, Growth, etc. Part I

Author, Year UI#	Demographics	Inclusion Criteria	Exclusion Criteria	Disease/Condition Type (N)	Study Design (Duration)

Casiro 1995 95264245	Location: Canada
	Years of Birth: 1988- 1990
	Mean GA f (range), wk:
	  Experiment: 25.8±1.6
	  Control: 24.8±1.1
	Mean BW (range), g:
	  Experiment: 652±64
	  Control: : 661±52
	Male:
	  Experiment: 40%
	  Control: 40%
	Race: White
	  Experiment: 6%
	  Control: 14%
	Enrolled: 113 (111 controls)
	Evaluated: 47 (42 controls)
	Number of sites: 13
		BW 500-749 g
		Informed consent
		Mechanical ventilation required
		within 24 hr. b/o RDS
		A/A PO2 ratio< 0.22
			"Exclusion criteria for this study were the same as those used in an earlier trial of synthetic surfactant" (Long W, Thompson T, et al., 1991)
			Died by age of 1 year
				Experiment:
				Exosurf (47)
				Control: Placebo (42)
					Randomized Controlled Trial

Evidence Table 2. Randomized Controlled Trials for LBW Infants and Multiple Outcomes: CNS, Eye, Lung, Growth, etc.
Part I

Author, Year UI#	Demographics	Inclusion Criteria	Exclusion Criteria	Disease/Condition Type (N)	Study Design (Duration)

Gerdes 1995 95264241	Location: US
	Years of Birth: 3/1989-4/1990
	Mean GA (range), wk:
	  Experiment 1: 27.2±1.7
	  Experiment 2: 27.2±1.8
	Mean BW (range), g:
	  Experiment 1: 907±121
	  Experiment 2: : 911±125
	Male:
	  Experiment 1: 55%
	  Experiment 2: 56%
	Race:
	  Experiment 1: White 55%, Black 37%,
	    Hispanic 4%, Other 5%
	  Experiment 2: White 60%, Black 30%,
	    Hispanic 5%, Other 5%
	Enrolled: 826
	Evaluated: 508
	Number of sites: 33
		Mothers who were expected to deliver premature infants with BW 700-1100 g	All exclusion prenatal.
			1) Proven fetal lung maturity
			2) Known malformation or chromosome anomaly
			3) Fetal growth retardation
			4) Hydrops
			5) Purulent amnionitis
			6) Maternal heroin addiction
			7) Obstetric decision not to support fetus
			Postnatal exclusions:
			1) Major malformation
			2) ≥3 minor anomalies
			3) Hydrops
				Experiment 1: One doses surfactant (244)
				Experiment 2: Three doses surfactant (264)
					Randomized comparison trial (1 year)

Evidence Table 2. Randomized Controlled Trials for LBW Infants and Multiple Outcomes: CNS, Eye, Lung, Growth, etc. Part I

Author, Year UI#	Demographics	Inclusion Criteria	Exclusion Criteria	Disease/Condition Type (N)	Study Design (Duration)
O'Shea 1998 98167528 98190123 *also in CNS table *overlapped sample as 98049056	Location: US Years of Birth: 1978-89; 1990-94 Mean GA (range), wk: Born in 1978-1989: Cases: 28(24-33) Unmatched controls: 29 (23-39) Matched controls: 28 (24-34) Born in 1990-1994: 28.0±2.9 Mean BW (range), g: Born in 1978-1989: Cases: 1021 (520-1500) Unmatched controls: 1150 (580-1490) Matched controls: 1095 (580-1490) Born in 1990-1994: 1039±291 Male: Born in 1978-1989: Cases: 54% Unmatched controls: 50% Matched controls: 51% Born in 1990-1994: 51% Race: Born in 1978-1989: Cases: 45% African-American Unmatched controls: 35% African-American Matched controls: 32% African-American Born in 1990-1994: 56% White Enrolled: 1978-1989 (1559); 1990-1994 (1264) Evaluated: 1978-1989 (80 cases, 240 controls); 1990-1994 (723) Number of sites: 2	BW 500-1500g, admitted to the 2 intensive care nurseries that served the 17 countries in NW N. Carolina. Birth at only tertiary OB center in region Survived to age 1 year corrected age Cases: diagnosis of any subtypes of cerebra palsy Controls: VLBW infants born closest in time to the respective case, who after examination at 1 year of age were felt to be free of any signs of cerebra palsy	Major congenital anomaly	Born in 1978-1989: Cases: CP (80) Unmatched controls (160) Matched controls (80) Born in 1990-1994: VLBW infants: 723	Case-control study (1 year corrected age)

99

Evidence Table 2. Randomized Controlled Trials for LBW Infants and Multiple Outcomes: CNS, Eye, Lung, Growth, etc.
Part I

Author, Year UI#	Demographics	Inclusion Criteria	Exclusion Criteria	Disease/Condition Type (N)	Study Design (Duration)
O'Connor 2001 21376723	Location: US Years of Birth: 1996-1998 Mean GA (range), wk: 29 (27-31) Mean BW (range), g: 1253 (965-1543) Male: 39% Race: ND Enrolled: 376 Evaluated: 246 (126 controls) Number of sites: 8	GA < 33 weeks and BW 750-1805 g Completed the study to 12 months' CA	Serious congenital abnormalities, major surgery prior to enrollment/ randomization. PVL/IVH > grade II Maternal Incapacity Liquid ventilation Severe asphyxia Uncontrolled systemic infection at enrollment	Sample 1: EHM-T fed infants (43), reference group only, not included in analyses At 12 months: Sample 2: AA+OHA (fish/fungal) (120) Sample 3: AA+DHA (egg-TG/fish) (126) Control: formula-fed infants (126)	Randomized controlled trial (12 months)

Evidence Table 2. Randomized Controlled Trials for LBW Infants and Multiple Outcomes: CNS, Eye, Lung, Growth, etc. Part II

Author, Year	Predictors	Predictor Measures	Outcomes	Outcome Measures
Casiro 1995 95264245	Cardiovascular/Pulmonary: Exosurf vs. placebo	ND	**CNS:** Motor delay Cerebral palsy Cognitive delay Severity impairment **Ophthalmology:** ROP **Growth:** Height, weight, head circumference **Other:** Re-hospitalization in 1st year of life	Bayley Scales of Infant Development: MDI and PDI The details of ophthalmologic examination, 1-year follow-up, health status evaluation were described in elsewhere (Courtney SE, Long W, et al., 1995)
Gerdes 1995 95264241	Cardiovascular or Pulmonary: Surfactant use	ND	**CNS:** Cerebral palsy Cognitive delay Mental retardation **Ophthalmology:** Visual impairment, Blindness **Audiology:** Hearing Disorder, Deafness **Pulmonary:** Asthma e/o CLD Respiratory support @ 1yr **Growth:** Height, Weight, HC **Other:** hospital re-admissions, h/o surgery	Mental retardation Bayley Scales MDI<69

101

Evidence Table 2. Randomized Controlled Trials for LBW Infants and Multiple Outcomes: CNS, Eye, Lung, Growth, etc.
Part II

Author, Year	Predictors	Predictor Measures	Outcomes	Outcome Measures
O'Shea 1998 98167528 98190123 *also in CNS table *overlapped sample as 98049056	General predictors: Birth weight GA CNS predictors: IVH White matter disorder Periventricular leukomalacia Ventriculomegaly/Ventricular dilation Other: Infectious disease Perinatal factors	Hemorrhage disease diagnosed by Cranial US finding	**CNS:** CP	CP including spastic hemiplegia (involvement of an arm and leg on the same side of the body), spastic diplegia (involvement of the both legs with minimal to no involvement of the arms); and, spastic quadriplegia (involvement of all four extremities)
O'Connor 2001 21376723	Other: Nutrition/growth	ND	**CNS:** Motor delay Cognitive delay Other: information processing languages **Ophthalmology:** Visual Acuity **Growth:** Weight Length Head circumferences	Bayley scales – PDI; MDI Teller visual acuity cards

Evidence Table 2. Randomized Controlled Trials for LBW Infants and Multiple Outcomes: CNS, Eye, Lung, Growth, etc.
Part III

Author, Year	Associations found	Potential Biases	Comments
Casiro 1995 95264245	Assessed at one year corrected age. No significant differences between placebo group and Exosurf group for: Bayley MDI (Placebo 79 ± 22 vs. Exosurf 87 ± 20) Bayley PDI (Placebo 73 ± 18 vs. Exosurf 81 ± 19) Percent of patients with Bayley MDI < 69 (22% vs. 21%) Percent of patients with Bayley PDI < 69 (29% vs. 19%) No significant differences between placebo and Exosurf groups for: No impairment (38% vs. 55%, Placebo vs. Exosurf) Any impairment (62% vs. 45%, Placebo vs. Exosurf) Serious impairment (41% vs. 32%, Placebo vs. Exosurf) No significant differences between placebo and Exosurf groups for: Bilateral sensorineural deafness: 7% vs. 9%, Placebo vs. Exosurf) Blindness: (7% vs. 2%, Placebo vs. Exosurf) No significant difference in height, weight or head circumference.	All patients had RDS requiring mechanical ventilation	No data on funding source

103

Evidence Table 2. Randomized Controlled Trials for LBW Infants and Multiple Outcomes: CNS, Eye, Lung, Growth, etc. Part III

Author, Year	Associations found	Potential Biases	Comments

Gerdes 1995 95264241	Severe ROP:
	  1 dose: 47(16) 3 dose: 35(11)
	Physical evidence of CLD:
	  1 dose: 43(18) 3 dose: 40(15)
	Medication for CLD:
	  1 dose: 35(14) 3 dose: 30(11)
	Medication for chronic neurologic disease:
	  1 dose: 12(5) 3 dose: 3(1)
	Index<2 SD (%):
	  1 dose: 29(15) 3 dose: 30(13)
	Impairment present:
	  1 dose: 106(44) 3 dose: 92(35)
	No impairment:
	  1 dose: 123(51) 3 dose: 155(59)
	Severity of impairment:
	Mild/moderate:
	  1 dose: 40(17) 3 dose: 39(15)
	Serious:
	  1 dose: 66(27) 3 dose: 53(20)
	Types of impairments:
	MDI<69:
	  1 dose: 40(16) 3 dose: 38(14)
	Moderate/severe CP:
	  1 dose: 22(9) 3 dose: 16(6)
	Bilateral sensorineural deafness:
	  1 dose: 5(2) 3 dose: 10(2)
	Deafness not requiring amplification:
	  1 dose: 5(2) 3 dose: 2(1)
	Bilateral blindness:
	  1 dose: 10(4) 3 dose: 4(2)
	Visual defect:
	  1 dose: 24(10) 3 dose: 22(8)
		25% loss to follow up, equal in both groups 1 year follow up does not predict long term outcome from all infants	No data on funding source
			
			"Prenatal and postantal exclusion criteria were identical to those used in an earlier prophylactic trial of this synthetic surfactant"
			Died by 1-year adjusted age
			Lost to follow-up

Evidence Table 2. Randomized Controlled Trials for LBW Infants and Multiple Outcomes: CNS, Eye, Lung, Growth, etc. Part III

Author, Year	Associations found				Potential Biases	Comments
		Dexamethasone	Placebo	P		
O'Shea 1998 98167528 98190123	Definite Cerebral Palsy:	12	3		(None)	Study was government funded
	Possible CP:	5	2			
	Overall CP:	17	5	0.006		
	Neuro exam severe					
*also in CNS table	Abnormal:	4	2			
	Mild abnormal:	16	6			
*overlapped sample as 98049056	Overall abnormal Neuro exam:	20	8	0.03		
	Authors analyze associations between prenatal factors and cerebral palsy in 80 infants with weights 500-1500g who were born in 1978-1989 to a resident of northwest region of Carolina. Factors that were strongly associated with increased risk of CP were: multiple gestation, chorioamnionitis, maternal antibiotics, antepartum vaginal bleeding, and labor lasting less than 4 hours. Pre-eclampsia and delivery without labor were associated with decreased risk of CP.					
O'Connor 2001 21376723	Growth (Wt, Ht, HC) no difference among the 4 pretem groups in terms of gm/kg/day for weight ; mm/wk for Ht and HC. Bayley at 12 months MDI range 92.2- 93.4 (no difference among 4 groups) PDI range 85.9-87.2 (no difference among 4 groups) For infants with BW<1250 gm Control group: PDI 81.8 which was sig less than PDI in AA-DHA (fish/fungal) (90.6)or AA-DHA (egg) (84.7) groups Language vocabulary comprehension at 14 mo. Comprehension: 97-101.6 (no difference among 4 groups) Production: 96.6-98.3 (no difference among 4 groups) Results support benefit in PDI of supplementing formulas for premature infants with AA+DHA from either fish/fungal or egg/fish source from first enteral feeding through 12 months in infants BW<1250 g				(None)	No data on funding source

105

Evidence Table 3. Studies Evaluating Association of LBW and Cerebral Palsy and Neurological Outcomes
Part I

Author, Year UI#	Demographics	Inclusion Criteria	Exclusion Criteria	Disease/Condition Type (N)	Study Design (Duration)
Leonard 1990 90204169	Location: US Years of Birth: 9/1/77- 9/1/82 Median GA (range), wk: 28.54±1.97 Mean BW (range), g: 1003±155 Male: 43% Race: ND Enrolled: 193 Evaluated: 129 Number of sites: 1	BW<1250 g Head CT between 5-6 days of life or head ultrasound days 3 and 10 after delivery	Died after discharge Lost to follow-up before reaching school age	VLBW infants (129): Without ICH (84), including 72 no parenting risk factor and 12 having parenting risk factor With ICH (45), including 38 no parenting risk factor and 7 having parenting risk factor	Prospective cohort (4.5 to 5 years)

Lucas 1992 92122860	Location: UK
	Years of Birth: 1982-1985
	Mean GA:
	  Sample 1: 31.4 ± 0.3
	  Sample 2: 31.4 ± 0.2
	Mean BW:
	  Sample 1: 1420 ± 30
	  Sample 2: 1440 ± 20
	Males:
	  Sample 1: 42%
	  Sample 2: 55%
	Race: ND
	Enrolled: 313
	Evaluated: 300
	Number of sites: 5
		Premature
		BW< 1850 g
			ND	Sample 1:
				Preterms- no mother's milk (mother's choice not to provide breast milk to her infant within 72 hrs from delivery) [90]
				
				Sample 2:
				Preterms- mother's milk (mother's choice to provide breast milk to her infant within 72 hrs from delivery) matched with sample 1 for :BW, GA, need for ventilation, ds of NICU stay, other diets [210]
					Prospective comparative longitudinal study (7.5-8 yrs)

106

Evidence Table 3. Studies Evaluating Association of LBW and Cerebral Palsy and Neurological Outcomes

Part I

Author, Year UI#	Demographics	Inclusion Criteria	Exclusion Criteria	Disease/Condition Type (N)	Study Design (Duration)
Robertson 1994 94181384	Location: Canada Years of Birth: 1990 Median GA (range), wk: ND Mean BW (range), g: 500-1500 Male: ND Race: ND Enrolled: 241 Evaluated: 163 → 157 Number of sites: 2	BW 500-1249 g, lived born in Alberta to Alberta parents	Corrected rates exclude infants with syndromes and / or CNS malformations Survived to 1- and 2-years of corrected age	VLBW infants survived to 1 year corrected age (163) → survived to 2 year corrected age (157)	Retrospective cohort (at 1 year and 2 year corrected age)
Spinillo 1994 94257064 *sample overlaps with Spinillo, 1997	Location: Italy Years of Birth: 1983-1989 Median GA (range), wk: Sample 1: 33.4±3.4 Sample 2: 31.6±4.3 Sample 3: 32.7±5.1 Controls: 32.7±4.0 Mean BW (range), g: Sample 1: 1800±458 Sample 2: 1641±570 Sample 3: 1768±633 Controls: 1748±569 Male: ND Race: ND Enrolled: 87 Evaluated: 77 (154 controls) Number of sites: 1	Cases: LBW infants with diagnosis of abnormal antepartum bleeding in mother's pregnancy Controls: two liveborn LBW infants of similar GA and free of malformations born immediately after each case	ND	Cases: Sample 1: Abruptio Placentae (40) Sample 2: Placenta Previa (22) Sample 3: Unclassified reason for antepartum bleeding (vaginal and cervical polyps, excessive blood show, and cervical lacerations) Controls (154)	Prospective cohort (2 year)

Evidence Table 3. Studies Evaluating Association of LBW and Cerebral Palsy and Neurological Outcomes
Part I

Author, Year UI#	Demographics	Inclusion Criteria	Exclusion Criteria	Disease/Condition Type (N)	Study Design (Duration)
Chen 1995 96009403	Location: Taiwan Years of Birth: 2/1990- 12/1991 Mean GA (range), wk: 30 (27-36) Mean BW (range), g: 1197 (625-1500) Male: ND Race: ND Enrolled: 74 Evaluated: 17 Number of sites: 1	VLBW preterm infants	ND	VLBW preterm infants (17): Group 1 - normal brain US (12) Group 2 - abnormal brain US (5, including 1 IVH grade I, 1 IVH grade III, and 3 PVL)	Prospective cohort (18-42 months) Left the hospital soon after birth at the request of their families (28) Families' refusal for further imaging studies (26 normal infants and 3 PVL infants)
Goetz 1995 96119489	Location: US Years of Birth: 1/1/1989 to 12/31/1992 Median GA (range), wk: ND Mean BW (range), g: 550-1100 Male: ND Race: ND Enrolled: 115 Evaluated: 14 Number of sites: 1	LBW < 1500 g Diagnosis of PVL	Death Transferred prior to being studied Not being followed-up	LBW infants with PVL (14)	Unclear (Retrospective or Prospective cohort, 11 months to 3 2/1 years)

108

Evidence Table 3. Studies Evaluating Association of LBW and Cerebral Palsy and Neurological Outcomes

Part I

Author, Year UI#	Demographics	Inclusion Criteria	Exclusion Criteria	Disease/Condition Type (N)	Study Design (Duration)
Speechley 1995 96356544	Location: Canada Years of Birth: 1978-1980 Mean GA: Sample 1: 37 (28-43) Sample 2: 40 (37-44) Mean BW: Sample 1: 2790 (850-4550) Sample 2: 3503 (2660-5170) Male: Sample 1: 56% Sample 2: 50% Race: Sample 1: whites : 90% Sample 2: whites: 90% (Original study: was a randomized interventional study of having a family volunteer visit the home on a regular base for 6 months) Eligible (for the original study): 828 Enrolled (for the original RCT): 312 Evaluated (at 12 yrs): 253 Number of sites: 1	All infants born at a tertiary care hospital in Ontario Born between 1978-1980 Transferred to NICU or Normal Neonatal Nursery (NNN)	Family residence more than 120 Km from hospital Newborn's survival was in question Language barrier Refused to participate to the original RCT.	Sample 1: Former NICU graduates: [116] Sample 2: Former NNN graduates [137]	Prospective, longitudinal, comparative, observational study (12 yrs)

Evidence Table 3. Studies Evaluating Association of LBW and Cerebral Palsy and Neurological Outcomes
Part I

Author, Year UI#	Demographics	Inclusion Criteria	Exclusion Criteria	Disease/Condition Type (N)	Study Design (Duration)
Wildin 1995 95385294 Wildin 1997 97422739 ***Data from same longitudinal study as Anderson, 1996 96314587 & Smith, 1996 97081985; overlapped sample**	Location: US Years of Birth: **1991-1992** Median GA (range), wk: Sample 1: 28.2±2.3 Sample 2: 30.8±2.2 Controls: 39.6±3.7 Median BW (range), g: Sample 1: 922±226 Sample 2: 1245±209 Controls: 3177±809 Male: Sample 1: 46% Sample 2: 42% Controls: 51% Race: African American Sample 1: 56% Sample 2: 56% Controls 3: 62% Enrolled: 370 Evaluated: 184 (114) Number of Setting: 2	(Sapme 1&2): BW< 1600g GA< 36wk Complete neurologic and developmental exams at 6 and 12 month corrected age. Controls: GA 37-42wks Apgar scores greater than 8 at 1 and 5 min Normal physical exam	"Significant" sensory impairment, meningitis, encephalitis, symptomatic congenital syphilis, congenital abnormality of brain, short bowel, HIV positive mother Primary care giver< 16y/o, drug abuser or did not speak English	Cases: preterm LBW infants (184): Sample 1: High risk (HR) (69) Sample 2: Low risk (LR) (115) Controls: Full Term (114)	Prospective cohort (at 6, and 12 months of age)

110

Evidence Table 3. Studies Evaluating Association of LBW and Cerebral Palsy and Neurological Outcomes

Part I

Author, Year UI#	Demographics	Inclusion Criteria	Exclusion Criteria	Disease/Condition Type (N)	Study Design (Duration)
Anderson 1996 96314587 Smith 1996 97081985 (CNS+All) *Data from same longitudinal study (U. of Texas Health Sciences Center in Houston and the U. of Texas Medical Branch in Galveston) as Wildin, 1995 & 1997; overlapped sample	Location: US Years of Birth: **1990-1992** Median GA (range), wk: Sample 1: 28.2±2.3 Sample 2: 30.8±2.2 Controls: 39.6±3.7 Mean BW (range), g: Sample 1: 922±226 Sample 2: 1245±209 Controls: 3177±809 Male: 50% Race: African American: Sample 1: 57% Sample 2: 62% Controls: 62% Caucasian: Sample 1: 25% Sample 2: 20% Controls: 25% Hispanic: Sample 1: 13% Sample 2: 15% Controls: 13% Other: Sample 1: 5% Sample 2: 3% Controls: 0% Enrolled: 368 Evaluated: 212 (128 controls) Number of sites: 2	(Sample 1&2): VLBW (<1600g) and GA<36 wk Female primary care giver completed both a 6 and 12 month home visit Controls: FT infants examined at 6 and 12 month corrected age	Infants with maternal substance abuse, major dysmorphisms, chromosomal anomalies, sensory impairment, meningitis, encephalitis, congenital syphilis, congenital abnormality of brain, cardiac abnormalities, NEC or HIV antibody positive Primary caregiver age < 16, drug abuser or not English-speaking (only in Smith, 1996)	Sample 1: High risk VLBW (89) Sample 2: Low risk VLBW (123) Controls: Full term (128)	Prospective cohort (6 and 12 months)

111

Evidence Table 3. Studies Evaluating Association of LBW and Cerebral Palsy and Neurological Outcomes
Part I

Author, Year UI#	Demographics	Inclusion Criteria	Exclusion Criteria	Disease/Condition Type (N)	Study Design (Duration)
Kato 1996 97182916	Location: Japan Years of Birth: 1984-1993 Median GA (range), wk: 28±2.8 Mean BW (range), g: 1031.3±271.7 Male: 48% Race: ND Enrolled: 305 Evaluated: 228 Number of sites: 2	VLBW singletons	Major anomaly Multiple gestation	VLBW infants (228)	Retrospective cohort (> 12 months)

Katz 1996 97145056	Location: UK
	Years of Birth: 5/83- 4/85
	Median GA (range), wk: 29.2±2.5 (26-34)
	Mean BW (range), g: 1227.5±341.4 (740-2240)
	Male:
	  Cases: 52%
	  Controls: 55%
	Race:
	  Cases: 75% White, 19% Black, 6% Asian
	  Controls: 75% White, 12.5% Black, 12.5% Asian
	Enrolled: 212
	Evaluated: 64 (40 controls)
	Number of sites: 2
		≤34 weeks, no major congenital anomaly, 3 cranial u/s in first week of life	Lost to follow-up
			Too impair due to multiple cognitive, sensory, or motor disabilities, to complete testing
				Cases: Preterm infants (64)
				Controls: Full-term comparison sample (40)
					Prospective cohort (6-8 years)

Evidence Table 3. Studies Evaluating Association of LBW and Cerebral Palsy and Neurological Outcomes
Part I

Author, Year UI#	Demographics	Inclusion Criteria	Exclusion Criteria	Disease/Condition Type (N)	Study Design (Duration)
Korkman 1996 96374730 Psy1996	Location: Finland Years of Birth: ND Mean GA: Sample 1: 30.8 ± 2.25 Sample 2: 28.8 ± 1.41 Sample 3: 39.7 ± 1.98 Sample 4: 40.0 ± 0.77 Mean BW: Sample 1: 1068.5 ± 151.2 Sample 2: 1212.2 ± 189.3 Sample 3: 3596.7 ± 705.0 Sample 4: 3469.9 ± 275.9 Males: Sample 1: 44% Sample 2: 49% Sample 3: 42% Sample 4: 55% Race: ND Enrolled: ND Evaluated: 158 Number of sites: 2	Born at OB/GYN dept of Univ Helsinki F/up at Children's Hospital and Children's Castle Hospital Had neuropsychological assessment between 5yrs-9 yrs. And specifically for each sample: Sample 1: VLBW: less than 1500 g And SGA (at least 2 SD below mean for their GA) Sample 2: VLBW and AGA Sample 3: Asphyxiated Term infants, GA> 34 weeks with: Umbilical arterial ph<7.05 Or Apgar scores at 5 min less than 6 (From a Birth Cohort of 982 deliveries that included all the term asphyxiated infants) Sample 4: Healthy term with normal delivery, AGA (within 1.5 SD), Umbilical artery pH: 7.18 or more Apgar score 1 min: 8 or more Neonatal period: uneventful Born in the same hospital from healthy mothers by a singleton uncomplicated pregnancy	Children with : Cerebral Palsy Mental retardation Visual impairment	Sample 1: VLBW and SGA [34] Sample 2: VLBW and AGA [43] Sample 3: Birth asphyxia group of term infants [36] Sample 4: Control Group [45]	Prospective comparative longitudinal study (5-9 yrs) (mean age: sample 1: 7.1 yrs, sample 2: 7.3 yrs, sample 3: 6.9 yrs, sample 4: 6.11 yrs)

113

Evidence Table 3. Studies Evaluating Association of LBW and Cerebral Palsy and Neurological Outcomes
Part I

Author, Year UI#	Demographics	Inclusion Criteria	Exclusion Criteria	Disease/Condition Type (N)	Study Design (Duration)

Lucas 1996 96302121	Location: US
	Years of Birth: 1988- 1991
	Median GA (range), wk:
	  Sample 1: 29.8±0.2
	  Sample 2: 29.8±0.2
	Mean BW (range), g:
	  Sample 1: 1306±28
	  Sample 2: 1263±26
	Male:
	  Sample 1: 47%
	  Sample 2: 47%
	Race: ND
	Enrolled: 275
	Evaluated: 275
	Number of sites: 2
		Breast feeding BW<1850; GA< 37, Survived to randomization at 48-72 hr; Received any breast milk	Not resident in UK and the present major congenital abnormalities (e.g. trisomy) known to influence neurodevelopment	Sample 1: Fortified breast milk (137)
				Sample 2: Minimally supplemented breast milk (138)
					RCT (9 and 18 months)

114

Evidence Table 3. Studies Evaluating Association of LBW and Cerebral Palsy and Neurological Outcomes
Part I

Author, Year UI#	Demographics	Inclusion Criteria	Exclusion Criteria	Disease/Condition Type (N)	Study Design (Duration)
Rieck 1996 Psy 1996 06905005	Location: Israel Years of Birth: ND Mean GA: ND Mean BW: ND Males: ND Race: Sample 1: whites 90%, asian-african10% Sample 2: whites: 94%, Asian-African: 5% Enrolled: Sample 1: 103 Evaluated: Sample 1: 103 Sample 2,3: ND Number of sites: ND	Sample 1: Premature VLBW < 1500 g Sample 2:: Children from middle socioeconomic class (MC) families Sample 3: Children from low socioeconomic class (LC) families	ND	Prospective longitudinal component: Sample 1: Premature VLBW <1500) [83] (mean age at assessment: 4.5 yrs) Cross-sectional comparative component: Sample 1 Premature VLBW < 1500 [83] Sample 2: Term children of middle class families [71] Matched with sample 1 only for mean age at assessment : 5.1 yrs Sample 3: Term children from low Class families [322] Matched with sample 1 only for mean age at assessment: 5.0 yrs	Longitudinal f/up study of children participating in a previous prospective longitudinal study (3-7 yrs) Cross sectional comparative component (3 arms: 2 control arms) (3- 7 yrs)

115

Evidence Table 3. Studies Evaluating Association of LBW and Cerebral Palsy and Neurological Outcomes
Part I

Author, Year UI#	Demographics	Inclusion Criteria	Exclusion Criteria	Disease/Condition Type (N)	Study Design (Duration)
Whitaker 1996 97040639	Location: US Years of Birth: 9/1/84-6/30/87 Median GA (range), wk: 31.5 Median BW (range), g: 1480.7 Male: 51% Race: White 74%, African-American 22%, Other 5% SES: middle class (19% of the families receiving public assistance) Enrolled: 685 Evaluated: 597 Number of sites: ND	BW 501-2000 g Survived to 6 years of age and participated in the study Home visit interview subjects	Families refusal (45) Unable to be located (143) Had been adopted (25)	Central New Jersey Neonatal Brain Hemorrhage study cohort LBW infants (597): Normal US finding (468) GM/IVH (83) PL/VE (46)	Prospective cohort (6 years)
Blitz 1997 97154301	Location: US Years of Birth: 1/90- 8/90 Mean GA (range), wk: 26.5±2.4 Mean BW (range), g: 775.9±138.4 Male: 36% Race: 40% White Enrolled: 248 Evaluated: 100 Number of sites: 1	Preemies, BW < 1001 g Maryland residents	Survived to hospital discharge Declined participation Serious congenital malformations, genetic disorder, diagnosed congenital syndromes with brain abnormality of known correlation with developmental disability, disorders secondary to prenatal toxic exposure with microcephaly, severe head injury after discharge Developed meningitis after discharge	ELBW preemies (100): Meningitis 6% PVL 10% Hydrocephalus 18% Seizures 7% IVH ≥ grade III 26% BPD 63% ROP 49% Retinopathy of prematurity 49%	Prospective cohort

116

Evidence Table 3. Studies Evaluating Association of LBW and Cerebral Palsy and Neurological Outcomes
Part I

Author, Year UI#	Demographics	Inclusion Criteria	Exclusion Criteria	Disease/Condition Type (N)	Study Design (Duration)
Cheung 1997 97310950	Location: Canada Years of Birth: 1988-1993 Median GA (range), wk: 26 (24-30) Mean BW (range), g: 891 (530-1180) Male: 67% Race: ND Enrolled: 52 Evaluated: 21 Number of sites: 1	Preterm neonates (GA < 30 weeks, BW < 1200 g) with severe respiratory failure treated with high frequency ventilation (HFO)	ND	Preterms with IVH (21)	Retrospective cohort
Ekert 1997 97251211	Location: Canada Years of Birth: 1988-1994 Median GA (range), wk: 27.6±2.1 Mean BW (range), g: 962±262g Male: 50% Race: ND Enrolled: 123 Evaluated: 123 Number of sites: 2	GA<32 wks informed parental consent	Congenital anomalies, meningitis, congenital infections, GBS disease, lack of consent	Patients entering study (123) → 104 left in analysis for outcome studies	Prospective cohort (seen at corrected age 4,8,12,18,24 months)

Evidence Table 3. Studies Evaluating Association of LBW and Cerebral Palsy and Neurological Outcomes
Part I

Author, Year UI#	Demographics	Inclusion Criteria	Exclusion Criteria	Disease/Condition Type (N)	Study Design (Duration)
Gerner 1997 97329414	Location: Sweden Years of birth: 1988-1993 Mean BW: 1047 ±258 g Mean GA: 28.2 ±2.7 wks Males: ND Race: ND Enrolled: 　Sample 1 and 2: 211 　Sample 3: ND Evaluated: 　Sample 1: 50 　Sample 2: 121 　Sample 3: 35 Number of sites: 2	Sample 1 and 2: Premature, VLBW infants<15000g From NICU of Karolinska Hospital and St Goran's Hospital in Stockholm Born between 9/1988 and 2/1993. Inborns and outborns included Had neurodevelopmental assessment at 10 months corrected age Sample 3: Full term infants Uneventful pregnancy and delivery Apgar score at 5 min: 10 No neonatal complications Born at Karolinska hospital During the same period Matched with cases for: sex, maternal age, maternal education and parity Had neurodevelopmental assessment at 10 months corrected age	ND	Sample 1: Preterm VLBW infants "healthy" without any risk factors [50] Sample 2: Preterm VLBW infants With one or more risk factors [Brain hemorrhage, white matter lesion, surgical closure of PDA, ventilator treatment or septicemia (except Staph epi) [121] (Risk factors and group definition were based on the risk factors that were statistically significantly correlated with outcome in the cohort of the 171 preterm VLBW infants) Sample 3: Full term " healthy" infants, born at Karolinska hospital, during the same period, and matched with the combined preterm VLBW cohort [35]	First component: Prospective observational cohort with 171 preterm VLBW infants (sample 1 and 2) Second component: Prospective comparative component : sample 1 vs sample 3 Third component: Prospective Comparative component: Sample 2 vs sample 1 [10 months]

118

Evidence Table 3. Studies Evaluating Association of LBW and Cerebral Palsy and Neurological Outcomes
Part I

Author, Year UI#	Demographics	Inclusion Criteria	Exclusion Criteria	Disease/Condition Type (N)	Study Design (Duration)
Koller 1997 97193708	Location: US Years of Birth: 1975-1989 Median GA (range), wk: 30.9 (25-37) Mean BW (range), g: 117±227 Male: 45% Race: 51% Black Enrolled: 203 Evaluated: 203 Number of sites: 3	GA <1500, data obtained at 4 follow-up data points	ND	VLBW infants (203)	Retrospective cohort

Murphy 1997 97192793	Location: Korea
	Years of Birth: 1984-1990
	Median GA (range), wk:
	  Cases: 28.6±2.3 (24-32)
	  Control: 29.9±1.9 (23-32)
	Median BW (range), g: ND
	Male:
	  Cases: 63%
	  Control: 57%
	Race: ND
	Enrolled: 638
	Evaluated: 59 (234 controls)
	Number of sites: 1
		GA<32 weeks Singleton
		Oxfordshire and West Berkshire resident
		Neonatal notes were available
			Multiple birth
			Died before discharged
				Cases: CP cases (59)
				Controls (234)
					Case-control study

119

Evidence Table 3. Studies Evaluating Association of LBW and Cerebral Palsy and Neurological Outcomes
Part I

Author, Year UI#	Demographics	Inclusion Criteria	Exclusion Criteria	Disease/Condition Type (N)	Study Design (Duration)
Schendel 1997 98033417	Location: US Years of Birth: 12/1/89 to 3/31/91 Mean GA (range), wk: Sample 1: 28.4 ±3.0 Sample 2: 35.6 ±2.8 Controls: 39.4 ±1.5 Mean BW (range), g: Sample 1: 1088±268 Sample 2: 2184±267 Controls: 3417±432 Male: Sample 1: 49% Sample 2: 46% Controls: 52% Race: Black Sample 1: 37% Sample 2: 37% Controls: 41% Enrolled: 920 (555 controls) Evaluated: 920 (555) Number of sites: 5	Singleton livebirths in MMIHS study population, survived to 1 year of age Cases: MLBW infants, BW 1500-2499g; VLBW infants, BW<1500g Controls: NBW infants randomly selected from the birth certificate files on the basis of frequency matching with cases by maternal race, age, and residence	ND	Sample 1: VLBW infants (367) Sample 2: MLBW infants (553) Controls: NBW infants (555)	Case-control study
Thompson 1997 97268338	Location: US Years of Birth: : 1986-1991 Median GA (range), wk: 28.36±2.11(24-33) Mean BW (range), g: 1100±2.11 (700-1500) Male: 46% Race: ND Enrolled: 111 Evaluated: 55 Number of sites: 1	Born at Duke BW<1500g Survived to discharge or to 6 mo. corrected age	ND	VLBW infants (55)	Prospective cohort (4 years) Death (12), lost to follow-up (34), incomplete data (4), invalid score (5)

120

Evidence Table 3. Studies Evaluating Association of LBW and Cerebral Palsy and Neurological Outcomes
Part I

Author, Year UI#	Demographics	Inclusion Criteria	Exclusion Criteria	Disease/Condition Type (N)	Study Design (Duration)
Victorian Infant Collaborative study Group 1997 98026322 *There are a series of Victorian articles in LBW-ALL. *This study will be combined in LBW-ALL table	Location: Australia Years of Birth: 1979-80, 1985-87, 1991-92 Median GA (range), wk: ND Mean BW (range), g: ND Male: ND Race: ND Enrolled: 453 (242 controls) Evaluated: 448 (242) Number of sites: 3	(Sample 1-3): ELBW infants, BW 500-999 g born in Victoria, Australia Survived to age of 2 years Controls: Normal birth weight (>2499 g) infants born in 1991-1992	Excluded infants born in 1979-1980 for current review	Cases: ELBW infants (448): Sample 1: born in 1985-1987 (212) Sample 2: born in 1991-1992 (241) Controls: Normal BW (>2499 g) infants (242)	Retrospective cohort
Battin 1998 99002694	Location: British Columbia, Canada Enrollment period: 1991-1993 Mean GA: ND (range: 23-25 wks) Mean BW: ND (Mean BW for the 333 live births during the study period : for GA of 23 wks: 581, for GA of 24 wks: 648, for GA of 25 wks: 764) Male: ND Race: ND Enrolled: 333 (total live births GA: 23-28 wks) Evaluated : 44 (out of 49 of GA 23-25 surviving to NICU discharge) Number of sites: 2	Prospective cohort: Birth at British Children's Hospital and British Womens' Hospital Born during 1991-1993 Extremely low gestational age (ELGA): 23-25 wks Had follow up at 18 mo of age Historical control group: Born at the same institution Born between 1983-1989 GA: 23-25 wks	Cases of therapeutic termination of pregnancies for lethal congenital anomalies Outborns	Prospective cohort of ELGA born during a period when antenatal steroids, surfactant and dexamethasone for BPD had become an accepted treatment [44]	Prospective observational cohort study and a comparative study with an historical control group (18 months)

121

Evidence Table 3. Studies Evaluating Association of LBW and Cerebral Palsy and Neurological Outcomes
Part I

Author, Year UI#	Demographics	Inclusion Criteria	Exclusion Criteria	Disease/Condition Type (N)	Study Design (Duration)
Bos 1998 98218970	Location: Netherlands Years of Birth: 1992-1994 Mean GA (range), wk: 26-34 Mean BW (range), g: 835-1780 Male: ND Race: ND Enrolled: 27 Evaluated: 27 Number of sites: ND	AGA GA <35 wks Lived within 60km of hospital Normal US findings	Major congenital anomalies Developed cystic PVL, or grade 3 or 4 IVH	Preterm infants with echodensities (27)	Prospective cohort

Cherkes-Julkowski 1998 98262696	Location: ND
	Years of Birth: ND
	Mean GA (range), wk: ND
	Mean BW (range):
	  Cases: 4.14±1.87 lbs
	  Controls: 7.30±1.87 lbs
	Male:
	  Cases: 61%
	  Controls: 50%
	Race: ND
	SES: "middle class"
	Enrolled: 48
	Evaluated: 28 (20 controls)
	Number of sites: 1
		Preterm:
		<38 wks, BW<5 lbs, no congenital disorders, no retrolenteal fibroplasia, discharge from hospital prior to 42 wks conceptional age, mother willing to participate
		Controls: participants were enrolled in a longitudinal study before their second month of age
			ND	Preterms (28)
				
				Controls: full term infants (20)
					Retrospective cohort

122

Evidence Table 3. Studies Evaluating Association of LBW and Cerebral Palsy and Neurological Outcomes

Part I

Author, Year UI#	Demographics	Inclusion Criteria	Exclusion Criteria	Disease/Condition Type (N)	Study Design (Duration)

Emsley 1998 98238139 (CNS+ All)	Location: US
	Years of Birth: 1984 to 1994
	Median GA (range), wk:
	  Sample 1: 24.5
	  Sample 2: 24.2
	Mean BW (range), g:
	  Sample 1: 751.7
	  Sample 2: 697.1
	Male:
	  Sample 1: 67%
	  Sample 2: 55%
	Race: ND
	Enrolled: 192
	Evaluated: 64
	Number of sites: 2
		GA 23-25 weeks	Survived until discharge	Sample 1: Cohort 1 Born 1984-1989 (24)
				
				Sample 2: Cohort 2 born 1990-1994 (40)
					Prospective cohort (3.3 –10.6 years)

Pasman 1998 98196839	Location: Netherlands
	Years of Birth: ND
	Median GA (range), wk:
	  Sample 1: 28.9±1.5 (25-30)
	  Sample 2: 32.5±1.1 (31-34)
	  Sample 3:
	  Sample 4: 30.1±1.6 (25-34)
	  Controls: 39.4±1.5 (38-42)
	Mean BW (range), g:
	  Sample 1: 1071±269
	  Sample 2: 1568±351
	  Sample 3:
	  Sample 4: 1317±299
	  Controls: 3144±516
	Male: ND
	Race: ND
	Enrolled: 81 (25 controls)
	Evaluated: 45 (18 controls)
	Number of sites: 2
		GA=25-34 weeks, admitted to university hospital	Dysgenetic brain lesions
			Major congenital anomalies
			Clinical syndromes
			Lost to follow-up
				Sample 1: Early preterms, low risk (15)
				Sample 2: Late preterms, low risk (21)
				Sample 3: Early high risk preterms (8)
				Sample 4: Late high risk preterms (9)
				Controls: Full term (18)
					Prospective cohort (followed to 5-7 years age)

123

Evidence Table 3. Studies Evaluating Association of LBW and Cerebral Palsy and Neurological Outcomes

Part I

Author, Year UI#	Demographics	Inclusion Criteria	Exclusion Criteria	Disease/Condition Type (N)	Study Design (Duration)

Redline 1998 99086405	Location: US
	Years of Birth: 1983-1991
	Median GA (range), wk:
	  Sample 1: 27.3 ±2.3
	  Sample 2: 27.5 ± 2.2
	Mean BW (range), g:
	  Sample 1: 978± 228
	  Sample 2: 1012±226
	Male: ND
	Race: African-American
	  Sample 1: 57%
	  Sample 2: 59%
	Enrolled: 72
	Evaluated: 60 (59 controls)
	Number of sites: 2
		Cases (Sample 1&2): Infants with major neurologic impairment at 20 months (strictly defined CP, loosely defined CP, hypertonia, Hypotonia) and those with NL neurologic exam at 20 months.
		Controls: infants born in the same year and matched for weight (±250 g), GA (±2 weeks), race, and sex who had a normal neurologic examination at 20 months.
			No placental reports and slides available	Cases: VLBW infants with major neurologic impairment at 20 months (60)
				Sample 1: Strict CP (42)
				Sample 2: Neurologic abnormalities (18)
				Controls (59)
					Case-control (at 20 months corrected age)

Rogers 1998 98438124	Location: US
	Years of Birth: 1988 to 1993
	Median GA (range), wk:
	  Sample 1: 27.9 ±2.0
	  Sample 2: 27.6 ±1.8
	Mean BW (range), g:
	  Sample 1: 1158±330
	  Sample 2: 1082± 290
	Male: ND
	Race: ND
	Enrolled: 41
	Evaluated: 41
	Number of sites: 1
		GA < 33 weeks live birth with unspecified IVH	ND	Sample 1: No growth failure (23)
				Sample 2: Growth failure (18)
					Retrospective cohort

124

Evidence Table 3. Studies Evaluating Association of LBW and Cerebral Palsy and Neurological Outcomes

Part I

Author, Year UI#	Demographics	Inclusion Criteria	Exclusion Criteria	Disease/Condition Type (N)	Study Design (Duration)
Spinillo 1998 98237382	Location: Italy Years of Birth: 1987 to 1993 Median GA (range), wk: Cases: 29.6 Controls: 30.5	GA 24–33 completed weeks Had a US scan done before 20 weeks' gestation	Severe malformations or chromosome abnormalities	Sample 1: Preterm infants with CP (40)	Prospective cohort (3, 6, 12, and 24 months)
Spinillo, 1997 98021316 & 97277958	Mean BW (range), g: Cases: 1317 Controls: 1451 Male: 52%			Sample 2: Preterm infants without CP (305)	
*have some overlapped sample with spinillo, 1994	Race: ND Enrolled: 461 Evaluated: 345 Number of sites: 2				
Tin 1998 99046171	Location: North of England Years of Birth: 1983, 1990-1991 Median GA (range), wk: ND Mean BW (range), g: ND Male: ND Race: ND Enrolled: 1983 (230); 1990-1 (566) Evaluated: 1983 (230); 1990-1 (566) Number of sites: 5	GA 23-31 weeks	ND	1983 cohort (230): Child reviewed without difficulty (204) Child traced with difficulty (14) Child seen with difficulty after child was traced (12) 1990 to 1991 (566): Child reviewed without difficulty (505) Child traced with difficulty (26) Child seen with difficulty after child was traced (35)	Prospective cohort *2 Cohorts of different time periods

125

Evidence Table 3. Studies Evaluating Association of LBW and Cerebral Palsy and Neurological Outcomes
Part I

Author, Year UI#	Demographics	Inclusion Criteria	Exclusion Criteria	Disease/Condition Type (N)	Study Design (Duration)
Burguet 1999 99126269	Location: France Years of Birth: : 10/1/90- 9/10/92 Mean GA (range), wk: 25-32 Mean BW (range), g: 8% BW>2000g Male: 51% Race: 86% Caucasian SES: 5% Family precariousness Enrolled: 203 Evaluated: 167 Number of sites: 20	All liveborn premature in 20 maternity hospitals in Franche-Comte region	Chromosomal or neurological congenital anomaly diagnosed in the neonatal period, discordance of 2 wks or more between pediatric and obstetrical or echographic determination of gestational age, triplets and more	Preemies (167): RDS 40% No RDS 60%	Prospective (93%) and retrospective (7%) cohort (followed until 2 years of age)
Cooke 1999 99257637	Location: UK Years of Birth: 1982-1993 Median GA (range), wk: ND Mean BW (range), g: ND Male: ND Race: ND Enrolled: 1722 Evaluated: 1187 Number of sites: 1	VLBW (not specifically defined) Have data at 3 years old	ND	VLBW infants (1187): 1982-19855 (411) 1986-1989 (387) 1990-1993 (398)	Retrospective cohort (followed until 3 years corrected age)
Cooke 1999 99380719	Location: UK Years of Birth: 1982-1993 Median GA (range), wk: 28.6±1.7 (24-35) Mean BW (range), g: 1103±203 (630-1500) Male: ND Race: ND Enrolled: 137 Evaluated: 87 (8 controls) Number of sites: 1	VLBW infants prospectively followed birth to age 13 with MRIs between age 15-17 yrs Controls: FT infants	ND	VLBW infants (87), with white matter disorder, PVL, Ventriculomegaly, MRI abnormality Controls: FT infants (8)	Prospectively cohort (15-17 years)

126

Evidence Table 3. Studies Evaluating Association of LBW and Cerebral Palsy and Neurological Outcomes
Part I

Author, Year UI#	Demographics	Inclusion Criteria	Exclusion Criteria	Disease/Condition Type (N)	Study Design (Duration)
Finer 1999 99436635	Location: UK Years of Birth: 1/1/94 to 12/31/96 Median GA (range), wk: 25 (24-28) Mean BW (range), g: 663 (440-968) Male: 50% Race: ND Enrolled: 177 Evaluated: 10 (10 controls) Number of sites: 1	Cases: Inborn infants BW < 1000g Received DR-CPR Survived until discharge Controls: Matched controls with similar mean BW and length of follow-up	Lethal congenital malformations	Cases: ELBW survived infants received DR-CPR (10) Controls (10)	Retrospective cohort (median 28 months)
Futagi 1999 99450356	Location: Japan Years of Birth: 1981-1986 and 1989 1993 Mean GA: Sample 1: 27.2±2.2 Sample 2: 26.8±2.4 Mean BW: Sample 1: 834.1±133.4 Sample 2: 786.0±133.2 Males: Sample 1: 38% Sample 2: 53% Race: ND Enrolled: 305 Evaluated: 276 Number of sites: 1	Presurfactant era cohort: BW less than 1000 gms Admitted to NICU Born during presurfactant era 1981-1986 Follow up for at least 3 years. Neurodevelopmental and Mental outcome documented in medical records Surfactant era cohort: same as above except Born during surfactant era, 1989-1993	Hereditary disorders Chromosomal abnormalities Follow up less than 3 years Absence of documentation of neurodevelopmental or mental outcome in medical records	Sample 1 Presurfactant cohort: Born during presurfactant era, between 1981-86 [107] Sample 2: Surfactant era cohort: Born during surfactant era, between 1989-1993 [169]	Retrospective comparative longitudinal study. Comparison done between 2 retrospective cohorts (pre-surfactant era cohort vs surfactant era cohort) [3-8.8 years, mean f/up: 6.0 ±1.3 yrs (not given per group)]

127

Evidence Table 3. Studies Evaluating Association of LBW and Cerebral Palsy and Neurological Outcomes
Part I

Author, Year UI#	Demographics	Inclusion Criteria	Exclusion Criteria	Disease/Condition Type (N)	Study Design (Duration)
Kim 1999 99416608	Location: UK Years of Birth: July 1996 to November 1997 Median GA (range), wk: Cases: 30.8±3.5 Control: 31.4± 2.2 Mean BW (range), g: Cases: 1557±252 Control: 1418±376 Male: Cases: 47% Control: 52% Race: ND Enrolled: 184 Evaluated: 17 (62 controls) Number of sites: ND	Preterm (GA<37 wks) infants and term infants with an Apgar score of less than 6 at 5 minutes, neonatal hyperbilirubinemia (total bilirubin concentration of 20 mg/dl or more) and bacterial meningitis BW<2000 g	Chromosomal abnormalities and congenital malformation	Cases: VLBW infants with CP or Developmental D (17) VLBW Controls (62)	Prospective cohort (at 2, 6, 12 months corrected age)
Krageloh-Mann 1999 99431017	Location: Denmark Years of Birth: 1986- 1989 Median GA (range), wk: 30.2 (27-34) Mean BW (range), g: 1461 (690-2655) Male: 66% Race: ND Enrolled: 40 Evaluated: 29 (57 controls) Number of sites:1	Preterm infants	Death (1), lost to follow-up (7), parental refusal (4), difficulties with sedation for MRI (1)	Cases: preterm infants (29) Controls: term-born pre-school children (57)	Prospective cohort

128

Evidence Table 3. Studies Evaluating Association of LBW and Cerebral Palsy and Neurological Outcomes

Part I

Author, Year UI#	Demographics	Inclusion Criteria	Exclusion Criteria	Disease/Condition Type (N)	Study Design (Duration)

Salokorpi 1999 99353226	Location: Finland
	Years of Birth: 1991 to 1994
	Median GA (range), wk:
	  Sample 1: 26.7 ±2.0
	  Sample 2: 26.7 ±2.4
	Mean BW (range), g:
	  Sample 1: 833±130
	  Sample 2: 817± 130
	Male:
	  Sample 1: 33%
	  Sample 2: 46%
	Race: ND
	Enrolled: 228
	Evaluated: 143
	Number of sites: 1
		Premature infants, BW < 1000 g, admitted to NICU	ND	Sample 1: CP present (27)
				Sample 2: CP absence (116)
					Prospective cohort
					
					Lost to follow-up (13) due to parent refusal or because had moved to remote areas
					Died by the age of 2 year (72)

Shepherd 1999 9165413	Location: Scotland Years of Birth: 2/95 to 2/97 Median GA (range), wk: 25.7-35 Mean BW (range), g: 570-3200 Male: ND Race: ND Enrolled: 81 (68 controls) Evaluated: 81 (68) Number of sites: 1	Preterm infants admitted to the special-care unit	Genetic or prenatal anomalies	Cases: preterms (81) Controls: term infants (68)	Prospective cohort

129

Evidence Table 3. Studies Evaluating Association of LBW and Cerebral Palsy and Neurological Outcomes
Part I

Author, Year UI#	Demographics	Inclusion Criteria	Exclusion Criteria	Disease/Condition Type (N)	Study Design (Duration)
Stathis 1999 99325758	Location: Australia Years of Birth: 1977-1986 Median GA (range), wk: 27.7(27.3-28.1) Mean BW (range), g: 860 (837-833) Male: 36% Race: ND Enrolled: 124 Evaluated: 87 Number of sites: 1	BW 500-999g survived to discharge Cared for in study NICU Enrolled in follow-up programs	ND	ELBW survived infants (87)	Prospective cohort (followed at 4, 8, 12, months)
Vohr 1999 99332101	Location: US Years of Birth: 1989-1992 Median GA (range), wk: Sample 1: 27.9±2 Sample 2: 28±2 Mean BW (range), g: Sample 1: 960±178 Sample 2: 965±179 Male: Sample 1: 59% Sample 2: 56% Race: Sample 1: Black 21%, Hispanic 3%, White 76% Sample 2: Black 20%, White 78%, Other 2% Enrolled: 392 Evaluated: 278 Number of sites: 3	BW 600-1250g Survived the first 3 years of life, and were seen for neurodevelopmental follow-up at 36 months CA	Non-English speaking home	Sample 1: Early IVH positive (29) Sample 2: Early IVH negative (249)	Unclear (Retrospective or prospective cohort, followed to 36 months corrected age)

Evidence Table 3. Studies Evaluating Association of LBW and Cerebral Palsy and Neurological Outcomes

Part I

Author, Year UI#	Demographics	Inclusion Criteria	Exclusion Criteria	Disease/Condition Type (N)	Study Design (Duration)
Agustines 2000 20279724	Location: US Years of Birth: 1990-1995 Median GA (range), wk: 25 (24-29) Median BW (range), g: 674 Male: ND Race: ND Enrolled: 63 Evaluated: 36 Number of sites: 1	BW: 500-750 g Born in Long Beach Hospital, between 1990 and 1995 (post corticosteroid, postsurfactant era) Survived to discharge Had follow up at 30 months	ND	VLBW infants (36)	Retrospective cohort (followed to 30 months CA) Lost to follow-up (27)
Breslau 2000 20298367	Location: US Years of Birth: 1983-1985 Mean GA (range), wk: ND Mean BW (range), g: ND Male: ND Male: ND Race: Sample 1 (urban) Blacks: 80% Sample 1 (suburban) Blacks:11% Sample 2 (urban) Blacks:74% Sample 2 (suburban) Blacks: 3% Enrolled: 1095 Evaluated: 823→717 Number of sites: ND	LBW cohort: <2500 g NBW cohort: Born between 1983-85, that were 6 yrs old during 1990-92; when the fieldwork took place From 2 major hospitals of South Michigan: one urban and one suburban (In each hospital, random samples of LBW and NBW children were drawn).	From the target sample: were excluded children with severe neurologic impairment: CP, MR, blindness From the analysis of incidence of severe attention problems were excluded children that already had severe attention problems at the assessment at 6 yrs	At 11 yrs (717): Sample 1: LBW (411) – Urban LBW (217) Suburban LBW (194) Sample 2: NBW (306) - Urban NBW)164) Suburban NBW (142)	Prospective cohort (11 years)
Bührer 2000 20280896	Location: Germany Years of Birth: 1/192- 12/31/97 Mean GA (range), wk: 28.7 (23.2-37.2) Mean BW (range), g: 1149 (430-1495) Male: ND Race: ND Enrolled: 455 Evaluated: 352 Number of sites: 1	VLBW, BW < 1500 g	ND	VLBW infants (352)	Prospective cohort (followed until 1 year CA)

131

Evidence Table 3. Studies Evaluating Association of LBW and Cerebral Palsy and Neurological Outcomes
Part I

Author, Year UI#	Demographics	Inclusion Criteria	Exclusion Criteria	Disease/Condition Type (N)	Study Design (Duration)

Grether 2000 20448692	Location: US
	Years of Birth: 1988-1994
	Median GA (range), wk:
	  Cases: : 27.1±2.4
	  Controls: 37.6±2.6
	Mean BW (range), g:
	  Cases: 1085±350
	  Controls: 1112±349
	Male:
	  Cases: 56%
	  Controls: 47%
	Race:
	  Cases: 47% White
	  Controls: 33% White
	Enrolled: 170 (280 controls)
	Evaluated: 170 (280)
	Number of sites: 22
		BW < 1500 g or BW 1500-1999g and <33 GA	Postural cause of CP identified.
			Congenital infection identified
				Cases: Cerebral palsy (170)
				Controls (288)
					Retrospective case-control study (2 years)

Katz-Salamon 2000 20332284	Location: Sweden
	Years of Birth: 1988-1993
	Median GA (range), wk:
	  Cases: : 26.1±2.0
	  Controls: 26.7±1.3
	Mean BW (range), g:
	  Cases: 874±183
	  Controls: 940±179
	Male: ND
	Race: ND
	Enrolled: 70
	Evaluated: 43 (43 controls)
	Number of sites: 1
		Cases:
		  VLBW
		  Survival with CLD
		Controls:
		  No IVH>2
		  No CLD
		  No PVL
		  VLBW
			Cases:
			  Unable to be examined because of other medical problems, including congenital cardiac malformation, hepatitis C, immobilization of the legs, severe visual defect, and severe cerebra infarction.
				Cases: VLBW infants with CLD (43)
				VLBW Controls (43)
					Prospective cohort

132

Evidence Table 3. Studies Evaluating Association of LBW and Cerebral Palsy and Neurological Outcomes
Part I

Author, Year UI#	Demographics	Inclusion Criteria	Exclusion Criteria	Disease/Condition Type (N)	Study Design (Duration)

Marlow 2000 20150342	Location: UK
	Years of Birth: 1990-1994
	Mean GA: ND
	(Median and Range)
	  Sample 1: 28 (26-31)
	  Sample 2: 28 (26-31)
	Mean BW: ND
	(Median and range)
	  Sample 1: 960 (600-2914)
	  Sample 2: 1026 (410-2814)
	Male: ND
	Race: ND
	Enrolled : 27
	Evaluated: 15
	Number of sites: 1
		For sensorineural hearing loss (SNHL) group
		GA: <33 wks
		Family resident of Greater Bristol area
		Records at Hearing Assessment Center of Royal Hospital for Sick children.
		Born during 1990-1994
		Diagnosis of SNHL of 50 dB
		
		For control group:
		Matched controls 2:1 to cases
		Admitted to the same NICUs as cases
		Matched for sex and GA and next and preceding matching children in the admission books of St Michael's and Sothmead hospitals
			ND	Sample 1:
				SNHL group [15]
				
				Sample 2:
				Control group [30]
				Matched with cases for sex, GA, admission dates in NICU
					Retrospective case control study with a longitudinal component (unclear if retrospective or prospective) (12 mo CA)

Palta 2000 20096107 (CNS+Eye)	Location: US Years of Birth: August 1988-June 1999 Median GA (range), wk: 28.54±1.97 Mean BW (range), g: 1003±155 Male: 43% Race: ND Enrolled: 626 Evaluated: 425 Number of sites: 6	Birth weight ≤1500 g Survived to 5 years of age Parental agreement to potential follow-up and provided recontact information before discharge.	Refusing participation at follow-up	VLBW infants (425)	Prospective cohort (followed to an average age of 5 years)

133

Evidence Table 3. Studies Evaluating Association of LBW and Cerebral Palsy and Neurological Outcomes
Part I

Author, Year UI#	Demographics	Inclusion Criteria	Exclusion Criteria	Disease/Condition Type (N)	Study Design (Duration)
Torrioli 2000 20275419 (CNS+Eye)	Location: Italy Years of Birth: 1991-1993 Median GA (range), wk: 32 (21-34) Median BW (range), g: 1120(560-1500) Male: 42% Race: ND SES: "medium and there was the same ethnic background" Enrolled: 86 Evaluated: 36 (ND on number of controls) Number of sites: 1	BW < 1500 gm Controls: born at term and without any perinatal or neonatal complication, matched for age, gender and socioeconomic condition including occupational status of the family and parents' educational status was performed by the same observers that examined the study group	Frankly disabling conditions (CP, MR, blindness, CNS infections, genetic syndromes, etc.); abnormal head ultrasound findings Refused to participate in the study	VLBW preterm infants (36)	Prospective cohort
Valkama 2000 20233239	Location: Finland Years of Birth: 11/1/1993-10/31/1995 Median GA (range), wk: 29.3±2.2 (24.9-33.7) Median BW (range), g: 1153±289 Male: 53% Race: ND Enrolled: 62 Evaluated: 51 Number of sites: 1	VLBW <1500g and <34 weeks	Congenital anomalies Died during neonatal period Parental refusal	VLBW preterm infants (51)	Prospective cohort (18 months)

Evidence Table 3. Studies Evaluating Association of LBW and Cerebral Palsy and Neurological Outcomes

Part I

Author, Year UI#	Demographics	Inclusion Criteria	Exclusion Criteria	Disease/Condition Type (N)	Study Design (Duration)
Vohr 2000 20295211	Location: US Years of Birth: 1/93-12/94 Median GA (range), wk: Mean BW (range), g: Male: Race: Enrolled: Evaluated: Number of sites: 12	Live born BW 401-1000 g	ND	1151 extremely low birth weight survivors cared for in the 12 participating centers of the National Institute of Child Health and Human Development Neonatal Research Network	Prospective cohort (18-22 months corrected age)
Dammann 2001 21334215	Location: Germany Years of Birth: July 1983-June 1986 Median GA (range), wk: ND Mean BW (range), g: ND Male: ND Race: ND Enrolled: 591 Evaluated: 324 Number of sites: 1	BW≤1500g	ND	LBW infants (324): SGA (92) AGA (232)	Prospective cohort (6 years) 7 non-BSCP cerebral palsy (no further explanation)

135

Evidence Table 3. Studies Evaluating Association of LBW and Cerebral Palsy and Neurological Outcomes
Part I

Author, Year UI#	Demographics	Inclusion Criteria	Exclusion Criteria	Disease/Condition Type (N)	Study Design (Duration)
Gaillard 2001 21221175	Location: UK Years of Birth:1994-1996 Mean GA: ND (only median and range given) Sample 1: 26 (23-34) Sample 2: 26 (23-33) Mean BW: ND (only median and range given) Sample 1: 852 (520-2710) Sample 2: 745 (580-1620) Male: Sample 1: 57% Sample 2: 50% Race: ND Enrolled: 100 Evaluated: 84 Number of sites: 1	Retrospective cohort : All infants born from 1/1/1994 to 12/31/1996 Born at Liverpool Women's Hospital Ventilated beyond 27 postnatal days	If transferred from another hospital after first postnatal week (mostly surgical referrals) If ventilated after 27 postnatal days after a surgical procedure requiring anesthesia	Sample 1 : Ventilated beyond 27 (but not 50) postnatal ds (56) Sample 2: Ventilated beyond 49ds (28)	First component: Retrospective longitudinal cohort with case-control design and cases defined based on exposure (length of ventilation). Unmatched. (3 years) Second component: Retrospective longitudinal cohort study With two historical control groups (3 years)
Horwood 2001 20574647	Location: US Years of Birth: 1/93 to 12/96 Median GA (range), wk: ND Mean BW (range), g: ND Male: ND Race: ND Enrolled: 413 Evaluated: 298 Number of sites: 1	VLBW infants admitted to neonatal unit still living in New Zealand at time of assessment, 7-8 years of age	Death 17 children could not complete IQ testing because of substantial disability	VLBW infants (298)	Prospective cohort

136

Evidence Table 3. Studies Evaluating Association of LBW and Cerebral Palsy and Neurological Outcomes

Part I

Author, Year UI#	Demographics	Inclusion Criteria	Exclusion Criteria	Disease/Condition Type (N)	Study Design (Duration)

Nadeau 2001 21163667	Location: Canada
	Years of Birth: 1987-1990
	Median GA (range), wk:
	  Cases: 27.4±1.1
	  Control: 39.8±1.6
	Median BW (range), g:
	  Cases: 1024.3±204.2
	  Control: 3453.4±497.8
	Male:
	  Cases: 51%
	  Control: 50%
	Race: ND
	Enrolled: 129
	Evaluated: 86 → 61 (50 controls)
	Number of sites: 1
		Cases: GA<29 weeks, BW<1500 g
		Controls: Normal BW children, born at the same hospital during the same time period
			Cases:
			Lost to follow-up at 5 years 9 months: families had moved away (33), parents' refusal (10)
			Lost to follow-up at age 7: families had moved away (10), parents' or school's refusal (13)
				Cases: EP/VLBW infants (86→61)	Prospective cohort (at 18 months, 5 years 9 months, and age 7)

Pierrat 2001 27221167	Location: France, Netherlands Years of Birth: 1990-1998 Median GA (range), wk: 28.54±1.97 Mean BW (range), g: 1003±155 Male: 43% Race: ND Enrolled: 72 Evaluated: 60 (59 controls) Number of sites: 2	GA < 32 weeks, admitted to Lille and Utrecht Diagnosis of grade II or III PVL	ND	Preterm infants with PVL (78): Grade II (39) Grade III (39)	Prospective cohort (1 year) Cysts on the first scan and therefore were considered to be of antenatal onset (7), admitted after the first month of life with evidence of cysts on the first scan (9); no definite classification could be achieved (2)

Evidence Table 3. Studies Evaluating Association of LBW and Cerebral Palsy and Neurological Outcomes
Part II

Author, Year	Predictors	Predictor Measures	Outcomes	Outcome Measures
Leonard 1990 90204169	*CNS Predictors:* Intracranial/ Intraventricular hemorrhage *Cardiovascular or Pulmonary Predictors:* Number of days on supplemental oxygen to help pO$_2$ > 50 *Other predictors:* Parenting risk factor Low socioeconomic status	Intracranial/ Intraventricular hemorrhage - Grades 0-IV by Papille; head CT if born before 1981, head U/S is born after 1981 Parenting risk factor - defined as referral by a physician, nurse, or health professional to child protective services for neglect or mild abuse (none were for severe abuse) Low socioeconomic status - one or both parents unemployed, mother not complete high school or health insurance through public assistance	**CNS:** Neurodevelopmental: 1) Cognitive delay 2) Neurologic abnormalities	Cognitive delay: measured by McCarthy Scales of Chilren's Abilities, Wechsler Intelligence Scale for Children (Revised), Wechsler Preschool and Primary Scale of Intelligence, and Stanford-Binet "mild" - score between 1-2 SD below the mean (69-83) "moderate to severe" - score >2 SD below the mean Neurologic abnormalities: abnormalities in muscle strength, tone, reflexes or movement that cause functional impairment, i.e. hemiplegia, ataxia, quadriplegia. Clumsiness or mild tremors not included.
Lucas 1992 92122860	Primary predictor: General: 1) Maternal choice to breast feed Secondary predictors: Others: 1) Received mother's milk 2) Social class 3) Maternal education 4) Gender 5) Days of ventilation	Social class: 4 categories: • Social class I or II • Non manual Social class III • Manual social class III • Social class IV or V Mother's education: 5 point scale From 1: no educational qualifications To 5: degree or higher performance qualifications	IQ score in Weschler Intelligence Scale for Children-Revised-Shortened version (WISC-R)-Anglicised. 1) Verbal scale 2) Performance scale 3) Overall IQ (Assessment at 9 mo, 18 mo, 7.5-8 yrs)	Not further specified

138

Evidence Table 3. Studies Evaluating Association of LBW and Cerebral Palsy and Neurological Outcomes
Part II

Author, Year	Predictors	Predictor Measures	Outcomes	Outcome Measures
Robertson 1994 94181384	Birth weight	ND	**CNS:** CP **Neurodevelopmental:** Motor delay Seizure disorder Multiple disabled **Ophthalmology:** Visual **Audiology:** Hearing	CP definition was that of Bax, "A disorder of movement and posture due to a defect or lesion of the immature brain", along with more recent guidelines by Levine using at least four of six clinical motor abnormalities leading to a constellation of findings of the cerebra palsy syndrome Mental retardation = scores Bayley mental scales. Initially by newborn screening; with subsequently tested repeatedly in a sound booth and/or by bristem audiological evoked response. Visual loss: acuity in the best seeing eye after correction, <20/60) including legal blindness (corrected acuity, <20/200) Hearing loss (loss of >= 30 dB binaurally)
Spinillo 1994 94257064 *have some overlapped sample with spinillo, 1997	Cause of antepartum bleeding **CNS:** Intracranial hemorrhage Periventricular leukolacia	Histological examination of detached placeta were used for confirmation of clinical classification Diagnosis of IVH and PVL according to US finding	**CNS:** CP **Neurodevelopmental:** Motor and cognitive delay Mental retardation Presence of grade 3-4 IVH or PVL	Amiel-Tison and Grenier Neonatal neurological Examination Major neonatal handicaps included definite CP such as spastic diplegia, hemiplegia or tetraplegia causing definite physical disability with moderate to severe interference with functioning, or mental retardation (Bayley Scale)

Evidence Table 3. Studies Evaluating Association of LBW and Cerebral Palsy and Neurological Outcomes
Part II

Author, Year	Predictors	Predictor Measures	Outcomes	Outcome Measures
Chen 1995 96009403	**CNS:** 1) Intracranial hemorrhage 2) Periventricular leukomalacia	ND	**CNS:** Motor delay CP	Development Screening test, modified for Chinese children Diagnosed by "complete neurological exams", including transient spasticity and spastic di-/ quardriplegia
Goetz 1995 96119489	PVL	ND	**CNS:** CP Neurodevelopmental: Motor and cognitive delay Seizure disorder **Ophthalmology:** Visual impairment	ND

Evidence Table 3. Studies Evaluating Association of LBW and Cerebral Palsy and Neurological Outcomes

Part II

Author, Year	Predictors	Predictor Measures	Outcomes	Outcome Measures
Speechley 1995 96356544	General: 1) Former NICU graduate (of any BW) 2) Gender	Not further specified	Physical health outcome at 12 yrs 1) Chronic physical health (mother's report) 2) Lifetime hospitalizations (mother's report) 3) Physical impairments (mother's report) 4) Perception of child's heath (child's report) 5) Perception of child's health (mother's report) Emotional and social well being at 12 yrs: 1) Internalizing problems (child's report) 2) Externalizing problems (child's report) 3) Social competence (child's report) 4) Social support (child's report) 5) Self esteem (child's report) 6) School performance (mother's report)	Based on responses on an interviewer administered and self-report questionnaire. Physical health outcome at 12 yrs 1) Chronic physical health (mother's report): Precoded 25 chronic illnesses 2) Lifetime hospitalizations (mother's report) 3) Physical impairments (mother's report):response to a question asking whether their child had any physical impairments 4) Perception of child's heath (child's report): 4-item scale 5) Perception of child's health (mother's report): 4-item scale Emotional and social well being at 12 yrs: 1) Internalizing problems (child's report) 3-item scale 2) Externalizing problems (child's report) 3-item scale 3) Social competence (child's report) 36-item scale 4) Social support (child's report) 24-item scale 5) Self esteem (child's report) 10-item scale 6) School performance (mother's report) 5-item scale

141

Evidence Table 3. Studies Evaluating Association of LBW and Cerebral Palsy and Neurological Outcomes
Part II

Author, Year	Predictors	Predictor Measures	Outcomes	Outcome Measures
Wildin 1995 95385294	CNS: 1) Neurological exam- 6 months - 12 months 2) Quantitative neurologic score	Based on Amiel-Tison examination done at 6 months corrected age	CNS: Neurodevelopmental: Motor delay Cognitive delay Rate of development	Stanford-Binet developmental test McCarthy Gross Motor subtests Bayley scale
Wildin 1997 97422739	Other: 1) Socioeconomic status 2) Medical risk category: High Risk (HR); Low Risk (LR)	High medical risk = severe medical complications of prematurity		
*Data from same longitudinal study as Anderson, 1996 96314587 & Smith, 1996 97081985; overlapped sample				

142

Evidence Table 3. Studies Evaluating Association of LBW and Cerebral Palsy and Neurological Outcomes
Part II

Author, Year	Predictors	Predictor Measures	Outcomes	Outcome Measures
Anderson 1996 96314587	Other Predictors: Illness Acuity – grouped into low-risk and high-risk.	Based on the severity of neonatoal complications grouping into High- and Low- risk groups: High risk: ≥1 severe neonatoal complications, including chronic lung disease (bronchopulmonary dysplasia), grade III or IV intraventricular hemorrhage, and periventicular leukomalacia Low risk: : ≥1 less severe neonatal complications, including transient respiratory distress, respiratory distress syndrome, and grade I or II intraventricular hemorrhage, and periventicular leukomalacia	**CNS:** Neurodevelopmental: Cognitive delay	Baley Mental and Psychomotor development indices (MDI, PDI) Neurologic scores based on scales developed by Amiel-Tison, Baird and Gordon, and Swaiman
Smith 1996 97081985 (CNS+All)	Maternal Behaviors: 1) warm sensitivity 2) Maintaining of infant interests and directiveness.	Maternal Behaviors - home observation with use of a rating scale.	**Audiology:** Language **Other:** Living skills	Sequenced mixture of communication development Daily living skills subscale from Adaptive Behavior Scale
*Data from same longitudinal study (U. of Texas Health Sciences Center in Houston and the U. of Texas Medical Branch in Galveston) as Wildin, 1995 & 1997; overlapped sample				
Kato 1996 97182916	VLBW GA Sex Perinatal factors (mat age, parity, preeclampsia, previa, PROM, fetal presentation,	VLBW= ND Small for Dates = ND PROM = ND	**CNS** CP: Neurodevelopmental: Mental retardation Seizure disorder Blindness Lump all together as major handicap	ND

143

Evidence Table 3. Studies Evaluating Association of LBW and Cerebral Palsy and Neurological Outcomes
Part II

Author, Year	Predictors	Predictor Measures	Outcomes	Outcome Measures
Katz 1996 97145056	General: GA CNS: 1) Intracranial/ Intraventicular hemorrhage 2) Periventricular leukomalcia (cystic PVD) 3) PVD (if unilateral or bilateral periventricular echogenic lesions present on at least 3 scans)	IA IVH: no lesion= consistently NC scans. Mild lesion = germinal hem or small IVH or PVD or mild vent dilation without hem. Severe lesion: blood distends the vents or in parenchyma, or multicystic PVC.	CNS: Neurodevelopmental: Attention IQ	Measured by CPT test (continuous Performance Test) measuring errors of omission or commission. Is also measured by CBCC (Child Behavior Check List); parents check off behavior related to n attention and hyperactivity. Measured by British Abilities Scale
Korkman 1996 96374730 Psy1996	Main predictors: General: 1) VLBW and AGA (surrogate for perinatal asphyxia in preterm) 2) VLBW and SGA (surrogate for ante-natal asphyxia in preterm) Secondary predictors General: 1) Apgar scores 2) Arterial PH at 2 hrs of life 3) Intrauterine growth retardation 4) BW Pulmonary: 1) RDS 2) Duration of ventilatory tx CNS: 1) IVH	1) VLBW: less than 1500 g 2) SGA: 2 SD below normal for GA 3) Birth asphyxia: Umbilical arterial ph<7.05 4) Or Apgar scores at 5 min less than 6	1) Psychometric Intelligence score. 2) Detailed Neuropsychological assessment score. 3) Neurological Disability status examination (Assessment between 5-9 yrs)	Psychometric Intelligence score: by Finnish standardized Revised version of the Wechsler Intelligence Scale for Children (WISC-R 1984) 1) FSIQ: Full Scale IQ 2) VIQ: Verbal IQ 3) PIQ: performance IQ Detailed Neuropsychological assessment score: 1) NEPSY test (a new test consisting of testing of attention, language, motor, sensory, visuospatial and memory subsets) 2) The Token test shortened version 3) The VMI test Established Finnish norms. Scores reported as SD scores (z scores) Sum scores in all 3 tests also calculated Neurological Disability status assessment: not specified

Evidence Table 3. Studies Evaluating Association of LBW and Cerebral Palsy and Neurological Outcomes
Part II

Author, Year	Predictors	Predictor Measures	Outcomes	Outcome Measures
Lucas 1996 96302121	General: 1) Full fortification for breast milk	Full breast milk Fortification vs Minim supplementation with minerals only, both groups received vitamins	CNS: 1) Neurodevelopmental: 2) Motor delay 3) Mental retardation Audiology: 1) Language Other: 2) Social development	At 9 month: Knobloch Developmental Inventory At 18 month: Knobloch; Bayley scales; Vineland test of social maturity

Evidence Table 3. Studies Evaluating Association of LBW and Cerebral Palsy and Neurological Outcomes
Part II

Author, Year	Predictors	Predictor Measures	Outcomes	Outcome Measures
Rieck 1996 Psy 1996 06905005	In prospective longitudinal component. General: 1) Perinatal factors: 2) BW 3) GA 4) SGA 5) Neurological complications in NICU 6) Sex Growth: 1) HC percentile CNS: 1) Developmental scores at 1-2 yrs of age Others: 1) Age at assessment 2) Parental (mother's and father's) age 3) Parental education 4) Country of origin Prospective comparative component. • VLBW vs Middle class term child And vs Low class term child	Neurologic complications in NICU: 1) Severe asphyxia 2) Loss of consciousness 3) Convulsions 4) IVH grade 3-4 5) CNS infections HC percentile: 1) > 20% 2) 3-20% 3) < 3% Country of origin: Israel Euro-American Asian-African	CNS: Neurodevelopmental outcome: 1) Scores in McCarthy 's 5 Scales of Children's Abilities test (MSCA) 2) General Cognitive Index (GCI) score (Assessment between 3-7 yrs of age)	MSCA: Translated in Hebrew Adapted to Israeli children 5 scales: 1) Verbal 2) Perceptual-Performance 3) Quantitative 4) Memory 5) Motor (GCI) scores: From subtests of the : 1) Verbal 2) Perceptual-performance and 3) Quantitative scales

146

Evidence Table 3. Studies Evaluating Association of LBW and Cerebral Palsy and Neurological Outcomes

Part II

Author, Year	Predictors	Predictor Measures	Outcomes	Outcome Measures
Whitaker 1996 97040639	General predictors: BW,GA, SGA/IUGR Chronic illness, Apgar score Sex CNS Predictor: IVH PL/VE Bronchopulmonary dysplasia Maternal-social disadvantage	Mat-Social Disadvantage: not high school graded; nonwhite race; income from public assist; <19 yrs; not married. According to US findings	**CNS:** Neurodevelopmental: Cognitive delay Mental retardation Memory **Ophthalmology** : Visual perceptual **Audiology:** Language	Test of language Development Stanford-Binet Intelligence Scale
Blitz 1997 97154301	Neonatal complications of ELBW infants, including meningitis, PVL, hydrocephalus, seizures, IVH, BPD, ROP, and whether the infant was discharged on oxygen	Diagnosis based on hospital course. IVH ≥ grade III	**CNS:** CP Neurodevelopmental Development outcome Neurologic Outcome **Ophthalmology:** Visual problems **Audiology:** Hearing loss Hearing loss Visual problem	BSID (Bayley Scale of Infant Development), MDI (Mental Developmental Index), PDI (Psychomotor developmental Index), CLAM (Clinical Linguisitc and Auditory Milestone Scale): Total (CLAM-T), Expressive (CLAM-E), and Receptive (CLAM-R) scores Neurodevelopmental examination, modified after Amiel –Tison and the Primitive Reflex Profile ND Strabismus, hyperopia, myopia, or retinal detachment
Cheung 1997 97310950	IVH grade III or IV	Diagnosed by US finding	**CNS:** Cognitive delay	Cognitive delay - Belay Mental and Psychomotor development indices (MDI, PDI) Normal neurodeveloplement: free of neurodevelopmental disability, with Bayley scores higher than 2 SD below the mean Neurodevelopmental disability: cerebral palsy or blindness or hearing loss

147

Evidence Table 3. Studies Evaluating Association of LBW and Cerebral Palsy and Neurological Outcomes
Part II

Author, Year	Predictors	Predictor Measures	Outcomes	Outcome Measures
Ekert 1997 97251211	General: 1) Birth weight 2) GA 3) Apgar score CNS: 1) Intracranial / Intraventricular hemorrhage 2) Periventricular leuko-malacia Cardiovascular/pulmonary: 1) Bronchopulmonary dysplasia other: a) ventilator days, b) 02 days Other: Hospital/health care resource (admission days) utilization.	Diagnosis of IVE or PVE according to US findings	**CNS:** Motor delay Cerebral palsy Cognitive delay	Motor and cognitive delays: Bayley score of < 84 (i.e., ≥1 SD below mean) or developmental quotient (developmental age divides by corrected age) of < 0.75 Evidence of hypertonicity and hyperreflexive in association with at least gross motor developmental delay

Evidence Table 3. Studies Evaluating Association of LBW and Cerebral Palsy and Neurological Outcomes
Part II

Author, Year	Predictors	Predictor Measures	Outcomes	Outcome Measures
Gerner 1997 97329414	General: 1) Prematurity (per se) 2) General maternal, obstetric, and perinatal predictors: ^ Maternal education ^ Maternal age ^ Parity ^ Maternal toxemia ^ Maternal septicemia ^ Placental bleeding ^ Sex, Gestational age, Birth weight, Intrauterine growth, Cardiotocography, Apgar score at 5 min 3) CNS: (Ultrasound findings) ^ Subependimal bleeding ^ Intraparenchymal lesions 4) Cardiovascular or Pulmonary: ^ PDA, RDS, Surfactant therapy, Days of Ventilatory tx, Chronic Lung Disease (CLD), Pneumothorax, 5) Other : ^ Age at time of test, Infantile septicemia.	Maternal education:3 levels Parity: 0 or more Maternal toxemia, Maternal septicemia, Placental bleeding: presence or absence Intrauterine growth: SGA or AGA Cardiotocography: normal or abnormal All cranial U/S findings classified according to the most advanced stage observed Subependymal bleeding: 3 grades: B1: isolated germinal matrix/ subependymal haemorrhage B2:IVH without ventricular dilatation B3:IVH with ventricular dilatation Intraparenchymal lesions: 4 grades: W1:Subtle or diffuse echodensity W2: Definite, distinct echodensity W3: perventricular cystic formation (PVL) Intraparenchymal W4: echodensity of haemorrhagic type or other gross pathology W1 – W2: correspond to non-cystic PVL B1-3 plus W1-4 PDA: none, spontaneous/ pharmacologic closure, Surgical ligation RDS: presence or absence CLD: according to Bacalari criteria Infantile septicemia: verified by blood culture: staph epi, candida, naerobic bacteria, other. (The other predictors were not specifically defined)	1) Griffith's Developmental Scale for Psychomotor development 2) Total Score (sum of subclasses scores) 3) Individual subclasses Scores (Assessment at 10 months of age)	Griffith's developmental scale, standardized for Swedish infants: 5 subclasses Scale A: locomotor function, Scale B: Personal-social competence, Scale C: hearing and speech Scale D: Hand and eye coordination: fine motor grasping Scale E: Performance: Perception and intelligence scale Scale Specificity of subclasses: limited when infants tested are immature/ Specificity increases with age.

149

Evidence Table 3. Studies Evaluating Association of LBW and Cerebral Palsy and Neurological Outcomes
Part II

Author, Year	Predictors	Predictor Measures	Outcomes	Outcome Measures
Koller 1997 97193708	General: 1) Birth weight 2) GA 3) Illness severity-neonatal health index 4) maternal education CNS: Neurological status at 1 year	Neurological status at 1 year corrected age: (1) abnormal, a severe abnormality, such as CP, global hypotonicity, chronic seizure, hydrocephaly, blindness, or severe sensorineural hearing loss, for which a diagnosis could be established (2) suspicious, some atypical or questionable signs in tone, reflexes, gait, or movement, but for which there is no definitive diagnosis or syndrome (3) Normal, based on a completely normal neurologic examination	**CNS:** Neurodevelopmental: Cognitive delay	Bayley MDI, Stanford-Binet IQ, Wechsler scale
Murphy 1997 97192793	General: GA, Apgar score CNS: Intracranial/Intraventricular hemorrhage White Matter Disorder Periventricular leukomalacia Ventriculomegaly/Ventricular diration. Seizures Cardiovascular: Bronchopulmonary dysplasia Preurmothora GI: Total Patenteral Nutrition Other: Infectious disease, Transfusion PDA, Prolonged ventilation.	Definitions not given for most predictors.	**CNS:** Cerebral palsy	Obtained diagnosis from regional registry of childhood impairments.

150

Evidence Table 3. Studies Evaluating Association of LBW and Cerebral Palsy and Neurological Outcomes
Part II

Author, Year	Predictors	Predictor Measures	Outcomes	Outcome Measures
Schendel 1997 98033417	*General Predictors* 1) Birth Weight- 3 groups VLBM (very low birth wt) MLBW (moderately low birth wt.) NBW (normal birth wt) *Other Predictors* 1) Other: married at birth 2) Other: Medicaid recipient	ND	**CNS:** Other: Developmental Delay **Pulmonary Outcomes** Birth weight	Developmental delay measured by Denver Developmental Screening Test II. "DELAY" defined by 9 measures of performance on Denver Developmental Screening Test II at age 15 months corrected.
Thompson 1997 97268338	Other predictors: 1) Neurobiological Risk Score (NBRS) 2) Hasseles Scale Score (HSS) → divided mothers into high and low risk; a "stress" score 3) Maternal variables	NBRS→weighted scored of medical events: ventilation, acidosis, seizures, IVH, PVL, sepsis and hypoglycemia	**CNS:** Neurodevelopmental: Cognitive delay	McCarthy scales at age 4 years Definition: not clear on how well validated either of the predictors are. Definitions of NBRS and Hasseles scores are probably OK, but I am not clear with these.
Victorian Collaborative study Group 1997 98026322 ***There are a series of Victorian articles in LBW-ALL. *This study will be combined in LBW-ALL table**	General: BW Other: period of time when born	Each sample were subdivided into BW=500-749 g and BW=750-999 g 1985-1987 vs. 1991-1992	**CNS:** Cerebral palsy Neurodevelopmental: Cognitive and motor delay Disability **Ophthalmology:** Blindness **Audiology:** Deafness or hearing aid	CP was not defined Bayley Scales of Infant Development DQ, using the published mean and SD Disability: "Sever" – bilateral blindness, cerebral palsy with the child unlikely ever to walk, or a DQ score <-3SD; "Moderate" – bilateral sensorineural deafness requiring hearing aids, cerebral palsy in children not walking at 2 but expected to walk, or a DQ score from –3SD to <-2 SD; "Mild" – cerebral palsy but walking at 2, or a DQ score form –2 SD to <-1 SD.

151

Evidence Table 3. Studies Evaluating Association of LBW and Cerebral Palsy and Neurological Outcomes
Part II

Author, Year	Predictors	Predictor Measures	Outcomes	Outcome Measures
Battin 1998 99002694	General: 1) GA (23-25 wks) In comparative component with Historical control group General: 1) Birth during a period with routine use of: antenatal steroids, surfactant and dexamethasone for BPD (vs birth in presurfactant, presteroid period)	ND	**CNS:** 1) Neurodevelopmental outcome 2) CP 3) Low MDI (below 2 SDs) **Ophthalmology- Audiology:** 1) Blind, Deaf	Neurologic exam Bayley scale: MDI, PDI Formal hearing test Ophthalmologic examination
Bos 1998 98218970	General predictors Quality of general movements CNS Head ultrasound finding of transient periventricular Echodensities	Diagnosed by US examination. The duration was determined for the frontal and the parieto-occipital region separately and classified according to four categories: (1) no echodensities, (2) echodensities between 1 and 6 d, (3) echodensities between 7 and 13 d, and (4) echodensities persisting for more than 14 d.	**CNS:** Neurodevelopmental CP Cognitive delay	Developmental trajectory of general movement quality, analyzed according to Prechtl's method. Movements were judged globally based on visual Gestalt perception. Normal general movements are characterized by complexity, variability, and fluency.
Cherkes-Julkowski 1998 98262696	General: GA Other: Mother perception of child competence	ND	**CNS:** Cognitive delay Neurodevelopmental School problem Neurological Impairment (NI) Attention Deficit Disorder (ADD) **Audiology:** Language	Cognitive delay, measured by Stanford-Binet School programs (school concerns = SC) Learning disabilities (LD) Neurological Impairment (NI) Attention deficit Disorder (ADD) Language impairment = LI – dx made by speech and language clinician

152

Evidence Table 3. Studies Evaluating Association of LBW and Cerebral Palsy and Neurological Outcomes
Part II

Author, Year	Predictors	Predictor Measures	Outcomes	Outcome Measures
Emsley 1998 98238139 (CNS+ All)	*General* 1) Birth weight 2) GA **CNS** 1) Other: significant cranial U/S findings (see page 1 for definition) *Other:* 1) Illness acuity – CRIB score 2) Other: male sex	CRIB score is determined by BW, GA< congenital malformations, max base excess in first 12 hours, minimum FIO$_2$ in first 12 hours and max FIO$_2$ in first 12 hours	**CNS :** CP Neurodevelopmental Behavioral disorders Learning disabilities Seizure disorder Developmental Delay **Ophthalmology :** Blindness Other Squint **Audiology:** Deafness Speech delay	ND "Normal" - No clinically apparent developmental abnormality causing functional disability "Mild Disability" - myopia, language delay, mild hearing loss, hyperactivity or clumsiness. "Moderate Disability" – Spastic diplegia, hemiplegia, moderate learning disability (DQ 50-69) "Severe Disability" – spastic quadriplegia, blindness, deafness (> 70 dB), uncontrolled epilepsy or severe learning disability (DQ < 50) and multiple disabilities. Not defined or how it is measured ND DQ <70 > 70 dB, dot defined or how it is measured ND
Pasman 1998 98196839	**CNS** 1) Other: Neurobiologic risk score (NBRS) 2) Neonatal Neurologic Inventory (NNI) table 1	13 items of NBRS 4 items of NNI	**CNS** Neurodevelopmental: Cognitive delay Mental retardation	Standardized testing: VMI Leiden diagnostic test WISC-R BWVR ADIT
Rogers 1998 98438124	Birth weight GA Periventricular Bronchopulmonary dysplasia Hospital/Health care resource utilization-length of stay	IVH according to discharge clinical record diagnosis	**CNS:** CP Neurodevelopmental: Growth failure	According to discharge clinical record diagnosis (quadriplegia, diplegia, or hemiplegia) Weight-for-age z score was more than 2 SD below the mean and subsequently fell below –2 SDS

153

Evidence Table 3. Studies Evaluating Association of LBW and Cerebral Palsy and Neurological Outcomes
Part II

Author, Year	Predictors	Predictor Measures	Outcomes	Outcome Measures
Spinillo 1998 98237382	General predictors: 1) Birth weight' 2) GA 3) SGA/IUGR 4) Maternal disease (diabetes, respiratory, cardiovascular, renal etc) 5) Antenatal steroids	Preeclampsia defined as: 1) Diastolic BP> 90 2) Systolic BP> 140 3) Proteinurea> 0.3 g Severe preeclampsia defined as: 1) Diastolic BP> 110 2) Systolic BP> 160 3) Proteinurea> 3 g	**CNS** CP Neurodevelopmental: Mental retardation	CP: Spastic diplegia, hemiplegia, tetraplegia , With moderate to severe interference with function, With or without mental retardation (MDI< 71) Bayley scales
Spinillo, 1997 98021316 & 97277958 *have some overlapped sample with spinillo, 1994	Other predictors: 1) Infectious disease 2) Dexamethasone 3) Perinatal factors (Socioeconomic factors, pregnancy variables, Delivery variables) 4) Meconum-stained amniotic fluid	Intrapartum Fetal HR abnormalities: ● Late decelerations 1) Variable decelerations 2) Bradycardia Tachycardia		
Tin 1998 99046171	General: GA (23-31 wks)	ND	**CNS:** Neurodevelopmental: 1) Mental retardation (IQ < 75) 2) Other; disability (severe, severe sensorimotor) 3) Other: development - assessed by Griffith's mental and developmental scales	Definition of "severe disability" and "severe sensorimotor disability" were not given in this article . They referred to the wrong reference for these definitions, therefore, I am unable to find the definitions. Reference population for Griffith's scales were "preterm babies in the study S serious sensorimotor disability"

Evidence Table 3. Studies Evaluating Association of LBW and Cerebral Palsy and Neurological Outcomes
Part II

Author, Year	Predictors	Predictor Measures	Outcomes	Outcome Measures
Burguet 1999 99126269	General Predictor: 1) Male gender Cardiovascular 1) Bronchopulmonary dysplasia Other predictor: 1) Infectious disease neonatal sepsis 2) Maternal hypertension 3) RDS 4) Outborn birth 5) Race 6) Urban residence 7) Family precariousness = father absent or both parents unemployed 8) PROM > 48 hours (preterm) 9) Monochorionic placentation 10) Singleton placentation 11) Dichorionic placentation	RDS diagnosed by chest radiography examination PROM = premature rupture of membrane	**CNS:** CP PVL	One or more of the following signs was observed – hemiplegia, diplegia, tetraplegia, dystonia, athetosis, blindness, or neurosensory deafness
Cooke 1999 99257637	General predictors: Antenatal steroids Period of birth CNS: IVH Periventricular leukomalacia Other: Surfactant use	ND	**CNS:** CP	Data from Regional Cerebral Palsy Register

155

Evidence Table 3. Studies Evaluating Association of LBW and Cerebral Palsy and Neurological Outcomes
Part II

Author, Year	Predictors	Predictor Measures	Outcomes	Outcome Measures
Cooke 1999 99380719	Birth weight CNS: white matter disorder, periventricular leukomalacia, ventriculomegaly, MRI abnormality, thinning of corpus callosum, povencephaly, Brain measurements (multiple)	ND	**CNS:** Motor delay Cerebral palsy Cognitive delay Mental retardation Behavioral disorders School problems Learning disabilities	IQ: WISC III Motor delay (motor disability): Movement of ABC scores Mental retardation Behavioral disorders School problems Learning disability: Suffolk Reading Scale. Basic Math and Spelling Test

Evidence Table 3. Studies Evaluating Association of LBW and Cerebral Palsy and Neurological Outcomes
Part II

Author, Year	Predictors	Predictor Measures	Outcomes	Outcome Measures
Finer 1999 99436635	*CNS Predictors:* Delivery room resuscitation (DR-CPR)	Defined as chest compressions and/or epinephrine used.	**CNS:** *Neurodevelopmental* 1) Motor delay 2) Post hemorrhagic hydrocephalus (PHH) 3) Apgar scores 4) IVH/echolucenies 5) Developmental 6) White matter injury	In the first year, neurodevelopmental assessment by Amiel-Tison Neurologic Screen. Thereafter, used Knoblick-Gesell Developmental Inventory. "Neuromotor Outcome - questionable": hypotonia, hypertonia, asymmetry "Neuromotor Outcome - abnormal": cerebral palsy "Developmental Outcome - normal": both mental and motor composite scores ▯86 "Developmental Outcome - questionable": either score 76-85 "Developmental Outcome - abnormal": either score <75 "Neurodevelopmental Outcome - normal" if both neuromotor and developmental evaluations are normal. "Neurodevelopmental Outcome - questionable" if either neuromotor or developmental evaluations are questionable. "Neurodevelopmental Outcome - abnormal" if either neuromotor or developmental evaluations are abnormal. "White matter injury": presence of grade 4 hemorrhage, echolucencies, or ventricular dilation unrelated to hemorrhage.

157

Evidence Table 3. Studies Evaluating Association of LBW and Cerebral Palsy and Neurological Outcomes
Part II

Author, Year	Predictors	Predictor Measures	Outcomes	Outcome Measures
Futagi 1999 99450356	General: 1) Birth in surfactant era 1989-1993 vs Birth in pre-surfactant era 1981-1986	Not specified further	1) Normal neurodevelopmental outcome 2) Cerebral palsy 3) Mental retardation 4) Borderline intelligence (Assessment between 3-8 yrs, mean age of assessment was 6 yrs)	1) Normal neurodevelopmental outcome: Absence of motor disturbances and developmental quotient and/or intelligence quotient more than 84. 2) Cerebral palsy: diagnosis based on Bax criteria (Outcome data also given for one child with spinal palsy: no definition given) 3) Mental retardation: DQ or IQ scores less than70 4) Borderline intelligence: DQ or IQ scores between 70-84, DQ and /or IQ scores: (of latest exam)according to Kyoto child guidance clinic development scale for children for subjects up to 7 yrs of age, Or according to the revised Wechsler Intelligence scale adapted for Japanese children for cases more than 7 yrs of age. (the results of gross motor skills in the former test were excluded for cerebral palsy children when computing DQs)
Kim 1999 99416608	Other Predictor-Perinatal factors	ND	**CNS:** CP **Neurodevelopmental:** Development delay	Non-progressive, often changing motor impairment syndromes secondary to lesions or anomalies of the brain arising in the early stages of development Delay in parameters for motor development of more than two months according to the stages of motor development by Vojta

158

Evidence Table 3. Studies Evaluating Association of LBW and Cerebral Palsy and Neurological Outcomes

Part II

Author, Year	Predictors	Predictor Measures	Outcomes	Outcome Measures
Krageloh-Mann 1999 99431017	CNS: 1) Intracranial/ Intraventricular hemorrhage 2) PVL 3) Cerebral blood flow 4) Cerebral oxygen delivery	CBF measured with ^{133}Xe clearance at 12.9 hours of life (range 1-48hr) Cerebral oxygen flow calculated as CBF x ART 02 content	CNS: Spastic CP **Neurodevelopmental**: Motor delay Mental retardation Anatomical abnormalities on MRI **Ophthalmology**: Visual blindness	Stott-Moyes-Henderson test - Spasticity of extremities with flexor hypertonicity, increased tendon reflexes and characteristic posturing Motor disability was graded as severe if the child could not walk unaided at the age of 5 y, otherwise as mild WISC
Salokorpi 1999 99353226	General: BW, GA, SGA/IUGR, Maternal disease CNS: IVH grade III or IV PVL Other: duration of ventilation, hypotension, hypocarbia, infectious disease	ND	CNS: CP Mortality by 2 years	A diagnosis of CP was confirmed when abnormal muscular tone, persistent or exaggerated primitive reflexes and major delay in motor development were found. The classification of CP syndromes was based on the definition by Hagberg et al.
Shepherd 1999 99165413	Ophthalmology : VEP (visual evoked potential)	One flash per second 20 cm from eyes. Each trial included 30 responses. 2 trials averaged. In preterms, VEP measured at 3 day of life in groups < 34 weeks, 34-36 weeks and 40 weeks, when 3,6-12 months.	CNS: Cerebral palsy	No definition of CP given
Stathis 1999 99325758	CNS Predictors 1) Other: head circumference category 2) Head growth velocity	Self-explanatory	CNS: **Neurodevelopmental**: Cognitive delay Behavioral disorders-ADHD School problems Learning disabilities	Academic problems--Answer questionnaires given to teacher ADHD--Dr. Paul rating scale McCarthy's scales

Evidence Table 3. Studies Evaluating Association of LBW and Cerebral Palsy and Neurological Outcomes
Part II

Author, Year	Predictors	Predictor Measures	Outcomes	Outcome Measures
Vohr 1999 99332101	Intracranial/Intraventricular hemorrhage	Cranial ultrasound finding	**CNS**: CP Neurodevelopmental: Cognitive and Motor delay	CP diagnosed by routine neurological exam. CP was based on the presence of hypertonicity, hyperreflexia, and dystonic or spastic movement quality in the affected limbs. Stanford-Binet Intelligence Scale PPVT-R
Agustines 2000 20279724	General predictors: 1) BW (500-750) 2) GA	ND	**Neurodevelopmental outcome:** Bayley scale 1) MDI 2) PDI 3) Overall neurodevelopmental outcome 4) Neurodevelopmental outcome stratified by GA (assessment at 30 months corrected age)	1) Normal development: Performance within 1 SD 2) Mild delay: Performance below 1 SD 3) Severe delay: Performance below 2 SD

160

Evidence Table 3. Studies Evaluating Association of LBW and Cerebral Palsy and Neurological Outcomes
Part II

Author, Year	Predictors	Predictor Measures	Outcomes	Outcome Measures
Breslau 2000 20298367	General: 1) LBW (vs Normal BW= NBW) 2) Urban (vs suburban setting) 3) Maternal smoking during pregnancy	ND	**CNS/Behavior** 1) Behavioral problems in 3 domains: Attention , Externalization Internalization 2) Severe attention problems (above a cutoff point of 67) Assessment at 11 yrs of age (assessment at 6 yrs: reported in another publication)	Mother's rating was done with: Child Behavior Checklist (CBCL) Teacher's rating was done with Teacher Report Form (TRF) (teachers were blind to the BW information of the child) Assessments at 11 yrs were conducted blindly to the results of assessments at 6 yrs (reported in another publication) Attention problem subscale; 20 items Externalization problem subscale: 2 subclasses Internalization problem subscale: 3 subclasses
Bührer 2000 20280896	CRIB score	Routinely measure on the first day of a baby's life. CRIB score determined from: BW, GA, congenital life-threatening malformations, worse base excess, min+max FIO2 in first 12 hrs of life	**CNS:** Neurodevelopmental	Griffith's test
Grether 2000 20448692	Received Magnesium sulfate	Chart review	**CNS:** CP	Mild, moderate, or severe CP assessed from record of 2 state agencies.
Katz-Salamon 2000 20332284	Cardiovascular or pulmonary predictors: chronic lung disease	1st week ⃞ acute lung injury; clinical signs; supplemental O$_2$ at 28 days; typical CXR	**CNS:** Neurodevelopmental: Cognitive delay CP	Griffith's development scale Movement assessment index (MAI): the original number of items was reduced to include only those reported to be the most valid as predictors of CP

161

Evidence Table 3. Studies Evaluating Association of LBW and Cerebral Palsy and Neurological Outcomes
Part II

Author, Year	Predictors	Predictor Measures	Outcomes	Outcome Measures
Marlow 2000 20150342	**General:** 1) Birth weight 2) Apgar score 3) Illness severity (CRIB) scores **CNS:** 1) Maximum bilirubin level 2) Abnormal cerebral US scan **Audiology:** 1) Sensorineural hearing loss **Cardiovascular/Pulomonary:** 1) Duration of intubation, respiratory support, oxygen, pH<7.2, base excess 2) Dopamine 3) Furosemide 4) Indomethacin use **Other:** 5) Netilmicin 6) Vancomycin 7) Positive blood cultures 8) Bilirubin >200 ꙴmol/l 9) Bilirubin>GA x 10 10) Creatinine >60 mmol/l 11) Netilmicin 12) Vancomycin combination of the above: 1) Bili.200 + acidosis 2) Bili> 200 + sepsis 3) Bili >200+ netilmicin 4) Bili> 200+ vancomycin 5) Bili>200+ furosemide 6) Peak bili+ acidosis 7) Peak bili+ sepsis 8) Peak bili+ netilmicin 9) Peak bili+ furosemide 10) Creatinine>60+ netilmicin or vancomycin or furosemide 11) Netilmicin+furosemide • Vancomycin+ furosemide	Not further specified	In case control component: **Audiology:** Sensorineural hearing loss (SNHL) of 50 dB within 9 months from birth In Longitudinal component: **CNS:** Cerebral palsy at 12 months of age in the 2 groups (SNHL and control group)	Cases of SNHL were identified if the hearing loss had been identified within 3 months of discharge home, (within 9 mo from birth); after excluding cases with conductive hearing loss, possible congenital cause, or had neonatal bacterial meningitis

Evidence Table 3. Studies Evaluating Association of LBW and Cerebral Palsy and Neurological Outcomes
Part II

Author, Year	Predictors	Predictor Measures	Outcomes	Outcome Measures
Palta 2000 20096107 (CNS+Eye)	General: 1) Birth weight 2)Antenatal steroids 3)Multiple birth CNS: Intracranial/ Intraventricular hemorrhage Ophthalmology: Retinopathy of Prematurity (ROP) Cardiovascular/ Pulmonary: 1)Surfactant administration 2)Respiratory score Other: 1)Multiple birth 2)Socioeconomics 3) Number days in NICU	BW ≤1500 gms VLBW -Baseline respiratory scores = disease 1st 3 days of life 0-100 based on increasing severity BPD: O2 use at 36 wks post conceptional age postnatal used corticosteroid use mechanical ventilation or both = severe BPD at 30 days	**CNS:** CP Neurodevelopmental: Functional assessments **Ophthalmology:** Visual impairment Blindness Standardized scores for **self care, mobility and social function**	CP: physician dx at parent interview and confirmed by clinic record abstraction as well as blindness and use of corrective lenses. Pediatric Evaluation of Disability Index (PEDI): standardized scores for self care, mobility and social function
Torrioli 2000 20275419 (CNS+Eye)	General: 1) Birth weight 2) GA 3) SGA/IUGR	ND	**CNS:** Neurodevelopmental: Motor delay Cognitive delay Behavioral disorder **Ophthalmology:** Visual impairment	For VMI &WISC measures, "abnormal" was defined as under the 5th%tile; "normal" was defined as over 15th %tile of a control group VMI Movement WISC Conner's relent symptom questionnaire
Valkama 2000 20233239	**General predictors:** Birth weight GA SGA/IUGR **CNS predictors:** IVH White matter disorder Periventricular leukomalacia MRI findings	IVH grading according to Papile PVL grading according to DeVries	**CNS:** Cerebral palsy	Infants whose motor development was delayed and who had abnormal muscle tone and motor function as an impairment or disability at a corrected age of 18 mo were defined as having CP in the sense of Hasberg et al.

Evidence Table 3. Studies Evaluating Association of LBW and Cerebral Palsy and Neurological Outcomes
Part II

Author, Year	Predictors	Predictor Measures	Outcomes	Outcome Measures
Vohr 2000 20295211	*General:* 1) Birth weight 2) Maternal disease (HTN) 3) Antenatal steroids *CNS:* 1) Intracranial/Intraventricular hemorrhage (GR 3 to $ IVH/PVL) *Cardiovascular or Pulmonary:* 1) Chronic lung disease (oxygen requirement at 36 weeks) 2) Other: postnatal steroids 3) Other: Surfactant *Gastrointestinal:* 1) Necrotizing "enterocolitis" *Other:* 1) Other: male sex 2) Other: Race (white) 3) Other: sepsis (early and late onset) 4) Other: maternal education	GR 3 to 4 IVH. PVL undefined sepsis undefined	**CNS :** Cerebral palsy Neurodevelopmental: 1) Motor delay (sitting, walking, pincer grasp, feeding) 2) Seizure disorder 3) Post hemorrhagic Hydrocephalus (PHH) and shunt 4) Other: Neurologic exam (normal; abnormal) 5) Development (MDI and PDI by Bayley II Scale) **Ophthalmology :** 1) Visual impairment (any) 2) Blindness (unilateral, bilateral) **Audiology:** 1) Hearing disorders	"normal Neurologic exam": no abnormalities on neurologic exams
Dammann 2001 21334215	*General Predictors:* 1) Birth weight 2) SGA/IUGR *CNS Predictors:* 1) Intracranial/ Intraventricular hemorrhage *Other predictors:* 1) Infectious disease 2) Perinatal factors - PTL, PROM, C-section	ND	**CNS:** CP	ND

164

Evidence Table 3. Studies Evaluating Association of LBW and Cerebral Palsy and Neurological Outcomes
Part II

Author, Year	Predictors	Predictor Measures	Outcomes	Outcome Measures
Gaillard 2001 21221175	In retrospective case-control component: **General:** 1) shorter length of ventilation beyond 27 (but not 50) postnatal ds vs more prolonged ventilation beyond 49 ds 2) Number of days "off" ventilator in the groups of 27-49 postnatal ds ventilation and the group of >49ds ventilation In retrospective cohort with historical control group component: **General:** 1) Birth in a period where Antenatal steroids and Surfactant were more routinely used vs birth in pre-surfactant pre-antenatal steroid period	Not further specified	**CNS:** Neurodevelopmental outcome: 1) Normal 2) Mild disability 3) Moderate disability 4) Severe disability	Normal neurodevelopmentally: no clinically apparent neurodevelopmental abnormality causing functional disability Mild disability: e.g. myopia, language delay, mild hearing loss, hyperactivity or motor clumsiness. Moderate disability: for example: spastic diplegia, hemiplegia or moderate learning disability (Developmental Quotient: 50-69) Severe disability: e.g. spastic quadriplegia, blindness, deafness (loss of 70 decibel or more), uncontrolled epilepsy, or severe learning disability (developmental quotient <50). Infants with multiple disabilities. (3 yrs CA)
Horwood 2001 20574647	Other: Breastfeeding duration	Retrospective questioning	**CNS:** Neurodevelopmental: Cognitive delay Mental retardation	WISC-R verbal and performance IQ scores at age seven years.

165

Evidence Table 3. Studies Evaluating Association of LBW and Cerebral Palsy and Neurological Outcomes
Part II

Author, Year	Predictors	Predictor Measures	Outcomes	Outcome Measures
Nadeau 2001 21163667	General: GA Other: Family adversity Index	Evaluated at 5 years 9 months, was developed using SES data such as the family status (two-parent, single-parent, blended), age of each parent, their respective levels of education, and professional occupations. 0=low ~ 7=high	**CNS:** Neurodevelopmental: Motor function Cognitive delay Behavioral disorders **Behavior**	Neuromotor development index: Huttenlocher neurological task test McCarthy Scales of Children's Abilities Behaviors were assessed by peers, teachers, and parents: RCP, TRF, parent's CBCL
Pierrat 2001 27221167	*CNS Predictors:* Periventricular leukomalacia (cystic) in ≤32 wk GA infants	Grade II - Transient periventricular densities, evolving into small cysts. Grade III - Transient periventricular densities, evolving into large cysts.	**CNS:** Neurodevelopmental: Motor delay Cerebral palsy	Motor delay - 12, 18, 24 month outcome as the protocol of Amiel-Tison and Stewart, and Touwen Criteria of Hagberg et al.

Evidence Table 3. Studies Evaluating Association of LBW and Cerebral Palsy and Neurological Outcomes

Part III

Author, Year	Associations found	Potential Biases	Comments
Leonard 1990 90204169	Neurologic abnormalities: Oxygen group (no IVH and no parenting risk): 0-29 days 9%, ≥ 50 days 0%, p=NS among oxygen groups, total 6% IVH (no parenting risk factor): none 6%, Gr 1-II 0%, Gr III-IV 21% Parenting risk (no IVH): absent 6%, Present 17%, p=NS Cognitive deficits: Oxygen (no IVH and no parenting risk): 0-29 days 18%, ≥ 50days 7%, total 17% IVH (no parenting risk factor): none 17%, Gr I-II 29%, Gr III-IV 50%, p < .005 between none and Gr III-IV groups Parenting risk (no IVH): Absent 17%, Present 75%, p<.001 NO cognitive risk factors: Low socioeconomic status with no parenting risk 74% Low socioeconomic status with parenting risk: 20% p<.02 Abnormal cognitive outcome (logistic regression): Oxygen: NS IVH: Grades 0-IV p= .0042, Gr I-II p=.18, Grade III-IV p=.003 Parenting risk with no IVH p= .0002 Low socioeconomic status p= .0107	Almost 30% dropout rate. Incomplete description of study groups No description of how neurodevelopmental assessment was done (who evaluated and were they blinded to the group). Conclusion that antenatal steroids and surfactant improves neurologic outcome is inappropriate since he had no control group that did not receive these treatments.	No data on funding source
Lucas 1992 92122860	Fortified breast-milk-fed vs. Minimally supplemented breast-milk-fed: Gross motor development/Knobloch scale: (Not significant) 102.7 ±1.8 ; 102.9+2 Language development/Knobloch scale: (Not significant) 92.6+0.9 ; 92.1+1.1 Social development: (Not significant) 104.6+1.1 ; 105.6+4 Motor development/Bayley: (Not significant) 92.3+1.6 ; 89.9+1.5 Mental development/Bayley: (Not significant) 106+2 ; 105.8+2 Social development/Vineland (Not significant) 118.9+1.7 ; 115.8+1.7	Not exclusively breast fed: in both groups total maternal intake was < 50 % breast milk with the Differential loss to follow up not reported-cannot determine BWT/GA of groups at follow-up	No data on funding source

167

Evidence Table 3. Studies Evaluating Association of LBW and Cerebral Palsy and Neurological Outcomes

Part III

Author, Year	Associations found	Potential Biases	Comments
Robertson 1994 94181384	**CP** 500 –749 g (20) 1/20; 750 –999 g (54) 6/59; 1000-1249 g (84) 4/84; 500-1249 g (163) 11/163 (6.7%) **Vision loss** 500 –749 g (20) 2/20; 750 –999 g (54) 0/59; 1000-1249 g (84) 0/84; 500-1249 g (163) 2/163 (1.2%) **Hearosensory** 500 –749 g (20) 1/20; 750 –999 g (54) 0/59; 1000-1249 g (84) 1/84; 500-1249 g (163) 2/163 (1.2%) **Mental retardation** 500 –749 g (20) 3/20; 750 –999 g (54) 0/59; 1000-1249 g (84) 0/84; 500-1249 g (163) 3/163 (1.8%) **Convulsive disorder** 500 –749 g (20) 0/20; 750 –999 g (54) 0/59; 1000-1249 g (84) 0/84; 500-1249 g (163) 0/163 (0%)	Does not give detailed characteristics of cohort	Study was private funded
Spinillo 1994 94257064 *have some overlapped sample with spinillo, 1997*	Studied outcome of LBW infants after 3rd trimester bleeding. Controls were LBW's without 3rd trimester bleeding. Abruption, n = 40; previa, n= 22; unclassified bleeding, n = 15; controls, n = 153.	Not all severe VLBW No information regarding frequenting of VLBW Bayley test score information no presented	No data on funding source

Group	Grade 3-4 IVH	Cystic PVL	Major handicap	Poor Outcome
Abruption	12.5%*	5%	11.1%+	OR = 3.9 (1.2, 2.1)
Previa	13.6%	0	0	OR = 0.9 (0.2, 3.6)
Unclassified	6.7%	0	0	OR = 0.6 (0.1, 0.3)
Control	3.9%	0.6%	0.7%	Reference group

*P = 0.02 vs. control
+P = 0.007 vs. control

168

Evidence Table 3. Studies Evaluating Association of LBW and Cerebral Palsy and Neurological Outcomes

Part III

Author, Year	Associations found	Potential Biases	Comments
Chen 1995 96009403	All of the LBW preterm infants with normal brain US finding (N=12) had "normal development". Two (17%) of them developed spastic CP. All of the LBW preterm infants with abnormal brain US finding (N=5) showed signs of spastic CP.	No reference of DDST Cases report without statistical analyses Vague or no definition of outcomes	No data on funding source
Goetz 1995 96119489	Tone abnormalities : (PVL) 12/12 Seizure disorder: (PVL) 1/12 Strabismus: (PVL) 3/12 Cognitive delay: (PVL) 6/12 mild 2/12 severe 4/12 They found cognitive delay in 6 of 12, seizures in 1 of 12 and strabismus in 3 of 12	Missing information Small sample	No data on funding source

Evidence Table 3. Studies Evaluating Association of LBW and Cerebral Palsy and Neurological Outcomes

Part III

Author, Year	Associations found	Potential Biases	Comments
Speechley 1995 96356544	**General Health outcome:** Among boys around 12 yrs of age: NICU graduates as opposed to normal boys: 1) Are living with more chronic health problems 2) Are more likely to have a physical impairment 3) And have been hospitalized more often. Among girls around 12 yrs of age: NICU graduates as compared to normal girls: No statistically significant differences in their physical health outcome. Among NICU graduates, boys were not different from girls in their long-term physical health outcomes. **Emotional and Social well being outcomes:** Among girls around 12 yrs of age: NICU graduates as opposed to normal girls: 1) Had significantly lower social competence 2) Lower social support 3) And Lower self-esteem. Among boys around 12 yrs of age: NICU graduates as compared to normal boys: 1) They had no difference in their emotional or social well being. There was no interaction between family's socioeconomic status and long term outcomes among NICU graduates. Analytically: The **physical health outcomes** at 12 yrs were (**Boys** NICU grads vs Boys NNN grads/ **Girls** NICU grads vs Girls NNN grads) • Chronic physical health (mother's report): 2.8 vs 1.8 (p<0.005)/ 2.4 vs 1.3 • Lifetime hospitalizations (mother's report): 2.5 vs 1.6 (p<0.005)/ 1.7 vs 0.4 • Physical impairments (mother's report): 0.29 vs 0.10 (p<0.005)/ 0.22 vs 0.06 • Perception of child's heath (child's report): 21.6 vs 22.2/ 21.1 vs 21.9 • Perception of child's health (mother's report): 16.9 vs 17.7/ 16.8vs 18.0 **Emotional and social well being at 12 yrs:** (Boys NICU grads vs Boys NNN grads, Girls NICU grads vs Girls NNN grads) • Internalizing problems (child's report):15.3 vs 15.5/ 18.2 vs 14.8 • Externalizing problems (child's report): 15.9 vs 16.0/ 14.3 vs 13.5 • Social competence (child's report): 109.1 vs 113.9 / 101.7 vs 115.7 (p<0.005 • Social support (child's report): 81.6 vs 83.2/ 79.9 vs 86.1 (p<0.005) • Self esteem (child's report): 31.9 vs 32.4/ 29.8 vs 32.5 (p<0.005) • School performance (mother's report): 4.5 vs 4.6/ 4.8 vs 5.3	1) There is an Inconsistency in Mother's appreciation of their child's physical health: mothers of NICU graduate boys reported that their children had more physical impairments than NNN boy graduates; however, their overall perception of their child's health status was not any different from NNN boys graduates. 2) Some of the outcomes 3) Collected are prone to recollection bias (e.g., frequency of lifetime hospitalizations).	1) In this NICU cohort, only 36% of infants had BW<2500 g and only 5% had BW < 1500 gs, reflecting more NICU populations in the 70s and early 80s, than the current ones. 2) It is unclear whether statistically significant differences in psychometric scales reflect clinically significant differences in the emotional and social wellbeing of these children. 3) Given the fact of many negative findings, post hoc power analyses demonstrated that the study had an 80% power to detect a 40% difference between the 2 groups. 4) The fact that girls ex NICU graduates had a more substantial psychological effect than boys may reflect that girls are further into adolescence than the boys, experiencing the sequelae earlier. Thus in order to determine whether the differences observed are a temporary effect/related to adolescence, this cohort had to be followed further into their teenage years

170

Evidence Table 3. Studies Evaluating Association of LBW and Cerebral Palsy and Neurological Outcomes
Part III

Author, Year	Associations found	Potential Biases	Comments
Wildin 1995 95385294	High risk (HR) preterms, low risk (LR) preterms and full term controls. Most infants who were classified as high risk were classified as such due to BPD. Bayley MDI and PDI at 12 months corrected age: Group n Bayley MDI Bayley PDI HR 49 92.8 (24.9) 89.8 (20.7) LR 92 103.8 (16.3) 99.1 (19.5) Control 114 108.2 (11.3) 108.5 (12.3)	Preterm HR (high risk) Group: 84% were HR because of BPD only, so this groups is really a BPD group Many exclusion criteria Full developmental evaluation only done on a subgroup; others only partly examined	No data on funding source
Wildin 1997 97422739			

*Data from same longitudinal study as Anderson, 1996 96314587 & Smith, 1996 97081985; overlapped sample	In Hierarchical linear models analyses:
	Cognitive/Bayley, Stanford-Binet
	Medical risk category LR (N=115) Hierarchical linear
	               HR (N=69) model P=0.02
	Rate of mental development/Bayley, Stanford-Binet
	Medical risk category LR (N=115)
	               HR (N=69) P=0.0004
	
	Socioeconomic status and cognitive/ Bayley Stanford-Binet association not significant.
	Medical risk category SES and rate of mental development/Bayley, Stanford-Binet association not significant.
	SES and rate of mental development/Bayley, Stanford-Binet association not significant.
	Motor development not significant
		Only analyzed infants retained through all 40 months
		Do not account for infants lost to follow-up
		Do not describe how group at 40 months differed in composition from group at enrollment.
		Use one-tailed test to achieve significance.	

171

Evidence Table 3. Studies Evaluating Association of LBW and Cerebral Palsy and Neurological Outcomes
Part III

Author, Year	Associations found	Potential Biases	Comments
Anderson 1996 96314587 Smith 1996 97081985 (CNS+All) *Data from same longitudinal study (U. of Texas Health Sciences Center in Houston and the U. of Texas Medical Branch in Galveston) as Wildin, 1995 & 1997; overlapped sample	Cognitive Development (Bayley MDI) at 6 and 12 months, respectively: VLBW high risk (N=58): 100.7 (24.9), 92.8 (19.2) VLBW low risk (N=96): 106.8 (19.5), 103.8 (16.3) FT (N=119): 113.6 (15.8), 108.2 (11.3) Motor Development (Bayley PDI) at 6 and 12 months, respectively: VLBW high risk (N=58): 100.7 (24.9), 92.8 (19.2) VLBW low risk (N=96): 106.8 (19.5), 103.8 (16.3) FT (N=119): 113.6 (15.8), 108.2 (11.3) All groups differed significantly on MDI and PDI at 6 months (p<.001). At 12 months, only the high-risk infants differed from the term infants (p<.001). The means for all three groups at 6 and 12 months were within the normal range. However, significantly more high-risk infants fell within the moderately and severely delayed ranged than low-risk and term infants did (data not given) Total neurologic score at 6 and 12 months, respectively: VLBW high risk (N=58): 0.30 (0.23), 0.16 (0.22) VLBW low risk (N=96): 0.16 (0.17), 0.08 (0.12) FT (N=119): 0.05 (0.07), 0.04 (0.05) All groups differed significantly on total neurologic score at both 6 and 12 months (p<.001). Total score significantly improved from 6 to 12 months of age in all groups (p<.001). Total score in high-risk group still remained abnormal after improvement, while the score in low-risk and term infants were normal at 12 months of age. Assessed risk status in relation to outcome in areas of development of cognitive skills, communication development and daily living skills. Mental Age and daily living skills data are in months and language data are in raw scores: <table><tr><td>Infant status</td><td>n</td><td>Mental Age</td><td>Daily living skills</td><td colspan="3">Language</td></tr><tr><td></td><td></td><td></td><td></td><td>Expressive</td><td>Receptive</td><td></td></tr><tr><td>High risk</td><td>88</td><td>11.6 (2.4)*</td><td>11.9 (2.65)</td><td>18.0 (5.4)#</td><td>14.2 (2.6)</td><td></td></tr><tr><td>Low risk</td><td>123</td><td>12.8 (1.7)*</td><td>12.97 (2.45)</td><td>20.5 (5.9)</td><td>15.3 (3.3)</td><td></td></tr><tr><td>Full term</td><td>128</td><td>12.9 (1.1)*</td><td>13.29 (2.0)</td><td>20.6 (4.7)#</td><td>15.3 (2.4)</td><td></td></tr></table> *p < 0.01 for High risk v. low risk and full term # p < 0.01 for high risk v. full term Other differences are not significant.	Some comparison scores not shown The overwhelming majority of HR VLBW's were HR because of BPD with or without IVH Low socioeconomic status, inner city population	Study was government funded Significantly more abnormal neurologic scores at 12 month of age in VLBW high-risk infants compared to FT controls. Higher abnormal scores suggest degree of abnormality at 12 months depending on level of risk as neonate.

172

Evidence Table 3. Studies Evaluating Association of LBW and Cerebral Palsy and Neurological Outcomes
Part III

Author, Year	Associations found	Potential Biases	Comments
Kato 1996 97182916	Independent predictors of CP/MR Fetal malpresentation vs. cephalic presentation (p<0.01) Use of tocolytics vs. no tocolytics (p<0.005) Umb cord artery pH<7.2 (p<0.05) Major handicap (CP/MR/Blindess) increased in VLBW infants delivered by breech/vag (25%) v. ceph/vag (0%) vs. Breech/c-section (5%) vs. cephalic/c-section (8.5%) (p<0.05)	Retrospective –completeness data (predictors/outcomes) not known. Predictors and outcomes poorly defined. No FT comparison.	No data on funding source
Katz 1996 97145056	**Attention deficit** is measured by the CPT test (error of omission). **Hyperactivity** and impulsivity is measured by the CPT test (error of commission). There were no differences among the preterm infants with mild, moderate and severe intracranial lesions. However, there was a significant increase in both errors of commission and omission in preterm with mild lesions compared to full term infants as well as in preterm with severe lesions compared to full term infants. With increasing severity of lesions in preterm infants, increasing percentage in each group commit errors of commission. Even in the absence of detectable intracranial lesions, preterm infants are still at higher risk for developing attention deficits than full term infants.	Exactly how FT controls were selected in an unbiased way is not described.	No data on funding source This study does not explore relationship of attention deficits identified with the CPT test with actual school performance and achievement in this group of preterm infants. This study includes older preterm 26-34 weeks and does not include the extremely preterm 24-25 wk infants.

173

Evidence Table 3. Studies Evaluating Association of LBW and Cerebral Palsy and Neurological Outcomes
Part III

Author, Year	Associations found	Potential Biases	Comments
Korkman 1996 96374730 Psy1996	Overall: the VLBW/SGA group had the poorest test results. The VLBW/AGA group was somewhat less impaired, whereas the birth asphyxia group performed at the control group level Impairment when present tended to be diffuse in all groups, affecting: psychometric intelligence, naming, visuo-motor performance, tactile finger discrimination, attention and phonological analysis. Predictors evaluation for **CNS outcome (Intelligence evaluation):** 1) VLBW/AGA was associated with poorer WISC-R score, when compared to healthy full term (FT) (p<0.05) 2) VLBW/SGA was associated with poorer WISC-R score, when compared to healthy FT (p<0.05) 3) VLBW/SGA was associated with poorer WISC-R score when compared to asphyxiated term infants (There was no difference in the scores between asphyxiated terms and healthy terms) Predictors evaluation for **CNS outcome (Neuropsychological evaluation):** 1) VLBW/SGA was associated with poorer NEPSY score (p<0.05) when compared to healthy FT 2) In the VLBW cohort, impairment when present tended to be diffuse (in all items examined). 3) VLBW/SGA was associated with poorer NEPSY score when compared to asphyxiated terms. Overall In the VLBW group (AGA and SGA) (n=77): 1) Apgar scores were not correlated with outcome measures 2) Arteria PH was correlated with FSIQ score 3) Intrauterine growth retardation correlated with NEPSY score 4) BW correlated with NEPSY score 5) There was no correlation between RDS, IVH, duration of ventilatory tx and cognitive dysfunction **Combined CNS / Ophthalmology outcome:** 1) VLBW/AGA: 21% (both mild and severe) 2) VLBW/SGA : 6/34 (18%) (mostly lids) 3) Birth asphyxial/ Term: 7/32 (22%) (mostly severe)	1) Cannot exclude potential selection bias (no description of patient flow in each group) 2) Cannot exclude diagnosis bias/no information on blinding of personnel evaluating developmental outcome component on PMHx. 3) The authors investigated associations between 7 predictors and many outcomes (the different subcomponents of WISC-R test and the NEPSY test)/ thus cannot exclude "multiple comparison" effect	Supported by non-governmental foundations

174

Evidence Table 3. Studies Evaluating Association of LBW and Cerebral Palsy and Neurological Outcomes

Part III

Author, Year	Associations found	Potential Biases	Comments
Lucas 1996 96302121	Predictor evaluation for **CNS outcomes**: (Unadjusted analysis) Mother's choice to breast feed was associated with higher IQ scores at 7 years: (No mother's milk group vs Mother's milk group) • WISC-R verbal scale (mean): 92.0 vs 102.1 (p<0.001) • WISC-R Performance scale : 93.2 vs 103.3 (p<0.001) • Overall IQ: 92.8 vs 103.0 (p<0.001) (Adjusted regression analysis for confounders) Mothers choice to Breast feed infant: N=210 babies • Higher Verbal scale scores: (p<0.001) • Higher Performance scale scores (p< 0.0001) • Higher Overall IQ: (p<0.0001) Successfully breast fed infants only: (Received breast milk) N=193 babies • Higher Verbal scale scores: (p<0.0001) • Higher Performance scale scores (<0.0001) • Higher Overall IQ: (p<0.0001) Overall (Regression analysis) • Whether Received breast milk: offered advantage of 8.3 points (p<0.001) • Social class: -3.5/class (p<0.004) • Mother's education: 2.0/ group (p=0.01) • Female sex (p=0.01) • Days of ventilation: -2.6/ week (p=0.02)	Cannot exclude false association due to unrecognized confounders between the 2 groups as this study was non-randomized (despite matching for BW, GA, need for ventilation, NICU stay and other diets ; there are still exist important unconsidered confounders)	

Evidence Table 3. Studies Evaluating Association of LBW and Cerebral Palsy and Neurological Outcomes
Part III

Author, Year	Associations found	Potential Biases	Comments
Rieck 1996 Psy 1996 06905005	In Prospective longitudinal component of the study: Predictor evaluation for **CNS** outcome: 1) Female Sex, HC percentile and Maternal education were independently associated with CGI score. (r^2= 0.41, p< 0.001) 2) Age at assessment, GA and HC percentile were independently associated with Verbal scale score. (r^2= 0.36, p< 0.001) 3) HC percentile was independently associated with Perception-performance score ($r2$= 0.12, p< 0.05) 4) Neurologic complication and HC percentile were independently associated with Quantitative scale score ($r2$= 0.30, p< 0.01) 5) Neurologic complications and HC percentile were independently associated with Memory scale score ($r2$= 0.36, p< 0.05) 6) HC's percentile were associated with higher scores in the 4 scales of McCarthy's test and in the GCI . (p<0.05) In Cross sectional component of the study: Predictor evaluation for **CNS** outcome: 1) VLBW children with normal IQ, score significantly lower than the Middle class group on many cognitive tasks, and may demonstrate more learning disabilities than Middle class children 2) VLBW and Low Class children had significantly lower score in all scales of McCarthy's test , as compared to Middle Class children. (p<0.01) 3) VLBW had no different scores from Low class children. 4) Evaluation of the change of scores with age revealed that from age 3-7 yrs, VLBW advanced significantly less than Middle class children in Word Knowledge, Conceptual grouping and Numerical Memory backwards. 5) The gap between the scores of the 2 groups increased with age.	1) There was no matching, except for the age between VLBW and MC, LC children. Thus, there was no control for possible confounders, 2) Selection bias might exists: As only those that had completed the test were analyzed. (Only 58% of VLBW children had completed the test) 3) Selection bias also might exist as no information is given in the selection process of the 103 VLBW infants that had participated in the original study	1) No data on the absolute size of the association between predictors and outcomes were given. 2) Statistically significant correlation does not always mean a clinically significant association.

176

Evidence Table 3. Studies Evaluating Association of LBW and Cerebral Palsy and Neurological Outcomes
Part III

Author, Year	Associations found	Potential Biases	Comments
Whitaker 1996 97040639	MR higher in LBW<2kg (5%) than in general pop distribution (2.5%) OR for MR vs Normal Intelligence: PVL/VE OR 65.83 (19.1-227.4) Isolated GMH/IVH OR 4.64(1.2-18.6) Verbal reasoning (Stanford-Binet area score) p<0.05 PVL/VE: 98.9 (10.8) GMH/IVH 102.9 (10.5) No abnormality 104.3 (10.9) Visual perception organization All abstract visual reasoning, visual-motor integration, and visual-perceptual stills were significantly (p<0.01 or p<0.005) were significantly lower for children who had PVL/VE compared to those with isolated GMH/IVH or No abnormality. 50% of MR attributable to PVL/VE independent of other factors.	(None)	Study was government and privately funded

177

Evidence Table 3. Studies Evaluating Association of LBW and Cerebral Palsy and Neurological Outcomes
Part III

Author, Year	Associations found	Potential Biases	Comments
Blitz 1997 97154301	Developmental outcome: The mean MDI, PID, CLAMS Total, Expressive, and Receptive scores were 99.7 (19.8), 88.9 (19.8), 94.9 (23.0), 90.8 (26.2), and 99.7 (21.3), respectively. MDI < 70 9% PDI < 70 18% Language delay (>1 SD below the mean) 34% Significant language delay (>2 SD below the mean)12% Multiple regression analysis showed BW and surfactant did not relate to developmental outcome. BPD, PVL, seizures and hydrocephalus account for 29.7% of the variance on the MDI scores (F=10.05, p<. 001). PVL, IVH, and BPD accounted for 23 % of the variance on the PDI scores (F=9.6, p < .001). For the total CLAMS score, 11% of the variance was accounted for by PVL and BPD (F= 7.1, p < .002) Neurologic outcome: Multiple regression analysis showed low BW was not associated with neurological impairment. On the contrary, BPD and PVL significantly increased the risk (14.8% if variance; F=8.4, p<. 001). No other individual variables reach the significance level. CP: present 24 %, suspect 27%, No CP 49% Audiology: Hearing loss 16%. None of the children were profoundly hearing-impaired. Visual problem 18%. None were clinically blind	36% declined or did not appear (possible selection bias). Language assessment at 2 years is too early to determine more subtle language delays. No control group.	No data on funding source
Cheung 1997 97310950	Of the 21 preterms with IVH treated with rescue HFO, 8 (38%) has neurodevelopmental disabilities. Of the 8 preterms with grade III or IV IVH treated with rescue HFO, 6 (75%) has neurodevelopmental disabilities.	The title is "High Frequency Oscillatory Ventilation" but the authors state that a high frequency flow interrupt ventilator is used in their nursery. These distinct modes of ventilation should not be confused 60% mortality among cohort meeting inclusion criteria Time of follow-up not well standardized	No data on funding source

178

Evidence Table 3. Studies Evaluating Association of LBW and Cerebral Palsy and Neurological Outcomes

Part III

Author, Year	Associations found	Potential Biases	Comments
Ekert 1997 97251211	Association between outcome (CP and/or developmental delay) and perinatal/neonatal variables: Multiple logistic regression analysis showed that only PVL was associated with abnormal outcome (PLV: p=0.0001)	(None)	Study was government funded

Evidence Table 3. Studies Evaluating Association of LBW and Cerebral Palsy and Neurological Outcomes
Part III

Author, Year	Associations found	Potential Biases	Comments

Gerner 1997 97329414	**Predictors evaluation for CNS outcome:**
	1) Healthy preterms did not differ significantly in psychodevelopmental outcome
	2) Prematurity was not associated with the sum score in the Griffith's test
	3) Prematurity was associated only with lower score Hand-Eye coordination scale
	4) The predictors associated with poor psychodevelopmental outcome in preterms were (univariate analysis):
	General predictors: Low GA: Pearson correlation coefficient r= 0.19 (171 pts) (p< 0.05); Low BW: Pearson correlation coefficient r= 0.25 (171 pts) (p< 0.001); Intraventricular hemorrhage (IVH) + ventricular dilatation: Pearson correlation coefficient r= -0.27 (p< 0.001)
	CNS predictors: Periventricular Cystic leukomalacia, (PVL) r= -0.24 (p< 0.01); B1-3 + W1-4 U/S findings, r= -0.27 (p< 0.001)
	Cardiovascular predictors: PDA (n=72 pts), r= -0.32 (p< 0.001)
	Pulmonary predictors: Prolonged ventilatory therapy (n-94 pts), r= -0.39 (p< 0.001); CLD: (n=56 pts), r= -0.26 (p< 0.001)
	5) Although the screening indicated that several risk factors were associated with adverse neurodevelopmental outcome- in the multiple regression model the contribution of individual variables was very low (less than 20%). 80% of the outcome variance still remained unexplained.'
	6) Only predictors independently associated with total sum score in Griffith's test were (multivariate analysis): combination contributed to outcome variance by 21%:
	Pulmonary predictors: Duration of ventilatory tx (r^2=16%) and CNS: PVL (r^2=5%)
	7) Predictors independently associated with scores of individual subscales:
	Locomotor subscale : combination contributed to outcome variance by 14%
	  • Duration of ventilatory tx (r^2=9%), PVL (r^2=5%)
	Personal-Social subscale: combination contributed to outcome variance by 17%
	  • BW (r^2=10%), PVL (r^2=7%)
	Hearing and speech subscale:
	  • Duration of ventilatory tx (r^2=13%)
	Hand and eye coordination subscale: combination contributed to outcome variance by 15%
	  • PDA requiring surgical ligation (r2=11%),
	  • Hemorrhage plus White matter lesions (r^2=4%)
	Performance subscale: combination contributed to outcome variance by 18%
	  • Duration of Ventilatory tx (r^2=12%) and White matter lesions (r^2=6%)
		1) In the comparative components (Group A vs C and Group B vs A), there was no control for possible confounders, as not appropriate matching was done between these compared groups
		2) Cannot exclude diagnosis bias as no information is given about blinding of personnel performing the neurodevelopmental assessment on the infants' risk factors
		3) Two many predictors investigated (28) for the total number of patients in the VLBW group (cannot exclude false associations found in the regression analysis)
		4) Cannot exclude false associations due to chance, as multiple subgroup analyses were done (subclasses of Griffith's test)
		5) The subclasses of Griffith's test have limited specificity, thus limited differentiating capacity at 10 months of age and especially for infants with neonatal complications as performance in one scale requires skills assessed in another scale.
			Supported by non-governmental Foundations.

180

Evidence Table 3. Studies Evaluating Association of LBW and Cerebral Palsy and Neurological Outcomes
Part III

Author, Year	Associations found	Potential Biases	Comments
Koller 1997 97193708	**Cognitive Development:** Birth weight: P <0.001 Gestational age: P<0.001 Neonatal health index: P<0.01 Neurological status @ 1 yr: P <0.001 Male gender: P <0.005 Maternal education: P<0.005	Selection bias-does not include all VLBW infants- only those for whom all follow-up data are available--how are these different from the ones who did not show for follow-up?	Study was government funded
Murphy 1997 97192793	Apgar score <3 at 5minutes - 5.3% cerebral palsy Patent ductus arteriousus - 2.0% cerebral palsy Hypotension - 2.2% cerebral palsy Transfusion - 3.2% cerebral palsy Prolonged ventilation - 2.7% cerebral palsy Pneumothorax - 3.4% cerebral palsy Sepsis - 2.8 % cerebral palsy Total parenteral nutrition – 3.0% cerebral palsy Hyponatremia - 6.8% cerebral palsy Chorioamnionitis and neonatal sepsis - 7.1% cerebral palsy Any maternal infection and neonatal sepsis - 4.2% cerebral palsy Seizure - 10.0% cerebral palsy Parenchymal damage - 32.0% cerebral palsy	Ascertainment of CP was from registry-- not examined as part of study Absence of CP was not obtained by exam as part of study Multiply definitions of predictor variables not reported Retrospective acquirement of risk factors- no standard definitions	Study was privately funded
Schendel 1997 98033417	Even apparently well VLBW with no overt physical impairment are consistently at higher risk for all measures of DELAY than MLBW or NBW infants. VLBW have DELAY in all areas of function with greatest risk for delay in gross motor domain. "**Abnormal**" – VLBW 10.9%, NBW 2.9%, p ≤ 0.001 Personal-Social ≥1 delays: VLBW 7.1%, NBW 2.2%, p = 0.001 **Language ≥ 1delays:** VLBW 8.8%, NBW 4%, p ≤ 0.01 **Fine motor-adaptive ≥ 1 delays:** VLBW 7.9%, NBW 2.2%, p ≤ 0.001 **Gross motor ≥1 delays:** VLBW 10.7%, NBW 1.8%, p ≤ 0.001	The people administering the Denver test were not blinded and were aware of degree of prematurity and this is a major source of bias. The adjusted age at f/u had very wide range 9-34 months	Study was government funded

181

Evidence Table 3. Studies Evaluating Association of LBW and Cerebral Palsy and Neurological Outcomes
Part III

Author, Year	Associations found	Potential Biases	Comments
Thompson 1997 97268338	Neurobiologic risk score (NBRS) investigated to determine predictive value for performance on McCarthy Scales at 4 years age. N = 55. McCarthy Scale — Mean (SD) — Range General cognitive index — 89 (20) — 49-126 Verbal — 44 (10) — 21-65 Perceptual-Performance — 44 (12) — 21-69 Quantitative — 46 (12) — 22-67 Memory — 46(10) — 21-67 Motor — 42 (12) — 20-70 Also: The NBRS was not found to be predictive of the McCarthy General Cognitive Index; in multiple regression analysis only birth weight, gestational age and gender were significantly related to the McCarthy scores.	One institution No control group Combined high NBRS and intermediate NRS patients into one group	Study was government funded
Victorian Infant Collaborative study Group 1997 98026322 *There are a series of Victorian articles in LBW-ALL. *This study will be combined in LBW-ALL table	Birth weight < 1000g; assessed at 2 years corrected age. Cohort — n — DQ <-3 SD — DQ -3 to -2 SD — DQ -2 to -1 SD — DQ >-1 SD '91-'92 — 237 — 5.9% — 6.3% — 13.9% — 73.4% '85-'87 — 211 — 6.2% — 4.3% — 14.2% — 75.4% Cohort — n — Mild CP — Mod. CP — Severe CP — Any CP — Blindness — Deaf '91-'92 — 237 — 3.8% — 1.7% — 3.8% — 9.3% — 2.1% — 0.8% '85-'87 — 211 — NS — NS — NS — 6.6% — 4.3% — 0.5% Cohort — No disability — Mild Disability — Moderate disability — Severe disability '91-92 n = 237 — 71.3% — 14.8% — 7.2% — 6.8% '85-'87 n = 211 — 71.6% — 15.6% — 6.2% — 6.6%	Incomplete reporting of demographic data, methods and results.	Study was government funded

Evidence Table 3. Studies Evaluating Association of LBW and Cerebral Palsy and Neurological Outcomes
Part III

Author, Year	Associations found	Potential Biases	Comments
Battin 1998 99002694	**CNS outcomes:** Major impairment was present in 36% of infants born at 23-25 wks GA, during 1991-1993 (N=44) 1) Cerebral palsy 9/44 (20%) 2) Low MDI 8/44 (18%) **Ophthalmology** outcome: 1) Blind 4/44 (9%) **Audiology** outcome: 1) Deaf 4/44 (9%) **Combined** outcome: 1) Overall impaired 16/44 (36%) 2) Multiple handicaps 6/16 (38%) Analysis of only 24-25 wks GA infants (N=43): Major handicaps: 15/44 (34%)	1) During 1991-93 period there is no concurrent control group for the comparative assessment of neurodevelopmental outcome 2) Group of infants of 23-25 wks GA, born during 1991-1993, was not matched to the historical control group born during 1983-1989. Possibility of confounders cannot be excluded. 3) No data were given on the number of infants in the historical control group that had f/up at 18 mo of age.	No report on source of funding
Bos 1998 98218970	The percentage of infants with major impairments and/ or multiple handicaps, for the 23-25 wks GA group, was the same in 1991-1993 and 1983-1989 periods (However, no data on the number of infants from this cohort that were actually followed up at 18 mo of age) The developmental course of the quality of general movements significantly correlated only with the duration of parieto-occipital echodensities (r=0.482, p<.02), while the duration of PVE frontal was not associated with the developmental outcome (r=0.241, NS)	No power estimates for defecting modest effects	No data on funding source
Cherkes-Julkowski 1998 9826696	No disorder identified: PT 25%, FT 75 % Attention deficit disorder: PT 17.8%, FT 7.1% Learning disability: PT 17.8%, FT 14.2% Language impairment: PT 3.5%, FT 0% Neurological impairment: PT 7.1%, FT 0% School concerns: PT 28.5%, FT 21.4% This group of only mildly preterm, seemingly healthy PT infants have significantly more disability than expected $\chi 2(5)$=62.577, p= .0001	Evaluators were people in the community and social system so that there may be significant variations in evaluations. Sample size too small for statistical analysis.	No data on funding source This study is more a study of predictability of the attention deployment test in identifying minimal brain dysfunction at 13 and 15 mos, rather than a study of predictors of long-term outcome.

Evidence Table 3. Studies Evaluating Association of LBW and Cerebral Palsy and Neurological Outcomes
Part III

Author, Year	Associations found	Potential Biases	Comments
Emsley 1998 98238139 (CNS+ All)	**Disability in 1st cohort 1984-1989 of 23-25 wks:** Any disability: 38% CP: 21% **Data on 2nd cohort 1990-1994 of 23-25 wks:** CP: 18% Blindness due to ROP: 18%, Myopia: 15%, Squint: 13% Developmental delay (DQ < 70): 15% Deafness: 3 % Epileptic seizures: 0 Speech delay: 15% Clumsy, learning difficulties, behavioral disorder: 3% Disability. Mild 38%, Moderate 13%, Severe 18% **Infants with disability have lower GA, worse CRIB** scores and significant cranial ultrasound findings. In comparing the 2 cohorts, increased survival is associated with increased disability but mostly mild disability. No significant change in %CP. High CRIB score assoc. with disability.	Sample numbers small. Does not state when the assessments were carried out and whether the evaluators were blinded to the GA and history of the infants.	No data on funding source

184

Evidence Table 3. Studies Evaluating Association of LBW and Cerebral Palsy and Neurological Outcomes
Part III

Author, Year	Associations found	Potential Biases	Comments
Pasman 1998 98196839	Assessment at 5 to 7 years of age. Full-term (FT) controls, neurologically normal low risk preterm (normal LR) infants, neurologically abnormal low risk preterm infants (abnormal LR), and high-risk preterm infants (HR). Risk classification was based on the neonatal neurologic inventory. Group / n / Total IQ / Verbal IQ / Performance IQ FT: / 18 / 114 (17) / 113 (18) / 111 (14) Normal LR w/ GA 25-30 weeks: / 15 / 108 (15) / 107 (16) / 106 (11) Normal LR w/ GA 31-34 weeks : / 21 / 113 (15) / 114 (18) / 107 (10) Abnormal LR w/GA 25-34 weeks: / 8 / 99 (12) / 104 (12) / 93 (14) HR w/ GA 25-34 weeks: / 9 / 78 (20) / 79 (19) / 81 (19) HR infants excluded from statistical analysis. Term infants vs. all low risk infants: Total IQ, no significant difference. Verbal IQ, no significant difference. Performance IQ P = 0.02.	Year of birth not given Small numbers in subgroups (e.g., 8,9) Incomplete reporting of results	Study was privately funded
Rogers 1998 98438124	There are no association between GA, BW, BPD Length of stay with growth failure P>0.05 Growth failure with CPVL 16/41 CP with CPVL 39/41	(None)	Study was privately funded

185

Evidence Table 3. Studies Evaluating Association of LBW and Cerebral Palsy and Neurological Outcomes
Part III

Author, Year	Associations found	Potential Biases	Comments
Spinillo 1998 98237382 Spinillo, 1997 98021316 & 97277958 *have some overlapped sample with spinillo, 1994	**CP prevalence** 12.3% in 24-33 wk preemies **Minor neurologic problems (abnormal tone or reflex but functionally normal) or borderline** (71-84) Bayley MDI: 16.1% **Factors assoc with increased CP:** PROM > 48 hrs OR 2.98 (1.12-7.96 CI 95th) Meconium-stained amniotic fluid OR 4.36 (1.69-11.2) Male sex OR 3.01 (1.32-6.71) Decreasing gestation: CP 22.2% in 24-25 wks, 23.1% in 26-27 wks, 14.5% in 28-29 %, 8.3% in 30-31 wks, 9.3% in 32-33 wk infants. <u>CP</u> Meconium-stained fluid (N=17) 41% (7/17%) Clear fluid (N=246) 13.4% (33/246) P=0.06 **CNS outcome:** 1) The incidence of cerebral palsy in this cohort of preterm infants was : 40/345: (12%), but this refer only to those survived: 391/450 (87%) and to those that completed the 2 yr f/up: 345/450 (77%) Predictors evaluation for **Survival at 2 yrs:** 1) Survival at 2 yrs was associated with higher GA (p<0.0001), higher BW, (p<0.0001) And History of fewer previous abortions. Predictors evaluation of **CNS outcomes:** (In a univariate analysis) From the maternal and neonatal characteristics and the pregnancy complication/predictors, those found to be associated with CP were Odds Ratio (95% CI) 1) Higher Maternal age 1.07 (1.0-1.15) 2) Lower GA 0.87 (0.76-0.99) 3) Lower BW 0.94 (0.87-1.00) 4) male gender 2.65 (1.28-5.50) 5) More Previous voluntary abortion (25% vs 7%) 4.51 (1.94-10.5) 6) Preeclampsia (5% vs 19%) 0.22 (0.05-0.94) In a multivariate regression model (including maternal age, BW Standard deviation score, GA and preeclampsia) only preeclampsia was independently associated with the risk of cerebral palsy: OR: 0.16 (0.04-0.74) The authors conclude a protective effect of preeclampsia against CP, in the absence of Mg sulfate utilization	1) Major confounding postnatal factors such as BPD, IVH, and PVL, which may be associated with CP, were not controlled for. 2) We cannot exclude selection bias. The associations found were relevant to the group of surviving infants with cerebral palsy who also had f/up at 2 yrs. A large number of infants were excluded from the analysis: 46 infants that were lost to f/up and 59 that had died.	No data on funding source

186

Evidence Table 3. Studies Evaluating Association of LBW and Cerebral Palsy and Neurological Outcomes
Part III

Author, Year	Associations found	Potential Biases	Comments
Tin 1998 99046171	**Result of 1983 cohort at 6 years:** *Severe disability:* Sample 1: 4.4%, Sample 2 : 2.1%, Sample 3: 50% *IQ < 75 without sensorimotor disability:* Sample 1 : 4.9%, Sample 2 : 0, Sample 3 : 25% *Severe sensorimotor disability:* Sample 1: 5.9%, Sample 2 : 21.4%, Sample 3 : 41.7% *Severe sensorimotor or cognitive disability:* Sample 1: 8.4% (5 - 13.1%, 95% CI) Sample 2 : 21.4% (4.7-50.8%) Sample 3: 41.7% (15.2-72.3%) **Result of 1990 cohort at 2 years:** *Severe disability:* Sample 1: 7.9%, Sample 2: 15.4%, Sample 3: 57.1% **High flu rate is critical because it may underestimate incidence of the outcome.**	No definitions of outcome, incomplete methods description, wrong reference	Study was privately funded
Burguet 1999 99126269	In univariate analysis: The prevalence of CP in LBW preemies with RDS (N=66) was 20%, compared to 9% in preemies without RDS (N=101). The difference was significant (p=0.04) Incidence of CP 7% in no PROM, 20% in PROM < 48 hrs, 30% in PROM 48h to 7 days, 11% in PROM >7 days, χ^2 trend: p= .004 In multivariate analysis: Controlling for environmental and maternal factors, the risk of CP was about 3 times in preemies with RDS, than preemies without RDS (adjusted OR 2.8, 95% CI 1.1-7.1). "The introduction of surfactant in the second stage of our study was not shown to have any impact on the incidence of CP among the children of this cohort." PROM ≥ 48 hours (OR 4.3, 95% CI 1.6-11.8), p= .005 Monochorionic twin placentation (OR 6.0, 1.7-21.3), p = .007 RDS (OR 2.8, 1.1-7.1) PROM +, PTL + (OR 7.5, 2.2-26.2), p= .001	8% BW>2000g Nonstandard definition of CP Suspected infant (mild hypotonia or delay to normal acquisition) were included in the normal group Evaluations done by community physician of parents' choice so, no standardization, and unblinded Used uncorrected age	No data on funding source Severe disability is common among extremely preterm infants of GA 22-25 wk

187

Evidence Table 3. Studies Evaluating Association of LBW and Cerebral Palsy and Neurological Outcomes
Part III

Author, Year	Associations found	Potential Biases	Comments
Cooke 1999 99257637	CP prevalences: 1982-5 (411) 45 10.9% 1986-9 (387) 42 10.9% 1990-3 (398) 29 7.3% P=0.046	ND	No data on funding source
Cooke 1999 99380719	MRI abnormality: VLBW group : 37/87 (42.5%) FT Control group: 0/8 (0%) Abnormal MRI not associated with ADHA, IQ, or motor coordination scores.	No statistical/ data analysis section Few controls (n=8) Disagree and interpretation (i.e. conclusion)	Study was privately funded Overall sample of LBW<2 kg had increased rate of MR compared to gen pop. PVL/VE was independently related to MR (OR 66) and to borderline IQ. Among children with nl IQ, those with PVL/VE vs. no PVL/VE performed more poorly on visual-perceptual organization. White matter injury is associated with adverse cognitive and visual perceptual disability.

188

Evidence Table 3. Studies Evaluating Association of LBW and Cerebral Palsy and Neurological Outcomes
Part III

Author, Year	Associations found	Potential Biases	Comments
Finer 1999 99436635	IVH: Sample 1: 70%, Sample 2 : 10%, p = .015. **Normal neuromotor outcome:** Sample 1: 70 %, Sample 2: 70%. *Abnormal neuromotor outcome:* Sample 1 : 20%, Sample 2: 0 *Normal developmental outcome:* Sample 1: 80%, Sample 2: 60% *Abnormal developmental outcome:* Sample 1: 20%, Sample 2: 20% *Normal neurodevelopmetal outcome:* Sample 1: 70%, Sample 2 60% No difference in developmental scores of following domains: composite mental, composite motor, adaptive, language, personal/social, fine motor, gross motor. They conclude that intact survival is possible for infants weighting <750 g who received CPR in the DR.	Very small sample size with 28% lost to f/u. Results are from a single center, difficult to generalize the results. Exact criteria for chest compressions and epinephrine not specified No information about the evaluators or whether they were blinded. Infants evaluated at wide range of ages where infants seen later may have done better or worse	No data on funding source Missing information Retrospective collection of breast feeding data

Evidence Table 3. Studies Evaluating Association of LBW and Cerebral Palsy and Neurological Outcomes
Part III

Author, Year	Associations found	Potential Biases	Comments
Futagi 1999 99450356	Predictor evaluation for **CNS outcome**: 1) Birth in surfactant era was not associated with neurodevelopmental outcome (good or poor prognosis) for infants of less than 1000 gms (Pre-surfactant era[107] vs surfactant era [169] • Neurodevelopmental outcome: 71/107 (66%) vs 100/169 (59%) • Cerebral palsy: 13/107 (12%) vs 18/169 (11%) • Mental retardation: 11/107 (10%) vs 16/169 (9.5%) • Borderline intelligence: 11/107 (10%) vs 35/169 (21%) 2) Birth in surfactant era was associated with higher incidence of borderline intelligence (20.6% in surfactant era vs 10.3% in pre-surfactant era) 3) Birth in surfactant era :was not associated with DQ or IQ scores in the individual neurodevelopmental categories (normal neurodevelopmentally, cerebral palsy, mental retardation, borderline intelligence) • Normal: 99.7 vs 100.1 • Cerebral palsy: 57.5 vs 62.5 • Mental retardation: 62.4 vs 55.1 • Borderline intelligence: 77.1 vs 77.6 4) Birth in surfactant era: was not associated with the distribution of subtypes of cerebral palsy.(spastic diplegia, spastic hemiplegia, spastic quadriplegia) 5) Birth in surfactant era was not associated with severity of cerebral palsy.(minimal, mild, moderate, severe)	1) Assessed the association between birth in the surfactant era and neurodevelopmental outcome and not of surfactant administration itself problems of ecological fallacy in that type of studies) 2) It is unknown if the results of this study could be generalized in other NICU populations where more than 50% of infants receive surfactant 3) The possibility of a masked association cannot be excluded due to existence of possible cofounders in the 2 groups. 4) Many subgroup exploratory analyses were performed that were not described in the Method section	Source of funding not reported
Kim 1999 99416608	Infants with BW < 2000g. Assessed at 12 months age. <table><tr><td>Risk Factor</td><td>CP</td><td>Devel. Delay</td><td>Both CP+DD</td><td>Neither</td></tr><tr><td>Neonatal sepsis</td><td>4/9*</td><td>1/8</td><td>5/17*</td><td>4/62</td></tr><tr><td>BPD</td><td>4/9*</td><td>3/8*</td><td>7/17*</td><td>9/62</td></tr><tr><td>IVH > grade 2</td><td>4/9*</td><td>1/8</td><td>5/17*</td><td>6/62</td></tr><tr><td>Days on ventilator</td><td>18.1 (25.1)*</td><td>11.3 (8.7)*</td><td>12.2 (19.6)*</td><td>3.3 (3.3)</td></tr><tr><td>Ventriculomegaly</td><td>5/9*</td><td>0</td><td>5/17</td><td>8/62</td></tr></table>P < 0.05 vs. neither CP/ DD Multivariate logistic regression, the following were not significant risk factors: Apgar score at 5 minutes, BPD, IVH, PDA, duration of mechanical ventilation, Sepsis	Study group as a whole is not described- only those infants developing CP CP infants are compared to "controls", but no description of how the control group was recruited or in what ways they were similar to or different from the study group. Concurrent? Historical? Matched for gestational age or birth weight? We are not told. Leaves open the possibility of massive bias/confounding.	In this cohort of preterm infants (BW 600-1250 grams) <1%blind or deaf; 1%- 3% had seizure disorder; and 7% had CP. Full scale IQ <80 occurred in 28% of total sample (BW 600-1250 grams) at 54 months follow-up

Evidence Table 3. Studies Evaluating Association of LBW and Cerebral Palsy and Neurological Outcomes

Part III

Author, Year	Associations found			Potential Biases	Comments

Kragelch-Mann 1999 99431017

	MRI normal (n=10)(%)	MRI abnormal (n=19)(%)	P
Preeclampsia	50	11	0.03
Placental abruption	0	32	0.07
Mechanical Ventilation>7d	0	42	0.03
ICH grades III + III	0	16	0.53
DO2 <ml O2/100g/min	12.5%	63%	0.03

Potential Biases:
1) Selection of preterm subject bias
2) No MRI of controls
3) Controls, "From Copewnagen suburb"- well matched with regard to SES, health-care measures, etc.?
4) Design is bizarre, complicated, and difficult to interpret.
5) Statistical analysis is not well described. It appears that they did not correct for multiple comparisons, which renders their positive findings suspect. They did not do a power analysis, which renders their negative findings suspect.
6) Much of the paper analyzes association between outcomes evident at 5-7 yrs f/u, for ex., association between abnormal MRI at 5 yr. And IQ at 5 yr.; this does not examine association between neonatal MRI+ IQ at 5 yr.

Comments: No data on funding source

Salokorpi 1999 99353226

Assessed selected risk factor in relation to cerebral palsy (CP) diagnosed at two years age.
CP present, n = 27; CP absent, n = 116.

Risk Factor	Odds ratio (CI)
Grade 3 or four IVH on head sonogram	7.94 (2.75, 22.95)
Hypotension	1.26 (0.47, 3.35)
Hypocarbia	2.20 (0.77, 6.31)

Also found no association between average duration of ventilation and CP.

Comments: Study was privately funded

191

Evidence Table 3. Studies Evaluating Association of LBW and Cerebral Palsy and Neurological Outcomes
Part III

Author, Year	Associations found	Potential Biases	Comments
Shepherd 1999 99165413	CP 9% in this group of preemies who were followed-up at least once after term age (N=53) Of the 5 infants with CP, 3 had abnormal VEP. Of those without CP, 4 had abnormal VEP. Sensitivity of VEP before term for CP = 60%. Specificity is 92%. Positive predictive value of abnormal VEP for CP is 43%. Negative predictive value is 96%.	CP not defined. CP evaluated by generalists with no uniform definition. Incomplete Methods and large number of missing information.	No data on funding source
Stathis 1999 99325758	Head circumference category at 8 months corrected age related to learning delay greater than one year when assessed at 6 years: HC Category / n / % with delay < 3rd percentile / 23 / 61% (39, 80) 3rd to 10th / 13 / 77% (46, 95) P = 0.004 > 10th / 40 / 30% (17, 47) Head circumference category at 12 months CA did predict McCarthy General Cognitive index at six years, but head circumference category at 24 months CA did not significantly predict McCarthy CGI at 6 years. Head circumference and head growth velocity was not shown to have a relationship with attention deficit hyperactivity disorder. Head circumference category < 10th vs. greater than 10th percentile at four and 8 months corrected age were significantly associated with McCarthy CGI at 6 years age	One nursery High rate of patients lost to follow-up (30%) Small numbers: limited ability to detect small differences; high chances of type 2 error	Study was privately funded

Evidence Table 3. Studies Evaluating Association of LBW and Cerebral Palsy and Neurological Outcomes
Part III

Author, Year	Associations found	Potential Biases	Comments
Vohr 1999 99332101	**Normal Neurologic Examination:** 75% CP overall: 17% but 29% in 401-500 g babies CP (quadriplegia): 6.4% CP (left hemiplegia): 0.45% CP (right hemiplegia): 0.91% CP (diplegia): 8.2% **Seizure disorder:** 5% Hydrocephalus with shunt: 4% Visual impairment (any): 9% Unilateral blindness: 1% overall but 7 % in 401-500g and 801-900g babies **Bilateral blindness:** 2 % overall but 14 % in 401-500 g babies Legally blind in one or both eyes: 3% Hearing impairment: overall 11 % Wearing hearing aids: overall 3 % **Sits unsupported:** 93% Sits well alone: 86% Walks: 83%, Walks fluently: 70% Independently feeds self: 80% **Bayley MDI** < 85 : 66%, Bayley MDI <70: 37% Bayley PDI <85: 57%, Bayley PDI <70: 29% Chronic lung disease, grades 3-4 IVH/PVL, steroids for CLD, NEC, and male gender associated with increased risk for morbidity	Poor f/u rate of 78% and this may significantly underestimate outcome.	

193

Evidence Table 3. Studies Evaluating Association of LBW and Cerebral Palsy and Neurological Outcomes
Part III

Author, Year	Associations found	Potential Biases	Comments
Agustines 2000 20279724	**Predictors for CNS outcome:** Rates of developmental delay at 30 months of corrected age, were significant among extremely VLBW infants 500-750 g	1) Long term f/up for only 57% (36/63 infants that had survived) Those who had f/up had less morbidity than those lost to f/up (incidence of RDS was 47% vs 92% in lost to f/up group)	Funding source not report
	Overall CNS outcomes in the 36 infants: 1) Normal MDI: 32% 2) Mild delay in MDI: 40% 3) Severe Delay in MDI: 28% 4) Combined mild and severe delay in MDI: 58% 5) Normal PDI: 42% 6) Mild delay in PDI: 16% 7) Severe delay in PDI: 42% 8) Combined mild and severe delay in PDI: 58%	2) There was no control group to compare outcomes of extremely VLBW with VLBW infants. 3) Stratified analysis for outcome in different GA subgroups had very few patients in each subgroup, thus the confidence intervals are very wide.	
	Stratified by GA: 24 wks 25 wks 26-29 (N=14) (N=14) (N=8) 1) Normal MDI: 11% 50% 33% 2) Mild delay in MDI: 55% 25% 50% 3) Severe Delay in MDI: 33% 25% 17% 4) Combined mild and severe delay in MDI: 88% 50% 67% 5) Normal PDI: 34% 50% 0% 6) Mild delay in PDI: 22% 0% 20% 7) Severe delay in PDI: 44% 50% 80% 8) Combined mild and severe delay in PDI: 68% 50% 100%	4) This study was not designed to compare outcomes of SGA vs AGA infants in the group of 500-750g; post hoc comparisons (most of the infants in the 26-29 GA group were SGA)	

Evidence Table 3. Studies Evaluating Association of LBW and Cerebral Palsy and Neurological Outcomes

Part III

Author, Year	Associations found	Potential Biases	Comments
Breslau 2000 20298367	1) Information from mothers and teachers on children's behavior problems at age 11 revealed that the effect of LBW on attention problems differed between urban and suburban settings. 2) LBW children had an excess of attention problems in the urban disadvantaged communities and not in the suburban middle class communities. 3) LBW infants in the urban setting had twice as high incidence of attention problems as more than twice as high in LBW than in NBW. 4) In Urban Setting LBW children had more than 2-fold severe attention problems than NBW children 5) In suburban setting there was no difference in severe attention problems between LBW and NBW children. 6) LBW children had externalizing problems both in the urban and suburban settings (this effect was mainly accounted for by maternal smoking in pregnancy) 7) No LBW effect was observed with respect to internalizing problems 8) Regardless of LBW status, maternal smoking during pregnancy was associated with an increase in externalizing problems 9) No association was found between maternal smoking during pregnancy and internalizing or attention problems **OVERALL SCORES** **MOTHER'S SCORES** Urban Attention scores Internalizing Externalizing LBW (n=217) 58.8 52.7 52.2 NBW (n=164) 55.8 51.5 50.4 Suburban LBW (n=194) 55.1 50.4 48.4 NBW (n=142) 53.8 48.6 46.3 **TEACHER'S SCORES** Urban LBW (n=186) 56.9 50.3 53.9 NBW (n=151) 54.7 48.8 48.5 Suburban LBW (n=180) 53.7 49.0 48.5 NBW (n=135) 54.0 48.7 48.3 1) According to mother's ratings: For attention, externalizing and internalizing problems: LBW scored higher (had more problems) than NBW children. 2) According to teacher's rating: Only for externalizing and internalizing problems: LBW scored slightly higher than NBW. 3) Urban children received higher scores than suburban children on all 3 domains, according to both mother" and teacher's ratings	1) Recollection bias: The Hx of maternal smoking during pregnancy was elicited when the child was 6 yrs old. This bias would have resulted in underestimation of the confounding effect of smoking during pregnancy. 2) Diagnosis bias: Although there was a correspondence of the findings of teachers' reports (who were blind to the LBW status of children) and the mothers' reports, mothers' reports could have been biased (worse scores from mothers of LBW infants)	Supported by grant from National Institute of Mental Health and National Institute of Drug Abuse

195

Evidence Table 3. Studies Evaluating Association of LBW and Cerebral Palsy and Neurological Outcomes
Part III

Author, Year	Associations found	Potential Biases	Comments
Bührer 2000 20280896	Major Neurodevelopmental impairment 22% Independent predictors of neurodevelopmental impairment (logistic regression): CRIB score: R =0.216, β =0.2233, SE =0.051 Maximum FIO2: R = 0.1201, β = 1.23, SE 0.4553 Griffith's general quotient ≤ 85 in this population: 21.6%.... A CRIB score of 6 or more has a sensitivity and specificity 27.6% and 91.3% for predicting neurologic impairment.	No information as to whether evaluators were blinded	No data on funding source

Grether 2000 20448692	Receipt of MgSO4 treatment:
	
	         CP Control
	    (N=170) (N=288)
	   98 (58%) 178 (62%)
	  OR: 0.84 95% CI: 0.56-1.26
	
	Total duration (HR): 51 ± 78 53 ± 72 NS
	(mean SD)
		Retrospective case control
		CP defined from chart review
			No data on funding source

Katz-Salamon 2000 20332284	Infants were assessed at 10 months corrected age. Authors used Griffith's Development Scale and the Movement Assessment Index (MAI, a surrogate for evolving CP) to assess children without high-grade IVH or PVL to determine whether chronic lung disease (CLD) itself was a risk factor for adverse outcomes. CLD was associated with significantly lower performance scores on each Griffith's subscale and with significantly higher MAI scores predicting a higher risk of CP. Even in the absence of high-grade IVH or PVL, CLD has a deleterious effect on early development.	One institution; small number of infants/group Oldest evaluation <10 months of age Used a surrogate measure, the MAI for CP	Study was privately funded Incomplete result data.

Evidence Table 3. Studies Evaluating Association of LBW and Cerebral Palsy and Neurological Outcomes
Part III

Author, Year	Associations found	Potential Biases	Comments
Marlow 2000 20150342	Pulmonary and Other predictors evaluation for **Audiology outcome.** Children with sensorineural hearing loss [15] as compared to control group[30] had longer periods of: 1) Intubation, (14 ds vs 2 ds) 2) Ventilation (34 ds vs 6 ds) 3) Oxygen therapy (57 ds vs 10 ds) 4) Acidosis (12 ds vs 0.5 ds), and 5) More treatments with dopamine (33% vs 7%)or 6) Furosemide (87% vs 53%) 7) Neither P/T of aminoglycosides 8) nor duration of jaundice 9) or level of bilirubin varied between the 2 groups. SNHL was more likely when : 1) netilmicin use coexisted with the peak of bilirubin (87% vs 14%)_ 2) when acidosis occurred when bilirubin was over 200 Đmol/l, (31% vs 4%) 3) when furosemide was used in the face of high creatinine levels (64% vs 27%) 4) when furosemide was used with netilmicin (67% vs 37%) **CNS outcome at 12 mo:** At 12 months of age evidence of cerebral palsy was present in 7/15 (47%) of children with SNHL vs 2/30 (7%) of children without SNHL.(p=0.022)	1) Very small sample size (cases with SNHL only 15) 2) Analyzed too many predictors and combination thereof, for very few outcomes. Very wide confidence intervals; and even those predictors found to be associated with the SNHL this may have been due to chance. 3) The association found between SNHL and cerebral palsy was not based on an adjusted analyses for possible confounders; 4) The 2 groups were different in many factors that were associated with both SNHL and CP	Did not report source of funding
Palta 2000 20096107 (CNS+Eye)	**CP 12.6%.** Independent predictors of CP and functional outcome: IVH OR 2.3 per grade (95 % CI 1.8-2.8) BPD OR 2.3 (95% CI 1.2-4.6) **Percent of the children scoring at least 2 SDs below** the normative means for the following functional outcomes: Self-care 11.7% Mobility 29.5% Social function 10.7%	(None)	Study was government funded No ophthalmology results were reported

Evidence Table 3. Studies Evaluating Association of LBW and Cerebral Palsy and Neurological Outcomes
Part III

Author, Year	Associations found	Potential Biases	Comments
Torrioli 2000 20275419 (CNS+Eye)	*Movement ABC:* Study: 15.58+7.96 Control: 7.08+4.61 — P<0.001 *Bell test rapidity:* Study: 19.08+7.92 Control: 22.02 + 7.36 — P<0.05 *Bell test rapidity:* Study: 57.34+19.67 Control: 69.08 + 18.10 — P<0.05 *Visual function (stereopsis %):* Study: 41.7 Control: 66.7 — P<0.05	Did not give the size of the control group. Baseline demographic data not presented.	Study was privately funded
Valkama 2000 20233239	51 BW < 1500g GA <34 wks: Severe CP: 5; Mod CP: 3; mild CP: 1 14 SGA: 2/14 CP (14%) 16 EVLBW<1000g: 6/16 CP (0.34) <29 wks : 12 CP Abnormal MRI 11/19 Delayed myelination 3/8	(None)	Study was privately funded
Vohr 2000 20295211	Studied effect of early IVH at 5 to 11 hours of age on IQ distribution and presence of cerebral palsy (CP). Assessed at 36 months CA. Later IVH had effect on Binet IQ similar to early IVH.	IVH rates seems high	No data on funding source

Vohr table:

	Early IVH present	Early IVH absent	P value
N	29	249	
Binet IQ	78.7 (25)	87.5 (20)	0.09
Binet IQ < 70	38%	19%	0.03
PPVT-R	76.6 (28)	86.0 (21)	0.15
CP at 36 months	25%	8%	0.01

198

Evidence Table 3. Studies Evaluating Association of LBW and Cerebral Palsy and Neurological Outcomes

Part III

Author, Year	Associations found	Potential Biases	Comments
Dammann 2001 21334215	CP prevalence: BW ≤ 1500g & AGA: 16% BW ≤ 1500g & SGA: 4% P=0.005 In this skewed population, 16 % of AGA infants and 4 % of SGA infants had CP at 6 years.	(None)	Study was privately funded
Gaillard 2001 21221175	**Predictors for Neurodevelopmental outcome:** 1) Shorter length of ventilation (beyond 27(but not 50) postnatal days) was associated with better neurodevelopmental outcome : 59% (33/56) neurodevelopmentally normal or only mildly disabled survivors vs 25% (7/28) with more prolonged ventilation(> 49 ds) *Ventilated beyond 27 (but not 50)ds vs Ventilated beyond 49 ds* Total: 56 vs 28 Survived: 48/56 (86%) vs 14/28 (50% Normal neurodevelopmentally: 26/48 (54%) vs 5/14 (36%) Mild disability: 7/48 (15%) vs 2/14 (14%) Moderate disability: 11/48 (23%) vs 4/14 (29%) Severe disability: 4/48 (8%) 3/14 (21%) 2) Number of days "off"" ventilator was not associated with the neurodevelopmental outcome at 3 yrs neither in the groups of 27-49 postnatal ds ventilation nor in the group of >49ds ventilation *Ventilated beyond 27 (but not 50)ds and O ds "off" ventilator vs 1-7 ds "off" ventilator vs > 7 ds off ventilator* Total: 18 vs 17 vs 21 Survived: 13 (72%) vs 15 (88%) vs 20 (95%) Neurodevelopmentally normal: 8 (44%) vs 7 (41%) vs 11 (52%) Mild disability: 2 (11%) vs 2 (12%) vs 3 (14%) Moderate disability: 3 (17%) vs 4 (24%) vs 4 (19%) Severe disability: 0 vs 2 (12%) vs 2 (10%) (In the second component: comparison of the retrospective cohort with the historical control) 3) Birth in a period where antenatal steroids and exogenous surfactant was more routinely used was associated with better neurodevelopmental outcome (69% vs 40% and 45% respectively in the 2 historical control cohorts)	In First component: retrospective cases control design: 1) the 2 groups were unmatched for possible confounders, thus cannot exclude false associations 2) Cannot exclude selection bias as only 62 survivors were analyzed from the 84 initially included in the 2 groups In the Second component: 3) Problems of confounders due to historical control group could be even greater Failed to report % of antenatal use in each group. Demographic data included babies that died prior to neurologic evaluation, possible source of bias. No information on comorbidities that may have led to prolonged intubation with no attempt to adjust for these	No data on funding source

199

Evidence Table 3. Studies Evaluating Association of LBW and Cerebral Palsy and Neurological Outcomes
Part III

Author, Year	Associations found	Potential Biases	Comments
Horwood 2001 20574647	Assessed influence of breastfeeding (BF) duration on outcome at 7-8 years age. IQ scores before adjusting for covariates. Group / n / Verbal IQ / Performance IQ Not BF / 76 / 94.4 (18.4) / 98.7 (19.6) BF < 4 mo / 99 / 97.2 (18.4) / 101.4 (15.6) BF 4-7 mo / 46 / 101.7 (17.3) / 101.1 (14.0) BF > 8 mo / 59 / 104.6 (14.7) / 104.9 (15.3) Adjustment for covariates of maternal education, two parent families, higher income families, non-smoking during pregnancy and non-Polynesian ethnicity did not change the hierarchy of results. Verbal IQ beta value = 0.12, $P < 0.05$ and performance IQ beta value 0.08 with $P > 0.15$	Retrospective collection of breast feeding data 17 children could not be tested because of sensorineural problems No information about perinatal medical condition Not clear if examiners were aware of feeding history	Study was government funded Goal of study was to assess predictive value of NBRS (neurobiologic risk score) and neonatal neurologic inventory, NNI, with respect to long-term neurodevelopment outcome of preterms between 25-34 weeks.
Nadeau 2001 21163667	EP/ VLBW, n = 61 and controls, n = 44. EP/ VLBW / Control / Significance Normal neuromotor function / 67% / 97% / NS Abnormal neuromotor function / 33% / 3% McCarthy IQ [mean (SD)] / 100.3 (19.1) / 112.8 (16.2) / $P < 0.01$ Behavioral ratings at 7 years age: Peers rated EP/ VLBW's as significantly more sensitive/ isolated than controls Teachers rated EP/ VLBW's as significantly more inattentive than controls Parents rated EP/ VLBW's as more hyperactive than controls Significantly = $P < 0.01$	(None)	No data on funding source Data on neuromotor and intellectual functioning only collected once Data on behavior collected once
Pierrat 2001 27221167	Overall, majority of premature infants with cystic PVL are not normal. Cystic-PVL (both Gr II and Gr III) is highly associated with CP. 29 of 30 infants with c-PVL + Ventriculomegaly at 40 wk PMA had CP. The following show differences in outcome based on whether the infant had cystic PVL (Grade II) or cystic PVL (Grade III): c-PVL (Gr II) / c-PVL (Gr III) No motor sequelae / 24% / 3% CP / 76% / 97% Independent walking / 22/29 / 3/26	(None)	No data on funding source

200

Evidence Table 4. Studies Evaluating Treatment Effects of LBW and Cerebral Palsy and Neurological Outcomes
Part I

Author, Year UI#	Demographics	Inclusion Criteria	Exclusion Criteria	Disease/Condition Type (N)	Study Design (Duration)
Als 1994 94358983 (CNS+ Pulmonary)	Location: US Years of Birth: ND Median GA (range), wk: Experiment: 27.1±1.6 Control: 26.5±1.4 Median BW (range), g: Experiment: 827±173 Control: : 862±145 Male: Experiment: 45% Control: 61% Race: Black Experiment: 40% Control: 17% SES I, II/III/IV, and V: Experiment: 45%, 20%, 35% Control: 56%, 17%, 27% Enrolled: 43 Evaluated: 38 Number of sites: 1	BW < 1250 g GA < 30 weeks and more than 24 weeks of estimated GA at birth Mechanical ventilation starting within the first 3 hrs after birth and lasting longer than 24 hrs in the first 48 hrs Alive at 48 hrs Absence of chromosomal or other major genetic anomalies, congenital infections, and known fetal exposure to drugs of addiction Singleton At least one family member with some English-language facility Telephone access Living within the greater Boston area	ND	Experiment: VLBW infants participated in individualized developmental care (20) Controls: VLBW infants received standard care (18)	Randomized controlled trial (2 weeks and 9 months)

201

Evidence Table 4. Studies Evaluating Treatment Effects of LBW and Cerebral Palsy and Neurological Outcomes
Part I

Author, Year UI#	Demographics	Inclusion Criteria	Exclusion Criteria	Disease/Condition Type (N)	Study Design (Duration)

Corbet 1995 95264244	Location; USA
	Years of Birth: 1986-1989
	Mean GA:
	  Sample 1: 27 ± 2
	  Sample 2: 27 ± 2
	Mean BW:
	  Sample 1: 934 ± 179
	  Sample 2: 931 ± 191
	Males:
	  Sample 1: 50%
	  Sample 2: 50%
	Race:
	  Sample 1: whites: 41%, blacks: 37%, others: 22%
	  Sample 2: whites: 46%, blacks: 36%, others: 18%
	Enrolled: 1046
	Evaluated: 597
	Number of sites: Multicenter
		Born alive
		Qualifying BW (not specified in this publication)
		That were intubated and assigned randomly to receive either synthetic surfactant or air placebo as part of their participation in 3 multicenter RCTS.
		Had follow up at 1 yr of age
			ND	Sample 1:
				Synthetic surfactant: [314]
				
				Sample 2:
				Air placebo [283]
					Combination of 3 multicenter, randomized, double blind studies of synthetic surfactant vs air placebo
					[1 yr]

Evidence Table 4. Studies Evaluating Treatment Effects of LBW and Cerebral Palsy and Neurological Outcomes
Part I

Author, Year UI#	Demographics	Inclusion Criteria	Exclusion Criteria	Disease/Condition Type (N)	Study Design (Duration)
Allan 1997 97336492 Ment 1996 97040638 Ment 2000 20164956 (CNS+All)	Location: US Years of Birth: 1989-1992 Median GA (range), wk: Experiment: 27.7±1.9 Control: 28.4±2.0 Median BW (range), g: Experiment: 945±191 Control: : 988±164 Male: Experiment: 56% Control: 57% Race: ND Enrolled: 505 Evaluated: 431 → 343 at 36 months → 337 at 54 months Number of sites: 3	BW 600-1250g Age< 6 hours No IVH presence at 6-12 hours	Died by age of 1 year Lost to follow-up Presence of IVH in sonogram between 6-12 hr of age Bilingual or non–English speaking at home	Experiment: Indomethacin group (173) Controls: Placebo (170) At 36 months: Experiment: Indomethacin group (173) Controls: Placebo (170) At 54 months: Experiment: Indomethacin group (170) Controls: Placebo (167)	Randomized Controlled Trial (36, and 54 months)

Evidence Table 4. Studies Evaluating Treatment Effects of LBW and Cerebral Palsy and Neurological Outcomes
Part I

Author, Year UI#	Demographics	Inclusion Criteria	Exclusion Criteria	Disease/Condition Type (N)	Study Design (Duration)
Van Wassenaer 1997 98103082	Location: Amsterdam Years of Birth: 1991-1993 Mean GA: ND Mean BW: Sample 1/subgr 1: 856 ±153 Sample 1/subgr 2: 1048 ± 195 Sample 1/subgr 3: 1140 ± 156 Sample 1/subgr 4: 1160 ± 246 Sample 2/subgr 1: 914 ± 111 Sample 2/subgr 2: 914 ± 137 Sample 2/subgr 3: 1173 ± 156 Sample 2/subgr 4: 1285 ± 236 Males: Sample 1/subgr 1: 54% Sample 1/subgr 2: 41% Sample 1/subgr 3: 44% Sample 1/subgr 4: 59% Sample 2/subgr 1: 56% Sample 2/subgr 2: 23% Sample 2/subgr 3: 38% Sample 2/subgr 4: 50% Race: ND Enrolled: 200 (100 in thyroxine group and 100 in placebo group) Evaluated: 158 Number of sites: 1	Premature : 25-30 wks Admitted to their NICU within first 24 hrs of life Admitted between 1991-1993	Congenital malformations Maternal endocrine disorders Maternal illicit drug use	Sample 1 Thyroxine (8 ìg/kg BW once daily) for the first 6 wks of life starting during the first 12-24 [82] Subgroup 1: 25-26 GA [13] Subgroup 2: 27 GA [17] Subgroup 3: 28 GA [23] Subgroup 4: 29 GA [29] Sample 2: Placebo [76] Subgroup 1: 25-26 GA [18] Subgroup 2: 27 GA [13] Subgroup 3: 28 GA [21] Subgroup 4: 29 GA [24]	Prospective comparative study (The initial study was a randomized, double blind, placebo-controlled trial but in the current comparative component the patients in the subgroups of different GA that were compared were no longer randomly assigned)

Evidence Table 4. Studies Evaluating Treatment Effects of LBW and Cerebral Palsy and Neurological Outcomes
Part I

Author, Year UI#	Demographics	Inclusion Criteria	Exclusion Criteria	Disease/Condition Type (N)	Study Design (Duration)
O'Shea 1999 99318938	Location: Korea Years of Birth: 1992-1995 Median GA (range), wk: Experiment: 25 (23-29) Control: 26 (23-31) Median BW (range), g: Experiment: 747 (420-1362) Control: 775 (495-1324) Male: Experiment: 48% Control: 51% Race: African-American Experiment: 34% Control: 49% Enrolled: 118 Evaluated: 95 Number of sites: 2	BW < 1501 g Age 15-25 days old Not wearing ventilator, no sepsis; no PDA, an echocardiogram indicating the absence of a patent ductus arteriosus	Parental refusal Survived to 1-year adjusted age	Experiment: Dexamethasone x 42 days (50) Controls: Placebo (45)	Randomized controlled trial (1 year)

Evidence Table 4. Studies Evaluating Treatment Effects of LBW and Cerebral Palsy and Neurological Outcomes
Part II

Author, Year	Predictors	Predictor Measures	Outcomes	Outcome Measures
Als 1994 94358983	Other: Participation in individualized developmental care staffing by specially educated nurses	The psychologist and clinical nurse specialist provided ongoing support for the care teams and parents of the infants in the experimental group in jointly planning and implementing individually supportive care and environments.	**CNS:** Neurodevelopmental: Cognitive delay **Pulmonary:** BPD severity	Baley Scale of Infant Development at 9 months of age Assessed by double-blind review of cranial US scans by a consultant senior radiologist

Evidence Table 4. Studies Evaluating Treatment Effects of LBW and Cerebral Palsy and Neurological Outcomes
Part II

Author, Year	Predictors	Predictor Measures	Outcomes	Outcome Measures
Corbet 1995 95264244	General: 1) Synthetic surfactant (single dose via ET tube of 5 mg/kg vs air placebo)	Not further specified	**Growth:** Growth status at 1 yr: 1) Weight 2) Height, 3) HC and percentiles distribution **Other:** Health status at 1 yr: 1) Surgeries 2) Readmissions to hospital 3) CLD, medications for CLD 4) Respiratory support on exam day 5) Medications for chronic neurologic disease 6) Asthma, Eczema **CNS:** Neurodevelopmental outcome 1) MDI 2) PDI 3) Impairments: Present absent 4) Severity of impairment 5) Type of impairment (MDI<69, MDI 69-84) 6) CP **Audiology** 1) B/L sensorineural deafness 2) Deafness not requiring amplification **Ophthalmology:** (worst exam and last) 1) B/L blindness 2) Visual defect 3) No ROP, mild/moderate ROP, severe ROP) 4) Treatment for ROP (surgery, cryotherapy)	Assessment at 1 yr of corrected age Not further specified

Evidence Table 4. Studies Evaluating Treatment Effects of LBW and Cerebral Palsy and Neurological Outcomes
Part II

Author, Year	Predictors	Predictor Measures	Outcomes	Outcome Measures
Allan 1997 97336492	General: SGA/IUGR, Antenatal steroids; Apgar score, Gender	Diagnoses according to radiologic assessments.	**CNS:** Cerebral palsy	Neurologic examination
	CNS: Intracranial/Intraventricular hemorrhage	The grading system for hemorrhages was: grade 1, blood in the periventricular germinal matrix	**Neurodevelopmental:** Cognitive delay	At 36 months: Stanford-Binet IQ PPVT-R
Ment 1996 97040638	Indomethacin Seizures Indomethacin	regions; grade 2, blood within the lateral ventricular system without ventricular dilation; grade 3, blood	Mental retardation Behavioral Disorders Seizure disorder	At 54 months: Cognitive delay: WPPSI-R or PPVT-R (Full scale IQ<70)
Ment 2000 20164956	Pulmonary: bronchopulmonary dysplasia Other: multiple birth, MgSO4, Surfactant	within and distending the lateral ventricles; and, grade 4, blood within the ventricular system and parencyhmal involvement.	**Ophthalmology:** Blindness **Audiology:** Deafness	Vineland adaptive checklist and child behavior checklist
(CNS+All)				

208

Evidence Table 4. Studies Evaluating Treatment Effects of LBW and Cerebral Palsy and Neurological Outcomes Part II

Author, Year	Predictors	Predictor Measures	Outcomes	Outcome Measures
Van Wassenaer 1997 9810382	Other/General: 1) Thyroxine administration during first 6 weeks of life (vs placebo) 2) GA	Thyroxine administration started at 12-24 hrs of life in a fixed dose of 8 ☐g/kg BW, once daily	**CNS** 1) Neurologic outcome 2) Developmental outcome (Assessment at 24 mo corrected age)	Neurodevelopmental outcome: Described in another publication Abnormal if: 1) Severe abnormality of tone 2) Severe abnormality of posture 3) Severe abnormality of movement Leading to functional impairment or Delay in motor development Suspect if: 1) Moderate abnormality of tone 2) Moderate abnormality of posture 3) Moderate abnormality of movement Leading to mild or moderate functional impairment or developmental delay MDI (Mental Development Index by Bayley) PDI (Psychomotor development index by Bayley) According to Dutch standards 1) Abnormal if: < 2 SDs below mean Or if score< 68 2) Suspect if < 1 SD or score: 68-84 3) Normal if score> 83

Evidence Table 4. Studies Evaluating Treatment Effects of LBW and Cerebral Palsy and Neurological Outcomes
Part II

Author, Year	Predictors	Predictor Measures	Outcomes	Outcome Measures
O'Shea, 1999 99318938	Other: Dexamethasone	ND	**CNS:** CP Neurodevelopmnetal: Cognitive delay Neurological exam	CP was diagnosed only if both a pediatrician and a physical therapist agreed with impaired motor function Bayley scale Based on subjective assessment of the physician and therapist, the neurologic exam was classified into no, mild, moderate, and severe abnormality. "Mild abnormality" – hypotonia (which typically was most prominent in the truncal musculature) but not CP No definition for moderate and severe abnormality.

Evidence Table 4. Studies Evaluating Treatment Effects of LBW and Cerebral Palsy and Neurological Outcomes
Part III

Author, Year	Associations found			Potential Biases	Comments
Als 1994 94358983	Studied effect of an individualized developmental care plan on Bayley score at 9 months age and occurrence and severity of BPD.			Small number of babies studied	Study was government funded
				Only one NICU	
				Only one neurodevelopmental assessment at 9 months of age	
	Experimental group	Controls	P value	Reported timing of IVH different from many other studies	
	N 20	18		High potential for contamination	
	Bayley MDI 118.30 (17.35)	94.38 (23.31)	< 0.001		
	Bayley PDI 100.6 (20.19)	83.56 (17.97)	< 0.01		
	No BPD 2/20	3/18			
	Mild BPD 13/20	7/18			
	Moderate BPD 5/20	2/18			
	Severe BPD 0	6/18	0.03		

Evidence Table 4. Studies Evaluating Treatment Effects of LBW and Cerebral Palsy and Neurological Outcomes
Part III

Author, Year	Associations found	Potential Biases	Comments
Corbet 1995 95264244	**GROWTH AT 1 YR:** Mean measurements of Height (74 cm), weight (9.1 kg) and HC (46 cm) and growth percentiles were equivalent in the 2 groups. **HEALTH STATUS AT 1 YR:** No difference in parameters between 2 groups 1) Surgeries (33% vs 34%) 2) Readmission to hospital (45% vs 39%) 2) CLD (11% vs 10%) 4) Medications for CLD (14% vs 14%) 3) Respiratory support (4% vs 2%) 4) Med. for chronic neurologic problems (1% vs 2%) 5) Asthma (this only was s/s : 9% vs 3%) 8) Eczema (2% vs 1%) **NEURODEVELOPMENTAL OUTCOME:** No difference in the outcomes between the 2 groups in these parameters. 1) Mean MDI (values <50= 49): 2) Mean MDI (only children with MDI>69) 2) Number of children with MDI<69: 4) Number of children with PDI<69 3) Mean PDI (values<50=49) 6) Mean PDI (only children with PDI>69) **CNS IMPAIRMENT:** No difference in any impairments between 2 groups 1) Present: 43% vs 37% 2) Absent: 57% vs 63% 2) Mild/moderate: 20% vs 14% 4) Severe:23% vs 23% 3) MDI<69: 17% vs 16% 6) MDI: 69-84: 18% vs 14% 4) CP mild: 8% vs 7% 8) CP moderate/severe: 7% vs 7% **Audiology:** 1) B/L sensorineural hearing deafness: 0% vs 1% 2) Deafness not needing amplification: 0% vs 1% **Ophthalmology:** 1) B/L blindness: 3% vs 2% 2) Visual defect: 8% vs 8% Worst examination 2) No ROP: 30% vs 33% 2) Mild/moderate ROP: 53% vs 52% 3) Severe ROP: 17% vs 15% 4) Surgical treatment for ROP:10% vs 12% 4) Cryotherapy for ROP: 5% vs 6% Last examination 5) No ROP: 69% vs 72% 2) Mild/moderate ROP: 26% vs 22% 6) Severe ROP: 5% vs 6% 4) Surgical treatment for ROP: 4% vs 4% 7) Cryotherapy for ROP: 2% vs 3% Infants who survived after treatment at birth with single-dose synthetic surfactant fare as well in terms of growth, development and late morbidities as infants who survive without treatment. No difference in medical history during first year of life, growth, incidence of visual or auditory defects, CP, neurodevelopmental delay at 1 yr adjusted age.	1) The incidence of severe impairment in the 19% of infants who did not return for evaluation at the age of 1 yr may be higher than in those who were evaluated.	Source of funding not reported. 1) The neurodevelopmental evaluation of infants at 1 yr may not be absolutely reliable for the estimation of later outcome. 2) The estimated mental retardation is likely to be low, and the estimated CP is likely to be high, compared to estimates at 2 and 3 yrs.

212

Evidence Table 4. Studies Evaluating Treatment Effects of LBW and Cerebral Palsy and Neurological Outcomes
Part III

Author, Year	Associations found				Potential Biases	Comments
Allan 1997 97336492	Antecedents of Cerebral Palsy (CP).				Stanford-Binet testing limited to monolingual, English-speaking families	Study was government funded
	Risk Factor		n	Percent with CP	P value		Study in a follow-up of originally randomized cohort; followed at 36 and 54 months age, corrected
	BPD	Yes	177	15%	< 0.001		
		No	203	4%			
Ment 1996	Surfactant	Yes	245	13%	0.003		
		No	136	4%			
97040638	Grade 3 or 4 IVH	Yes	15	53%	< 0.001		
		No	366	8%			
Ment 2000	PVL	Yes	25	53%	< 0.001		
		No	352	6%			
20164956	Ventriculomegaly	Yes	17	59%	< 0.001		
		No	328	7%			

(CNS+All)

Assessed at 36 months corrected age:
No significant differences between placebo and indo. for: Presence of CP/
abnormal neurologic exam (8% vs. 8%, Placebo vs. Indo); Blindness (1% in
each); Deafness (1% in each); Stanford-Binet IQ (85.0±20.8 vs. 89.6±18.9,
Placebo vs. Indo)
Presence of IVH was associated with a significant decrease in Stanford-Binet
IQ: IVH absent, 84.4 ± 19.6 vs. IVH present 80.2 ± 20.9 (P = 0.03)
Assessed at 54 months corrected age:

	Indomethacin	Placebo	P-value
N	170	167	
Blind	1 (<1%)	1 (<1%)	ns
Deaf	1 (<1%)	1 (<1%)	ns
Seizures	1 (1%)	5 (3%)	ns
CP	7%	7%	ns
WPPSI Full IQ<70	9%	17%	0.035
WPPSI Full IQ 70-80	12%	18%	
PPVT-R IQ<70	12%	26%	0.02
PPVT-R IQ70-80	19%	6%	
N	119	114	

Vineland Total Score   *There was no significant difference between groups:
    Communication; Daily living skills; Socialization; Motor skills
For CBCL results, children in Indo. group has significant lower score in
Withdrawn subscale than children in Placebo group (52.7 vs. 54.6, p=0.02).
    There is no significant difference found in the other subscales of CBCL.

213

Evidence Table 4. Studies Evaluating Treatment Effects of LBW and Cerebral Palsy and Neurological Outcomes
Part III

Author, Year	Associations found	Potential Biases	Comments
Van Wassenaer 1997 9810382	1) In infants of 25-26 wks GA, thyroxine administration during the first 6 weeks after birth is associated with an improvement in mental developmental outcome/MDIs. (p<0.01) 2) Thyroxine administration does not improve and might even harm mental (but not psychomotor/PDIs or neurological) outcomes in infants 27-20 wks. 3) There was also a trend towards a better psychomotor and neurologic outcome (normal, suspect, abnormal).	1) In this study, many pot hoc exploratory subgroup analyses were done: Small number of patients in each subgroup and although the patients were randomly assigned in the original 2 groups, this does not continue to be the same for the subgroups of different GA analyzed. 2) Thus association proposed for beneficial effect of T4 particularly for the subgroup of infants less than 27, weeks and only for the MDI scores; and not for the PDI scores or the neurological outcomes; must be viewed cautiously. 3) Except for Thyroxine and GA the effect of the other covaraties/predictors included in the linear regression model was not discussed.	It should be taken into consideration that the initial RCT with 200 infants less than 30 wks had shown no clear association between thyroxine administration and neurodevelopmental outcome.
O'Shea, 1999 99318938	(None)		Study was government funded

	Dexamethasone (N=50)	Placebo (N=45)	P
Definite Cerebral Palsy:	12	3	
Possible CP:	5	2	
Overall CP:	17	5	0.006
Neuro exam severe Abnormal:	4	2	
Mild abnormal:	16	6	
Overall abnormal Neuro exam:	20	8	0.03

214

Evidence Table 5A. Studies Evaluating Association of LBW to Speech and Language Disorders
Part I

Author, Year UI#	Demographics	Inclusion Criteria	Exclusion Criteria	Disease/Condition Type (N)	Study Design (Duration)
Wood 2000 20373840	Location: UK and Ireland Years of Birth: 1995-1996 Mean GA (range), wk: 22-25 Mean BW (range), g: ND Male: ND Race: ND Enrolled: 314 Evaluated: 283 Number of sites: 276	GA 20-25 weeks survivors	ND	Preterm infants (283)	Prospective cohort (30 [28-40] months)
Lefebvre 1998 98387703	Location: Canada Years of Birth: 1987-1992 Mean GA (range), wk: 27.0±1.2 Mean BW (range), g: 961±179 (585-1450) Male: 52% Race: ND Enrolled: 139 Evaluated: 121 Number of sites: 1	GA<28 weeks 3 or more cranial ultrasounds Survival to discharge	ND	Preterm infants (121): Low risk (50) Moderate risk (37) High risk (34)	Prospective cohort (CA 18.6±1.2 [17-19] months)

Evidence Table 5A. Studies Evaluating Association of LBW to Speech and Language Disorders
Part I

Author, Year UI#	Demographics	Inclusion Criteria	Exclusion Criteria	Disease/Condition Type (N)	Study Design (Duration)
Wolke 1999 10075095	Location: Germany Years of Birth:1985-1986 Description of group: Sample 1: VLBW Sample 2: Full term/ controls Sample 3: Normative sample Mean GA (range), wk: VLBW: 29.5± .2 (29.3-29.7) Control: 39.6± .1 (39.5-39.7) Mean BW (range), g: VLBW: 1288±42 (1247-1330) Control: 3407±58 (3351-3463) Male (%): VLBW: 56.4% Control: 56.4% Normative: 51% Race: ND Enrolled: VLBW: 560 Control: 916 Normative: 311 Evaluated: VLBW: 264 Control: 264 Normative: 311 Number of sites: 17 (hospitals)	Cases: 1) Requiring admission to 1 of 17 hospitals in S. Bavaria within first 10 days. 2) Assessments at 5 and 20 months, 4 years 8 months, and 6 years 3 months. 3) VLBW (very preterm) GA≤ 32 weeks at birth. Controls: 1) Control group (full term) GA>36 weeks at birth. For all groups: German-speaking	ND	Cases: Sample 1: VLBW (or very preterm): 264 Controls: Sample 2: Full term/ controls: 264 Sample 3: Normative: 311	Non-randomized comparison trial

216

Evidence Table 5A. Studies Evaluating Association of LBW to Speech and Language Disorders
Part I

Author, Year UI#	Demographics	Inclusion Criteria	Exclusion Criteria	Disease/Condition Type (N)	Study Design (Duration)
Smith 1996 97081985	Location: US Years of Birth: 1990-1992 Description of group: Sample 1: High risk VLBW Sample 2: Low risk VLBW Sample 3: Full term (controls) Mean GA (range), wk: HR VLBW: 28± 2 LR VLBW: 30.9±2 FT: 39.1±5.9 Mean BW (range), g: HR VLBW: 930±233 LR VLBW: 1263±202 FT: 3187±767 Male (%): HR VLBW: 50% LR VLBW: 41% FT: 50% Race (% African-American): HR VLBW: 57% LR VLBW: 62% FT: 62% Enrolled: HR VLBW: 89 LR VLBW: 123 FT: 128 Evaluated: HR VLBW: 88 LR VLBW: 123 FT: 128 Number of sites: 2	Cases: 1)VLBW≤1600 g 2)Female primary caregiver 3)Completed both a 6 and 12 mos. home visit. 4)GA≤ 36 weeks at birth. Sample 1: HR VLBW: one or more severe medical complications: bronchopulmonary dysplasia (BPD) defined as need for O2 for more than 28 days, severe IVH with progressive dilitation defined as a Grades III or IV subependymal hemorrhage, and/or periventricular leukomalacia characterized by ischemic lesions. Sample 2: LR VLBW: one or more less severe medical complications, including transient respiratory distress where O2 is required for less than 28 days and/or mild IVH without dilitation- Grades I and II. Controls: Sample 3: FT: GA: 37-42 weeks with normal pregnancy history and physical examination at birth.	1) Primary caregiver age<16, drug abuser, or not English-speaking. 2) Sensory impairment, meningitis, encephalitis, congenital syphilis, congenital abnormality of the brain, cardiac abnormalities, NEC or HIV antibody positive.	Cases: Total VLBW: 211 Sample 1: HR VLBW: 88 Sample 2: LR VLBR: 123 Controls: Sample 3: Full-term infants: 128	Non-randomized comparison trial

217

Evidence Table 5A. Studies Evaluating Association of LBW to Speech and Language Disorders
Part I

Author, Year UI#	Demographics	Inclusion Criteria	Exclusion Criteria	Disease/Condition Type (N)	Study Design (Duration)
Sajaniemi 2001 11227991	Location: Finland Years of birth:1989-1991 Description of group: VLBW Mean GA (range), wk: 29.4± 3 Mean BW (range), g: 1246±472 Male: ND Race: ND Days of mechanical ventilation: 12.3±26 Enrolled: 138 Evaluated: 63 Number of sites: 1	Cases: 1) Mothers referred to University Central Hospital in Helsinki for threatened pre-term delivery 2) Assessments at 2 and 4 months, 3) VLBW (very preterm) GA≤ 29.4± 3 weeks at birth.	Major disabilities (CP or mental retardation)	Cases: VLBW (or very preterm): 63 No control group	Prospective (single arm) cohort
Briscoe 1998 98300800	Location: UK Years of Birth: 7/91- 7/92 Mean GA (range), wk: 28±1.9 (26-32) Mean BW (range), g: 1206±345 (815-1985) Male: ND Race: ND Enrolled: 26 (26 controls) Evaluated: 26 (26) Number of sites: 1	Cases: Preterm infants, GA<32 weeks, from an Avon Premature Infant Project, Marlow, 1997. Free of major and minor physical impairment at 2 years of age Controls: Children age between 3years 7 months and 4 years 5 months born full-term, GA>37 weeks.	ND	Cases: Preterm infants (26) Controls: Full term infants (26)	Case-control study

218

Evidence Table 5A. Studies Evaluating Association of LBW to Speech and Language Disorders
Part I

Author, Year UI#	Demographics	Inclusion Criteria	Exclusion Criteria	Disease/Condition Type (N)	Study Design (Duration)
Saigal 2001 21376729	Location: Canada Years of Birth: 1977-1982 Mean GA (range), wk: Cases: 27±2 Controls: "Term" Mean BW (range), g: Cases: 835±124 Controls: 3401±481 Male: Cases: 31% Controls: 36% Race: ND SES: middle class Cases: 30% Controls: 30% Enrolled: 179 (145 controls) Evaluated: 154 (125) Number of sites: 1	ELBW survivors, BW= 501-1000g Controls: term infants recruited at 8 years of age from a random list obtained through the directors of 2 school boards and matched for gender, age, and SES to each case	ND (Died after discharge (10) Lost to follow-up (8) Refusal (5) Unable to be reached (2) Controls: Lost to follow-up (10) Refusal (8) Unable to be reached (2))	Cases: ELBW infants (154) Controls: Term infants (125)	Prospective cohort (followed to 12-16 years age)

Evidence Table 5A. Studies Evaluating Association of LBW to Speech and Language Disorders
Part I

Author, Year UI#	Demographics	Inclusion Criteria	Exclusion Criteria	Disease/Condition Type (N)	Study Design (Duration)

Schendel 1997 98033417	Location: US
	Years of Birth: 12/1/89 to 3/31/91
	Mean GA (range), wk:
	  Sample 1: 28.4 ±3.0
	  Sample 2: 35.6 ±2.8
	  Controls: 39.4 ±1.5
	Mean BW (range), g:
	  Sample 1: 1088±268
	  Sample 2: 2184±267
	  Controls: 3417±432
	Male:
	  Sample 1: 49%
	  Sample 2: 46%
	  Controls: 52%
	Race: Black
	  Sample 1: 37%
	  Sample 2: 37%
	  Controls: 41%
	Enrolled: 920 (555 controls)
	Evaluated: 920 (555)
	Number of sites: 5
		Singleton livebirths in MMIHS study population, survived to 1 year of age
		Cases: MLBW infants, BW 1500-2499g; VLBW infants, BW<1500g
		Controls: NBW infants randomly selected from the birth certificate files on the basis of frequency matching with cases by maternal race, age, and residence
			ND	Sample 1: VLBW infants (367)
				Sample 2: MLBW infants (553)
				Controls: NBW infants (555)
					Case-control study

220

Evidence Table 5A. Studies Evaluating Association of LBW to Speech and Language Disorders
Part II

Author, Year	Predictors	Predictor Measures	Outcomes	Outcome Measures
Singer 2001 21163669	Cardiovascular or pulmonary predictors: 1) Bronchopulmonary dysplasia General: : BW, Neurologic risk Other: Race, Socioeconomic status	BPD: preterm, <1500g BW, oxygen for >28 days with radiographic evidence of CLD	**CNS outcomes:** Cerebral palsy Cognitive delay Mental retardation **Ophthalmology outcomes:** Visual impairment **Audiology outcomes:** Hearing disorders Speech Language Communication disorder	Bayley scale of infant development Language (speech/communication) measured by Battelle Developmental Communication Subscale Domain→ receptive, expressive and total communication scores converted to DQ mean 100 and SD 15.
Wood 2000 20373840	*General:* 1) GA 2) Gender Other: Perinatal Factors→ Multiple gestation	ND	**CNS:** Motor delay Cognitive delay Seizure disorder Overall development **Ophthalmology:** Visual impairment Blindness **Audiology:** Hearing disorders Deafness Speech Communication disorder **Other:** Severely disabled Other disability No disability Disability of hearing, vision, or communication	Bayley scales Severe disability = need of physical assistance to perform daily activities. If disability didn't fit into this category = "other disability"

221

Evidence Table 5A. Studies Evaluating Association of LBW to Speech and Language Disorders
Part II

Author, Year	Predictors	Predictor Measures	Outcomes	Outcome Measures
Lefebvre 1998 98387703	Other: Neurobiologic risk score (NBRS)	Items in NBRS: ventilation, PH, surgeries, IVH< PVL, infection, hypoglycemia-items scored zero or greater in progression	**CNS:** Cerebral palsy Cognitive delay- Other: neurodevelopmental impairment **Ophthalmology:** Blindness **Audiology:** hearing disorders-free fetal audiogram	Neurologic exam Griffith's mental development scale Mental retardation-Griffith's mental development scale 1) Global developmental quotient (DA) 2) Mild/moderate: DA 80-89 or CP 3) Severe: DA<80, severe CP unilateral blindness or severe hearing defect 4) Normal: more of the above Areas of Griffith's Developmental Scales: - Locomotor - Personal-social - Hearing and speech - Eye and hand coordination - Performance Control mean DA=110+or- in literature

Evidence Table 5A. Studies Evaluating Association of LBW to Speech and Language Disorders
Part II

Author, Year	Predictors	Predictor Measures	Outcomes	Outcome Measures
Wolke 1999 10075095	General predictors: GA	Gestational age GA≤32 for VLBW, GA>36 weeks for full term control group.	Audiology outcomes: 1) Language development 2) Prereading skills 3) Cognitive status	I. Language development: a) Heidelberger Sprachentwicklungstest (HSET) (German test) II. Prereading skills: a) Rhyming and sound-to-word-matching tasks III. Cognitive status: a) Kaufman Assessment Battery for Children (K-ABC) for cognitive assessment. Intelligence was measured with the Mental Processing Composite (MPC); simultaneous and sequential information processing subtests (SGD and SED), and The Achievement Score (AS)
Smith 1996 97081985	General predictors: Illness acuity, grouped into LR VLBW and HR VLBW, and maternal behavior, warm sensitivity and maintaining of infants interests and directiveness.	Gestational age GA≤ 36 weeks at birth.	Audiology outcomes: 1) Cognitive skills 2) Language development 3) Living skills	I. Cognitive skills: a) Bayley Scales of infant Development expressed as mental age II. Language development: a) Sequenced Inventory of Communication Development III. Living Skills: a) Daily Living Skills subscale from the Vineland Adaptive Behavior Scale

223

Evidence Table 5A. Studies Evaluating Association of LBW to Speech and Language Disorders
Part II

Author, Year	Predictors	Predictor Measures	Outcomes	Outcome Measures
Sajaniemi 2001 11227991	General predictors:	Gestational age GA≤ 29.4± 3	Audiology outcomes: 1) Temperamental characteristics (at 2 years of age) 2) Behavioral characteristics (at 2 years of age) 3) Cognitive precursors (at 2 and 4 years of age) 4) Neuropsychological assessment (at 4 years of age)	I. Temperamental characteristics: a) Toddler Temperament Questionnaire (TTQ), measuring activity, rhyhmicity, approach, adaptability, intensity, mood, persistence, distractability, and sensory threshold. II. Behavioral characteristics: a) Infant Behavior Record (IBR) of the Bayley Scales, measuring fearfulness, emotional tone, activity, attention span, and goal directness. III. Cognitive precursors: a) Mental Development Index (MDI) from the Bayley Scales of Infant Development was used to measure cognitive level at 2 years. a) Wechsler Preschool-Primary Scale of Intelligence (WPPSI) (Finnish version) was used at 4 years of age. IV. Neuropsychological assessment: a) pre-standard version of the Finnish Neuropsychological Investigation for Children (NEPSY-r, extended version)

Evidence Table 5A. Studies Evaluating Association of LBW to Speech and Language Disorders
Part II

Author, Year	Predictors	Predictor Measures	Outcomes	Outcome Measures
Briscoe 1998 98300800	General predictors: GA	Gestational age < 32 weeks based on expected date of delivery	Audiology outcomes: 1) Language 2) Short-term memory 3) General non-verbal ability	II. Vocabulary knowledge: a) British picture vocabulary scales b) Oral vocabulary component of McCarthy scales of Children's Abilities c) Bus Story test of Continuous speech tested expressive language ability (retelling story using pictures as on aid) III. Phonological short-term memory: a) Digit span: set of pseudo-random numbers to repeat b) Non-word repetition IV. Non-verbal ability: a) Raven's Progressive Coloured Matrices adapted for use here under 5 years of age V. Early Development Assessment: a) Griffith's mental development scales

Evidence Table 5A. Studies Evaluating Association of LBW to Speech and Language Disorders
Part II

Author, Year	Predictors	Predictor Measures	Outcomes	Outcome Measures
Saigal 2001 21376729	Birth weight GA	ELBW=500-1000 g	**CNS:** Motor delay Cognitive delay Other: neurosensory impairment **Ophthalmology:** Visual impairment **Growth:** Height Weight Head circumferences BMI (wt/ht2) **Other:** Health status and problems; current and past Extra health care expenses Utilization and health care resources	Reported previously in the authors' other paper Growth reference population was using the age- and gender-specific reference data provided by the NCHS growth chart
Schendel 1997 98033417	**General Predictors** 1) Birth Weight- 3 groups VLBM (very low birth wt) MLBW (moderately low birth wt.) NBW (normal birth wt) **Other Predictors** 1) Other: married at birth 2) Other: Medicaid recipient	ND	**CNS:** Other: Developmental Delay **Pulmonary:** Birth weight	Developmental delay measured by Denver Developmental Screening Test II. "DELAY" defined by 9 measures of performance on Denver Developmental Screening Test II at age 15 months corrected.

226

Evidence Table 5A. Studies Evaluating Association of LBW to Speech and Language Disorders
Part III

Author, Year	Associations found	Potential Biases	Comments
Singer 2001 21163669	Evaluation at 36 months corrected age. VLBW, VLBW with BPD, full term (FT). Bayley MDI % with MDI below 70 VLBW 90 + 16 (38-126) 11% VLBW w/ BPD 84 + 24 (10-116) 21% FT 96 + 12 (57-127) 4% P = 0.001 for VLBW vs. VLBW w/ BPD Bayley PDI % with PDI below 70 VLBW 98 + 20 (33-122) 9% VLBW w/ BPD 84 + 29 (8-127) 9% FT 103 + 15 (58-128) 1% P = 0.001 for VLBW vs. VLBW w/ BPD At 3 years BPD predicted poorer motor outcome but not poorer mental outcome. **Receptive DQ:** BPD < VLBW < Term, p < 05 **Receptive DQ < 85:** BPD 49%, VLBW 34%, Term 30%, BPD < VLBW + Term p < .05 **Expressive DQ:** BPD < VLBW + Term, p < .05 **Expressive DQ<85:** BPD 44%, VLBW 25%, Term 25% BPD < VLBW + Term p < .05 **Communication DQ:** BPD < VLBW + Term, p < .05 **Communication DQ < 85:** BPD 43%, VLBW 31%, Term 28%, NS Rank order listing of risk factors in order of magnitude of effect and the number of communication DQ lowered by the risk factor: PDA lowered DQ by 13 points, Minority race by 6 points, lower socioeconomic status by 5 points, and higher neurologic risk by 5 points. p .001 **Bayley Scales MDI:** BPD 83.7 ± 24, VLBW 90 ±16, Term 96.4 ± 12, BPD < VLBW < Term, p< 0.05 **Bayley Scales PDI:** BPD 84.1 28, VLBW 97.4 19, Term 102.8 14 BPD < VLBW + Term, p< .05 **ROP:** BPD 43%, VLBW 4%, p= .001 **Seizures:** BPD 7%, **Neurologic score:** BPD 1.3 ± 2, VLBW 58 ± 1, p < .001	Single region, but at least it is a region Unclear if examiners were blinded to groups' status	Study was government funded
Wood	Infants 22-25 weeks GA developmentally assessed at median 30 months	(None)	Severe disability common

227

Evidence Table 5A. Studies Evaluating Association of LBW to Speech and Language Disorders
Part III

Author, Year	Associations found	Potential Biases	Comments

2000 20373840	• 138/283 had disability (49%:64 met criteria for severe disability)
	  49% no disability
	• 53/283 severely delayed 19%(Bayley below 3 SD)
	• 32/283 2-3 below SD 11%
	• 28 severe neuromotor disability 10%; 7 blind or perceived light only 2%
	• 8 hearing loss that was uncorrectable or required hearing aids 3%
	  Survived without overall disability
	  22 wks--------0.7 %
	  23 wks--------5%
	  24 wks--------12%
	  25 wks--------23%
	  Severe disability at 30 months
	  22 ------------0.7%
	  23 ------------3%
	  24 ------------6%
	  25 ------------9%
	• no relation between morbidity pattern and either gestational age &multiple birth; boys were likely to be disabled than girls
			Children born extremely premature

Lefebvre 1998 98337703	Assessed at 18 months corrected age. Divided into low, moderate and high risk group based on Neurobiologic risk score (NBRS). Tested with Griffith's Developmental Scales. Griffiths Developmental Score Category 	Risk Group	n	Severe impairment, <80	All < 80
Low	50	0%	12%
Moderate	37	22%	24%
High	34	50%	71% | Significance: for severe or any delay the NBRS was predictive, P < 0.0001 | Risk Group	n	Severe CP (+)	Any CP
Low	50	0%	4%
Moderate	37	13%	19%
High	34	26%	41%	 Significance: NBRS predictive of CP, severe CP, P < 0.0009, any CP P < 0.0001	(None)	Study was privately funded
Wolke	• Preterm birth is significantly associated with deficits in wide range of	Drop-out rate <25%.	Internal validity: A

Evidence Table 5A. Studies Evaluating Association of LBW to Speech and Language Disorders
Part III

Author, Year	Associations found	Potential Biases	Comments
1999 10075095	abilities including all measures of cognition, language comprehension and expression, articulation, and prereading skills compare to full-term controls. • Specific intellectual deficit is in simultaneous central information processing • Specific language deficits include problems with grammatical rules, detecting semantically incorrect sentences, motor aspects of speech, articulation, and pronunciation • Specific prereading skills deficits include problems with rhyming tasks, sound-to-word matching and naming or number/letters. • Deafness 0% in the preterm group		
Smith 1996 97081985	• HR infants have a significantly lower mental age (cognitive skills) at 6 and at 12 mos. then either FT controls or LR infants. • HR infants scored lower in living skills at 6 mos. than FT's but not LR infants. There was no difference between groups at 12 mos. • HR infants scored lower for language development at 6 and 12 mos. than FT controls	The overwhelming majority of HR VLBW's were HR because of BPD with or without IVH. Low socioeconomic status, inner city population	Study was privately funded
Sajaniemi 2001 11227991	• Cognition, behavior and temperament as early as 2 year of age predicted impaired language functioning at age 4 years in infants without major disabilities. • Preterm children were temperamentally less active, less persistent, and less goal-directed with passive attitude toward environmental stimulus. • Preterm infants were less cooperative and highly distractable.	No full-term controls	Internal validity B
Briscoe 1998 98300800	When comparing short-term memory and language outcomes, across all measures, preterm infants performed at a lower level, typically one half SD lower. • 2/3 of preterm infants had normal cognitive profiles. • "at risk" subgroup of preterms for language impairment can be identified using an expressive screening tool at an early age (less than 5 yrs) when intervention can be effective(Bus Story Test). • Meta-analysis 80 studies, preterm IQ lower than full terms but still in the normal range.	No difference in regard to social class, maternal education or single parent status. No GA less than 26 weeks Small sample made effect of IVH/PVL difficult to interpret "Most" children were recruited through friends and relatives (excluding siblings) of the preterm children in order to minimize social and economic disparity	Study was privately funded
Saigal 2001	Neurosensory Impairment:: ELBW 28%, FT Controls 2%, p= 0.001 Growth: Weight: diff. between ELBW and FT (mean z scores) –5.78	Didn't specify exclusion criteria but these are implied based on clear industry criteria units;	Study was privately funded

Evidence Table 5A. Studies Evaluating Association of LBW to Speech and Language Disorders
Part III

Author, Year	Associations found	Potential Biases	Comments

21376729	(p<0.0001)
	Visual Problems: ELBW 57%, FT Controls 21%, p=<0.001 (OR 5.1, CI 2.89-9.05)
	
	Current Health Problems (multiple/patient): ≥3 Health Problems: ELBW 35%, FT Controls 7%, p<0.0001
	Past Health Problems:
	  Seizures: ELBW 11%, FT Controls 2%, p<0.005
	  Asthma: ELBW 25%, FT Controls 14%, p=0.05
	  Recurrent bronchiolitis/pneumonia: ELBW 14%, FT Controls 3%, p=0.005
	Current (at 12-16 yr age) Functional Limitation (Table 4 page 411) (multiple/patient)
	  Visual difficulty: ELBW 57%, FT Controls 21%, p<0.001
	  Hearing Difficulty: ELBW 7%, FT Controls 5%, ns.
	  Emotional problems: ELBW 4%, FT Controls 1%, ns
	  Mental problems: ELBW 4%, FT Controls 1%, ns.
	  Clumsiness: ELBW 25%, FT Controls 1%, p<0.001
	  Developmental Delay: ELBW 26%, FT Controls 1%, p<0.001
	  Learning Disability: ELBW 34%, FT Controls 10%, p<0.001
	  Hyperactivity: ELBW 9%, FT Controls 2%, p=0.04
	  Reduced self-abilities: ELBW 5%, FT Controls 0%, p=0.02
	Limitation in school or in normal activity: ELBW 31%, FT Controls 9%, p<0.002
	Any functional limitation: ELBW 81%, FT Controls 42%, p<0.001
	Functional limitation/child [Mean (SD)]: ELBW 2.0 (1.8), FT Controls 0.6 (0.8), p<0.001
	Utilization of Health Care Resources:
	  Pediatrician: ELBW 34%, FT Controls 14%, p<0.0002
	  Ophthalmologist: ELBW 62%, FT Controls 34%, p<0.0001
	  Ear/nose/throat: ELBW 14%, FT Controls 6%, p<0.05
	  Occupational therapist: ELBW 7%, FT Controls 1%, p=0.002
	  Speech therapist: ELBW 8%, FT Controls 0%, p<0.002
	  Special Education: ELBW 48%, FT Controls 10%, p<0.0001
	  Prescription Glasses: ELBW 36%, FT Controls 10%, p<0.001
		to generalizability: different era of natural care 2 white race 3 access to universal health care in Canada	

230

Evidence Table 5A. Studies Evaluating Association of LBW to Speech and Language Disorders
Part III

Author, Year	Associations found	Potential Biases	Comments
Schendel 1997 98033417	Even apparently well VLBW infants with no overt physical impairment are consistently at higher risk for all measures of DELAY than MLBW or NBW infants. VLBW have DELAY in all areas of function with greatest risk for delay in gross motor domain. "Abnormal" – VLBW 10.9%, NBW 2.9%, p ≤ 0.001 Personal-Social ≥1 delays: VLBW 7.1%, NBW 2.2%, p ≤ 0.001 Language ≥ 1delays: VLBW 8.8%, NBW 4%, p ≤ 0.01 Fine motor-adaptive ≥ 1 delays: VLBW 7.9%, NBW 2.2%, p ≤ 0.001 Gross motor ≥1 delays: VLBW 10.7%, NBW 1.8%, p ≤ 0.001	The people administering the Denver test were not blinded and were aware of degree of prematurity. The adjusted age at f/u had very wide range 9-34 months	Study was government funded

Evidence Table 5B. Studies Evaluating Association of LBW to Audiology Outcomes
Part II

Author, Year UI#	Demographics	Inclusion Criteria	Exclusion Criteria	Disease/Condition Type (N)	Study Design (Duration)
Northern Neonatal Nursing Initiative Trial Group 1996 96304894	Location: UK Years of Birth: 1990-1992 Mean GA (range), wk: 29 (27-31) Mean BW (range), g: 1253 (965-1543) Male: 39% Race: ND Enrolled: 776 Evaluated: 776 Number of sites: 16	GA <32 weeks; resident in northern UK	ND	Experiment 1: fresh frozen plasma treatment (257) Experiment 2: gelatin plasma substitute (261) Glucose controls (258)	Randomized controlled trial (2 years)

Hack 1996 97066007	Location: US
	Years of Birth: 7/1982-6/1988, 1/1990-12/1992
	Mean GA (range), wk:
	  Sample 1: 25.9±2 (22-31)
	  Sample 1: 25.7±2 (22-31)
	Mean BW (range), g:
	  Sample 1: 688.6±73 (560-740)
	  Sample 2: 670.6±56 (502-742)
	Male:
	  Sample 1: 28%
	  Sample 2: 29%
	Race: White
	  Sample 1: 31%
	  Sample 2: 37%
	Enrolled: 280
	Evaluated: 280
	Number of sites: 1
		BW 500-759 g
		Survived to 20 months corrected Age
			ND	Sample 1: VLBW survived infants born in 1990-1992 (surfactant/dex era) (114)
				Sample 2: VLBW survived infants born in 1982-1988 (surfactant and less dex. era) (166)
					Prospective cohort (followed to 20 months corrected age)

Hack 2000 20358826	Location: US Years of Birth: : 1/1/1992-2/31/1995 Mean GA (range), wk: 26.4±1.8 Mean BW (range), g: 813±125 Male: 43% Race: ND Enrolled: 333 Evaluated: 221 Number of sites: 1	BW<1000g	Major congenital malformations	VLBW infants (221)	Prospective cohort

232

Evidence Table 5B. Studies Evaluating Association of LBW to Audiology Outcomes
Part II

Author, Year UI#	Demographics	Inclusion Criteria	Exclusion Criteria	Disease/Condition Type (N)	Study Design (Duration)
Wood 2000 20373840	Location: UK and Ireland Years of Birth: 1995-1996 Mean GA (range), wk: 22-25 Mean BW (range), g: ND Male: ND Race: ND Enrolled: 314 Evaluated: 283 Number of sites: 276	GA 20-25 weeks survivors	ND	Preterm infants (283)	Prospective cohort (30 [28-40] months)

Singer 1997 98049057
 	
Singer 2001 21163669
	Location: US
	Years of Birth: 1989-1991
	Mean GA (range), wk:
	  Sample 1: 27±2
	  Sample 2: 30±2
	  Controls: 40±2
	Mean BW (range), g:
	  Sample 1: 956±248
	  Sample 2: 1252±178
	  Controls: 3451±526
	Male:
	  Sample 1: 52%
	  Sample 2: 43%
	  Controls: 50%
	Race: White
	  Sample 1: 55%
	  Sample 2: 48%
	  Controls: 51%
	SES: Hollingshed classification:
	  Sample 1: 3.5±1
	  Sample 2: 3.6±1
	  Controls: 3.6±1
	Enrolled: 464
	Evaluated: 206 (123 controls)
	Number of sites: 3
		Cases (sample 1&2): premature infants, BW < 1500g
		Controls: term infants with no diagnosed medical illness or abnormalities at birth, >36 weeks, GW>2500g
			Major congenital abnormality
			Drug exposure
			Maternal illness
			HIV
			Maternal mental retardation
			>2 hours driving time from hospital
				Sample 1: VLBW infants with BPD infants (122)
				Sample 2: VLBW without BPD (84)
				Sample 3: Full term infants (123)
					Prospective cohort (followed to 3 years corrected age)

233

Evidence Table 5B. Studies Evaluating Association of LBW to Audiology Outcomes
Part II

Author, Year UI#	Demographics	Inclusion Criteria	Exclusion Criteria	Disease/Condition Type (N)	Study Design (Duration)
Schmidt 2001 21298249	Location: Canada, USA, Australia, New Zealand, Hong Kong Years of Birth: 1996-1998 Mean GA: 　Sample 1: 25.9 ±1.8 　Sample 2: 26 ±1.9 Mean BW: 　Sample 1: 782 ±131 　Sample 2: 783 ± 130 Male: 51% Race: Sample 1:White: 69%, black: 13%, Asian: 5%, other: 12% Sample 2: White: 67%, black: 14%, Asian: 7%, other: 12% Enrolled: 2756 Evaluated: 1202 Number of sites: 32	BW: 500-999g 2 hrs old Born in 1 of the 32 participating centers in Canada, USA or Australia. Born during 1/1996-3/1998	Excluded total 981 (not eligible) Unable to administer study drug within 6 hrs of birth , n=469 Structural heart disease Renal disease or both, or strongly suspected (n=24) dysmorphic feature or congenital abnormalities likely to affect life expectancy or neurologic development or to be associated with structural heart disease or renal disease (n=49) Maternal tocolytic therapy with indomethacin or another prostaglandin inhibitor within 72hr before delivery (n=245) Overt clinical bleeding at more than one site (n=8) Platelet count <50.000 (n=25) Hydrops (n=9) Not considered viable (n=171) Unlikely to be available for f/up (n=31)	Sample 1: Indomethacin group [574] Sample 2: Placebo group [569]	Randomized, multicenter, placebo/controlled, double-blind trial [18 mo CA]

234

Evidence Table 5B. Studies Evaluating Association of LBW to Audiology Outcomes
Part II

Author, Year UI#	Demographics	Inclusion Criteria	Exclusion Criteria	Disease/Condition Type (N)	Study Design (Duration)
Battin 1998 99002694	Location: British Columbia, Canada Enrollment period: 1991-1993 Mean GA: ND (range: 23-25 wks) Mean BW: ND (Mean BW for the 333 live births during the study period : for GA of 23 wks: 581, for GA of 24 wks: 648, for GA of 25 wks: 764) Male: ND Race: ND Enrolled: 333 (total live births GA: 23-28 wks) Evaluated : 44 (out of 49 of GA 23-25 surviving to NICU discharge) Number of sites: 2	Prospective cohort: Birth at British Children's Hospital and British Womens' Hospital Born during 1991-1993 Extremely low gestational age (ELGA): 23-25 wks Had follow up at 18 mo of age Historical control group: Born at the same institution Born between 1983-1989 GA: 23-25 wks	Cases of therapeutic termination of pregnancies for lethal congenital anomalies Outborns	Prospective cohort of ELGA born during a period when antenatal steroids, surfactant and dexamethasone for BPD had become an accepted treatment [44]	Prospective observational cohort study and a comparative study with an historical control group (18 months)
Vohr 2000 20295211	Location: US Years of Birth: 1/93-12/94 Median GA (range), wk: Mean BW (range), g: ND Male: ND Race: ND Enrolled: ND Evaluated: ND Number of sites: 12	Live born BW 401-1000 g	ND	1151 extremely low birth weight survivors cared for in the 12 participating centers of the National Institute of Child Health and Human Development Neonatal Research Network	Prospective cohort (18-22 months corrected age)

235

Evidence Table 5B. Studies Evaluating Association of LBW to Audiology Outcomes
Part II

Author, Year UI#	Demographics	Inclusion Criteria	Exclusion Criteria	Disease/Condition Type (N)	Study Design (Duration)
Piecuch 1997 98012134	Location: US Years of Birth: 1990-1994 Mean GA (range), wk: 　Sample 1: 24 　Sample 2: 25 　Sample 3: 26 Mean BW (range), g: 　Sample 1: 668±91 (450-850) 　Sample 2: 790±115 (550-1000) 　Sample 3: 842±158 (505-1260) Male: 　Sample 1: 50% 　Sample 2: 73% 　Sample 3: 50% Race: ND SES: high social risk 　Sample 1: 89% 　Sample 2: 43% 　Sample 3: 68% Enrolled: 94 Evaluated: 86 Number of sites: 1	24, 25 or 26 week GA Non-anomalous Born at University of California, San Francisco	ND (Died after discharge (2) Accidental severe central nervous system insult after discharge (1) Lost to follow-up (5)}	Sample 1: GA 24 weeks (18) Sample 2: GA 25 weeks (30) Sample 3: GA 26 weeks (38)	Prospective cohort (at 12 months, 18 months, 2 ½ years, 4 ½ years. 7-8 years)
Victorian Infant Collaborative study Group, 1997 97466059	Location: Australia Years of Birth: 1979-80, 1985-87, 1991-92 Mean GA (range), wk: ND Mean BW (range), g: ND Male: ND Race: ND Enrolled: 36 Evaluated: 35 Number of sites: 3	ELBW infants, BW 500-999 g born outside the level III perinatal centers in Victoria, Australia survived to age of 2 years	Excluded infants born in 1979-1980 for current review	ELBW infants (36): 　Sample 1: born in 1985-1987 (19) 　Sample 2: born in 1991-1992 (16)	Retrospective cohort (2 years)
Ambalavanan 2000 21031370	Location: US Years of Birth: 1/1990 to 12/1994 Mean GA (range), wk: 26±2 Mean BW (range), g: 829±123 Male: 45% Race: African-American 66% Enrolled: 218 Evaluated: 218 Number of sites: 1	ELBW infants, BW <1000 g	ND	ELBW infants (218)	Retrospective cohort (followed to 18 months of age)

236

Evidence Table 5B. Studies Evaluating Association of LBW to Audiology Outcomes
Part II

Author, Year UI#	Demographics	Inclusion Criteria	Exclusion Criteria	Disease/Condition Type (N)	Study Design (Duration)

Cheung 1999 99146391	Location: Canada
	Years of Birth: 1990-1993
	Mean GA (range), wk:
	  Sample 1: 25 (22-29)
	  Sample 2: 26 (24-30)
	  Sample 3: 28 (23-32)
	Mean BW (range), g:
	  Sample 1: 660±56
	  Sample 2: 873±73
	  Sample 3: 1127±71
	Male: total 57%
	Race: ND
	Enrolled: 187
	Evaluated: 164
	Number of sites: 2
		BW<1250 gm
		GA < 32 weeks
		Mild or no significant respiratory disease (O₂ < 30%, RR < 70)
			Major congenital abnormalities, syndromes
			Infants with neurologic insult after discharge from NICU.
				Sample 1:
				BW 500-749 g (26)
				Sample 2:
				BW 750-999 g (63)
				Sample 3:
				BW 1000-1249 g (75)
					Prospective cohort (followed to 24 months adjusted age)

Doyle 2001 21326609 Victorian Infant Collaborative study Group, 1997 97290716	Location: Australia Years of Birth: 1991-92 Mean GA (range), wk: 23-27 Mean BW (range), g: ND Male: ND Race: ND Enrolled: 225 Evaluated: 225 (265 controls) Number of sites: 1	Cases: GA 23-27 weeks, survived to 2 and 5 years of age Controls: randomly selected Contemporaneous normal birth weight controls (BW > 2499 g)	ND	Sample 1: Pretem survivors (N= 401) Controls: Randomly selected contemporaneous normal birth weight controls (BW>2499 grams) (N=265)	Prospective cohort (Doyle - 5 years; Victorian – 2 years)

*some subjects were overlapped with 20307288 (stated in text)
*possibly overlapped with 98026322

237

Evidence Table 5B. Studies Evaluating Association of LBW to Audiology Outcomes
Part II

Author, Year UI#	Demographics	Inclusion Criteria	Exclusion Criteria	Disease/Condition Type (N)	Study Design (Duration)

Corbet 1995 95264244	Location; USA
	Years of Birth: 1986-1989
	Mean GA:
	  Sample 1: 27 ± 2
	  Sample 2: 27 ± 2
	Mean BW:
	  Sample 1: 934 ± 179
	  Sample 2: 931 ± 191
	Males:
	  Sample 1: 50%
	  Sample 2: 50%
	Race:
	  Sample 1: whites: 41%, blacks: 37%, others: 22%
	  Sample 2: whites: 46%, blacks: 36%, others: 18%
	Enrolled: 1046
	Evaluated: 597
	Number of sites: Multicenter
		Born alive
		Qualifying BW (Not specified in this publications)
		That were intubated and assigned randomly to receive either synthetic surfactant or air placebo as part of their participation in 3 multicenter RCTS.
		Had follow up at 1 yr of age
			ND	Sample 1:
				Synthetic surfactant: [314]
				
				Sample 2:
				Air placebo [283]
					Combination of 3 multicenter, randomized, double blind studies of synthetic surfactant vs air placebo [1 yr]

Gerdes 1995 95264241	Location: US
	Years of Birth: 3/1989-4/1990
	Mean GA (range), wk:
	  Experiment 1: 27.2±1.7
	  Experiment 2: 27.2±1.8
	Mean BW (range), g:
	  Experiment 1: 907±121
	  Experiment 2: : 911±125
	Male:
	  Experiment 1: 55%
	  Experiment 2: 56%
	Race:
	  Experiment 1: White 55%, Black 37%, Hispanic 4%, Other 5%
	  Experiment 2: White 60%, Black 30%, Hispanic 5%, Other 5%
	Enrolled: 826
	Evaluated: 508
	Number of sites: 33
		Mothers who were expected to deliver premature infants with BW 700-1100 g	All exclusion prenatal.
			1) Proven fetal lung maturity
			2) Known malformation or chromosome anomaly
			3) Fetal growth retardation
			4) Hydrops
			5) Purulent amnionitis
			6) Maternal heroin addiction
			7) Obstetric decision not to support fetus
			Postnatal exclusions:
			1) Major malformation
			2) ≥3 minor anomalies
			3) Hydrops
				Experiment 1: One doses surfactant (244)
				Experiment 2: Three doses surfactant (264)
					Randomized comparison trial (1 year)

Evidence Table 5B. Studies Evaluating Association of LBW to Audiology Outcomes
Part II

Author, Year UI#	Demographics	Inclusion Criteria	Exclusion Criteria	Disease/Condition Type (N)	Study Design (Duration)
Marlow 2000 20150342	Location: UK Years of Birth: 1990-1994 Mean GA: ND (Median and Range) Sample 1: 28 (26-31) Sample 2: 28 (26-31) Mean BW: ND (Median and range) Sample 1: 960 (600-2914) Sample 2: 1026 (410-2814) Male: ND Race: ND Enrolled : 27 Evaluated: 15 Number of sites: 1	For sensorineural hearing loss (SNHL) group GA: <33 wks Family resident of Greater Bristol area Records at Hearing Assessment Center of Royal Hospital for Sick children. Born during 1990-1994 Diagnosis of SNHL of 50 dB For control group: Matched controls 2:1 to cases Admitted to the same NICUs as cases Matched for sex and GA and next and preceding matching children in the admission books of St Michael's and Sothmead hospitals	ND	Sample 1: SNHL group [15] Sample 2: Control group [30] Matched with cases for sex, GA, admission dates in NICU	Retrospective case control study with a longitudinal component (unclear if retrospective or prospective) (12 mo CA)
Lee 1998 9842293	Location: Canada Years of Birth: 1990-1995 Mean GA: ND Mean BW: Sample 1: 763 ±157 Sample 2: 807±176 Male: ND Race: ND Enrolled: ND (total N not given, data only for enrolled cases with candidemia: N= 29) Evaluated: 50 Assessed for outcome: 35 (14 cases and 21 controls) Number of sites: 2	For cases: Prematures with BW<1250 g Admitted in the NICU s of UAH and RAH from 1990-1995 Diagnosis of candidemia: by at least one positive blood culture Diagnosis of candidal meningitis: By isolation of candida in the CSF or >45x10 ^{6} WBCs in the CSF and candidemia. For controls: Prematures with BW <1250 g Admitted to the same NICUs during the same period without candidal infection	*Neonates with major congenital anomalies*	Sample 1: Premature infants <1250 with candidemia and/ or candida meningitis (25) Sample 2: Premature neonates with BW <1250 matched with cases for BW, GA, sex and admission dates, without candidal infection (25)	Retrospective longitudinal comparative study with case control design and cases defined based on exposure to candidemia and matched controls (f/up between 37 and 70 mo CA) Average age at assessment: for cases :31 ±19 mo, and for controls: 28 ±20 mo

Evidence Table 5B. Studies Evaluating Association of LBW to Audiology Outcomes
Part II

Author, Year UI#	Demographics	Inclusion Criteria	Exclusion Criteria	Disease/Condition Type (N)	Study Design (Duration)
DeReginer 1997 98041177	Location: US Years of Birth: 1987-1991 Mean GA (range), wk: Sample 1: 28.0±1.5 Sample 2: 27.1±1.2 Sample 3: 27.5±1.7 Mean BW (range), g: Sample 1: 1030±140 Sample 2: 1007±122 Sample 3: 1007±140 Male: ND Race: ND Enrolled: 174 Evaluated: 164 Number of sites: 2	BW ≤1500 g survived until Discharged Able to match to a patient in other two respiratory groups	Presence of independent of chronic lung disease known to adversely affect neurodevelopment, sensory, or growth, i.e. severe intracranial abnormalities, congenital anomalies or viral infections, etc. Unable to match to a patient in other groups Died after discharged (6) Lost to follow-up (4)	Sample 1: No chronic lung disease (58) Sample 2: Mild chronic lung disease (58) Sample 3: Severe chronic lung disease (58)	Retrospective chart review with marched subject group (1 year of adjusted age)
Kurkinen-Raty 1998 98387235 (All+Lung) *sample from the same big population as 20284814	Location: Finland Years of Birth: 1990-1996 Mean GA (range), wk: Cases: 28.2 (23.8- 37.2) Controls: 28.4 (22.9-36.9) Mean BW (range), g: Cases: 1138.3±434 Controls: 1272.4±547.2 Male: ND Race: ND Enrolled: 78 (78 controls) Evaluated: 78 (78) Number of sites: 1	Preterm PROM between 17-30 weeks gestation; singleton; delivered > 2 hr after rupture Controls: preterm no PROM; spontaneous preterm delivery matched for GA and year of delivery.	Rupture unconfirmed or transient	Sample 2: Preterm rupture (78) Sample 2: Preterm delivery no rupture (78)	Retrospective cohort
Kurkinen-Raty, 2000 20284814 *sample from the same big population as 98197235	Location: Finland Years of Birth: 1990-1997 Mean GA (range), wk: Cases: 30.5±2.1 Controls: 30.4±2.1 Mean BW (range), g: Cases: 1294±469 Controls: 1605±427 Male: ND Race: ND Enrolled: 103 (103 controls) Evaluated: 103 (103) Number of sites: 1	Casarean delivered singleton, GA 24-33 weeks Controls: spontaneous delivered singleton after regular contractions and/or preterm rupture of the membranes no more than 24 hrs before. The mothers were matched one-to-one by gestational age at delivery plus or minus 1 week.	ND	Sample 1: Indicated preterm (i.e., preterm birth 'indicated' for maternal/fetal reasons (103) Sample 2: Spontaneous preterm delivery due to preterm labor (103)	Retrospective cohort

240

Evidence Table 5B. Studies Evaluating Association of LBW to Audiology Outcomes
Part II

Author, Year UI#	Predictors	Predictor Measures	Outcomes	Outcome Measures
Northern Neonatal Nursing Initiative Trial Group 1996 96304894	Cardiovascular or Pulmonary Predictors: use of FFP or plasma substitute to expand vascular volume prophylactically	ND	**CNS Outcomes:** Motor delay Cerebral palsy Seizure disorder Post hemorrhagic hydrocephalus **Ophthalmology:** Visual impairment Blindness **Audiology Outcomes:** Hearing disorders Speech **Other outcomes:** Blind, deaf, or unable to walk – combined outcome No severe disability – combined outcome Overall developmental quotient – Griffith's	Motor delay: Griffith's gross motor quotient >350 below mean Griffith's quotient for speech + hearing >350 below mean
Hack 1996 97066007	General: Birth Weight	500-750 gm	**CNS:** Cerebral palsy Motor and cognitive delay **Ophthalmology:** Blindness **Audiology:** Deafness	Neurosensory status BSID: MDI, PDI

241

Evidence Table 5B. Studies Evaluating Association of LBW to Audiology Outcomes
Part II

Author, Year UI#	Predictors	Predictor Measures	Outcomes	Outcome Measures
Hack 2000 20358826	General: 1) Birth weight 2) GA 3) SGA/IUGR 4) Antenatal steroids 5) Jaundice CNS: 1) Intracranial/Intraventricular Hemorrhage 2) Periventricular leukomalacia 3) Ventriculomegaly/ ventricular dilation Cardiovascular/Pulmonary: Chronic lung disease Gastrointestinal: Necrotizing "entroclitis" Other: 1) Infectious Disease 2) Dexamethasone 3) Perinatal factors (chorioamnionotis) 4) Multiple birth 5) C-section 6) Social risk 7) Male sex	ND	**CNS:** Cerebral palsy Motor delay Cognitive delay MDI score<70 Post hemorrhagic Hydrocephalus **Ophthalmology:** Blindness **Audiology:** Deafness	Neurologic abnormality- includes: CP, hypotonia, hypertonia Shunt-dependent hydrocephalus

Evidence Table 5B. Studies Evaluating Association of LBW to Audiology Outcomes
Part II

Author, Year UI#	Predictors	Predictor Measures	Outcomes	Outcome Measures
Wood 2000 20373840	*General:* 1) GA 2) Gender Other: Perinatal Factors→ Multiple gestation	ND	**CNS:** Motor delay Cognitive delay Seizure disorder Overall development **Ophthalmology:** Visual impairment Blindness **Audiology:** Hearing disorder Deafness Speech Communication disorder **Other:** Severely disabled Other disability No disability Disability of hearing, vision, or communication	Bayley scales Severe disability = need of physical assistance to perform daily activities. If disability did not fit into this category = "other disability"
Singer 1997 98049057	Cardiovascular or pulmonary predictors: 1) Bronchopulmonary dysplasia General : BW, Neurologic risk Other: Race, Socioeconomic status	BPD: preterm, <1500g BW, oxygen for >28 days with radiographic evidence of CLD	**CNS outcomes:** Cerebral palsy Cognitive delay Mental retardation	Bayley scale of infant development
Singer 2001 21163669			**Ophthalmology outcomes:** Visual impairment **Audiology outcomes:** Hearing disorders Speech Language Communication disorder	Language (speech/communication) measured by Battelle Developmental Communication Subscale Domain→ receptive, expressive and total communication scores converted to DQ mean 100 and SD 15.

243

Evidence Table 5B. Studies Evaluating Association of LBW to Audiology Outcomes
Part II

Author, Year UI#	Predictors	Predictor Measures	Outcomes	Outcome Measures
Schmidt 2001 21298249	1) Prophylactic indomethacin administration : 0.1 mg/kg Q24 hrs X 3 days (vs NS placebo) in VLBW infants, during first 6 hrs of life	Nor further specified	Primary outcomes at 18 months of age: 1) Composite outcome: death or impairment 2) Death before 18 mo corrected age 3) Cerebral palsy 4) Cognitive delay (MDI<70) 5) Hearing loss requiring amplification 6) Bilateral blindness Secondary long term outcomes outcomes: 1) Hydrocephalus, necessitating the placement of shunt 2) Seizure disorders 3) Microcephaly (HC<3 d %)	1) Death before a corrected age of 18 months or documentation in survivors of one of the following: CP, Cognitive delay, Hearing loss requiring amplification, B/L blindness 2) Cerebral palsy diagnosed if had nonprogressive motor impairment with abnormal muscle tone and decreased range or control of movements. 3) Cognitive delay: as MDI less than 70 (2SD below the mean of 100) on the Bayley scale between 85-114: classified as normal, Scores below 70: marked cognitive delay. 4) Documentation of composite primary outcome: required documentation that the infant had died or had survived with one of the 4 types of impairment. A single missing component of the f/up assessment would result in designation of missing for primary outcome. A priori criteria for definitions of presence or absence of component of the primary outcome. 5) In cases it was difficult to obtain Audiologic test results, deafness requiring amplification was assumed to be absent if no such indication was present during the Bayley test. (n=27) 6) Blindness: a corrected visual Acuity of less than 20/200. F/up evaluation around 18 mo: allowed range 18-21 mo. (Home visits were permitted when necessary)

Evidence Table 5B. Studies Evaluating Association of LBW to Audiology Outcomes
Part II

Author, Year UI#	Predictors	Predictor Measures	Outcomes	Outcome Measures
Battin 1998 99002694	**General:** 1) GA (23-25 wks) In comparative component with historical control group **General:** 1) Birth during a period with routine use of: antenatal steroids, surfactant and dexamethasone for BPD (vs birth in presurfactant, presteroid period)	ND	**CNS:** Neurodevelopmental outcome CP Low MDI (below 2 SDs) **Ophthalmology- Audiology:** Blind, Deaf	Neurologic exam Bayley scale: MDI, PDI Formal hearing test Ophthalmologic examination
Vohr 2000 20295211	**General:** 1) Birth weight 2) Maternal disease (HTN) 3) Antenatal steroids **CNS:** 1) Intracranial/Intraventricular hemorrhage (GR 3 to $ IVH/PVL) Cardiovascular or Pulmonary: 1) Chronic lung disease (oxygen requirement at 36 weeks) 2) Other: postnatal steroids 3) Other: Surfactant Gastrointestinal: 1) Necrotizing "enterocolitis" Other: 1) Other: male sex 2) Other: Race (white) 3) Other: sepsis (early and late onset) 4) Other: maternal education	GR 3 to 4 IVH. PVL undefined sepsis undefined	**CNS :** Cerebral palsy **Neurodevelopmental:** Motor delay (sitting, walking, picer grasp, feeding) Seizure disorder Post hemorrhagic Hydrocephalus (PHH) and shunt Other: Neurologic exam (normal; abnormal) Development (MDI and PDI by Bayley II Scale) **Ophthalmology :** Visual impairment (any) Blindness (unilateral, bilateral) **Audiology:** Hearing disorders	"normal Neurologic exam": no abnormalities on neurologic exams

245

Evidence Table 5B. Studies Evaluating Association of LBW to Audiology Outcomes
Part II

Author, Year UI#	Predictors	Predictor Measures	Outcomes	Outcome Measures
Piecuch 1997 98012134	General predictors: 1) GA CNS predictors: 1) intracranial/ intraventricular hemorrhage 2) periventricular leukomalacia *Cardiovascular or pulmonary predictors:* 1) chronic lung disease *Other predictors:* 1) social risk: economic 2) social risk: substance abuse	CLD - at 36 weeks PCA, requirement for supplemental O_2 IVH grade 3 or 4 & PVL, according to sonogram Social risk economic - maternal education <12 grade; complete unemployment in household; or government assistance for health insurance Social risk substance abuse - positive toxicology screens or confirmed history of drug or alcohol abuse	**CNS outcomes:** Cerebral palsy Cognitive delay **Ophthalmology outcomes:** Visual impairment **Audiology outcomes:** Hearing disorders	Visual – Near point tests or Snellen eye charts Audiologic- behavioral testing followed by BAER or pure tone audiometry. Cognitive outcome - Bayley scales at 12 and 18 months; Stanford-Binet at 2.5-4 years; McCarthy scales at 4-6 years. Abnormal neurological outcome – CP, quadriplegia, dysplegia, hemiplegia Suspicious neurological outcome - clumsiness, tremors Severe neurosensory abnormalities – Bilateral hearing loss, blindness Mild neurosensory abnormalities - high frequency hearing loss without hearing aids, visual deficit without glasses
Victorian Infant Collaborative study Group, 1997 97466059 Arch Dis Child	Other: time period of birth	ND	**CNS:** Cerebral Palsy Cognitive delay Post Hemorrhagic Hydrocephalus (PHH) Ophthalmology: Blindness **Audiology:** Deafness **Other:** Sensorineural disability: severe, mental, moderate, none.	CP neurologic exam Bayley MDI, PDI scores Blindness-not stated Deafness-not stated Degrees of sensorineural delay are defined as an aggregate measure and are approximated.
Victorian Infant Collaborative study Group, 1997 98026322	General: BW Other: period of time when born	Each sample were subdivided into BW=500-749 g and BW=750-999 g 1985-1987 vs. 1991-1992	**CNS:** Cerebral palsy Neurodevelopmental: Cognitive and motor delay Disability **Ophthalmology:** Blindness **Audiology:** Deafness or hearing aid	CP was not defined Bayley Scales of Infant Development DQ, using the published mean and SD Disability: "Sever" – bilateral blindness, cerebral palsy with the child unlikely ever to walk, or a DQ score <-3SD; "Moderate" – bilateral sensorineural deafness requiring hearing aids, cerebral palsy in children not walking at 2 but expected to walk, or a DQ score from –3SD to <-2 SD; "Mild" – cerebral palsy but walking at 2 , or a DQ score form –2 SD to <-1 SD.

246

Evidence Table 5B. Studies Evaluating Association of LBW to Audiology Outcomes
Part II

Author, Year UI#	Predictors	Predictor Measures	Outcomes	Outcome Measures
Ambalavanan 2000 21031370	General: BW, GA, Antenatal steroids, Apgar score Other: Race, Gender Multiple gestation, Maternal education, Maternal age CNS: Intracranial hemorrhage Periventricular/Ventricular Dilation Bronchopulmonary dysplasia GI: Necrotizing "entrocolitis" Interinal perforation, Chorioamnionitis Multiple gestation Maternal education Maternal age	Extensive list of the 21 predictor variables	**CNS:** Motor delay Cerebral palsy Cognitive delay Mental retardation PHH Neurologic exam Major handicap **Ophthalmology:** Visual impairment Blindness **Audiology:** Hearing disorders Deafness	Bayley scales Major handicap-presence of one or any poor outcome (i.e. CP, deadness, blindness), Mental retardation (MDI or PDI <70), PHH requiring sheet
Cheung 1999 99146391	*General predictors:* 1) BW 2) GA 3) Apgar score *CNS predictors:* 1) intracranial/ intraventricular hemorrhage *Cardiovascular or pulmonary predictors:* 1) days of ventilation 2) days of O_2 use *Other predictors:* 1) frequency of apnea 2) mean desaturation of apnea 3) mean frequency of apnea 4) Blisten index (socioeconomic status)	ND	**CNS outcomes:** Motor delay Cerebral palsy Cognitive delay Mental retardation Seizure disorder Neurodevelopmental disability **Ophthalmology outcomes:** Blindness **Audiology outcomes:** Hearing disorders **Growth outcomes:** Weight > 2 SD below the mean Height > 2 SD below the mean HC > 2 SD below the mean	Bayley scores Stanford-Binet Intelligence Scale Peabody Developmental Motor Scale Neurodevelopmental disability: "children with 1 or more of a) cerebral palsy b) legal blindness c) hearing loss d) convulsive disorder e) cognitive delay

Evidence Table 5B. Studies Evaluating Association of LBW to Audiology Outcomes
Part II

Author, Year UI#	Predictors	Predictor Measures	Outcomes	Outcome Measures
Doyle 2001 21326609	*General predictors:* 1) GA 2) SGA/IUGR 3) antenatal steroids 4) gender (female) 5) postnatal age	1) SGA/IUGR - BW ratio <0.8 2) intracranial/ intraventricular hemorrhage - Papille system 3) periventricular leukomalacia - cystic lesions in PVWM dx < discharge	**CNS:** Motor delay Cerebral palsy Cognitive delay Mental retardation	1) motor delay, cognitive delay - WPPSI-R and alternative IQ tests 2) cerebral palsy - not walking or walking with difficulty 3) mental retardation - IQ < 2 SD below mean for NBW group
Victorian Infant Collaborative study Group, 1997 97290716	*CNS predictors:* 1) intracranial/ intraventricular hemorrhage 2) periventricular leukomalacia	4) bronchopulmonary dysplasia - ROS + O$_2$ Rx after 28 days age 5) dexamethasone - postnatal steroid use	**Ophthalmology outcomes:** Blindness	
*some subjects were overlapped with 20307288 (stated in text)	*Cardiovascular or pulmonary predictors:* 1) bronchopulmonary dysplasia		**Audiology outcomes:** Hearing disorders Deafness	

*possibly overlapped with 98026322	*Other predictors:*
	 1) dexamethasone
	 2) perinatal factors
	   a) multiple birth
	   b) cesarian section
	 3) socioeconomic variables
	   i) Asian mother
	   ii) higher SEC
	   iii) no English-speaking at home
	 4) surgery in primary hospital
	 5) patient with no adverse events
			Other:
			 Survival without major disability at 5 years age
			 Survival with major neurosensory disability at 5 years age	

248

Evidence Table 5B. Studies Evaluating Association of LBW to Audiology Outcomes
Part II

Author, Year UI#	Predictors	Predictor Measures	Outcomes	Outcome Measures
Corbet 1995 95264244	**General:** 1) Synthetic surfactant (single dose via ET tube of 5 mg/kg vs air placebo)	Not further specified	**Growth:** Growth status at 1 yr: 1) Weight 2) Height, 3) HC and percentiles distribution **Other:** Health status at 1 yr: 1) Surgeries 2) Readmissions to hospital 3) CLD,Medications for CLD 4) Respiratory support on exam day 5) Medications for chronic neurologic disease 6) Asthma, Eczema **CNS:** Neurodevelopmental outcome 1) MDI 2) PDI 3) Impairments: Present absent 4) Severity of impairment 5) Type of impairment (MDI<69, MDI 69-84) 6) CP **Audiology** 1) B/L sensorineural deafness 2) Deafness not requiring amplification **Ophthalmology:** (worst exam and last) 1) B/L blindness 2) Visual defect 3) No ROP, mild/moderate ROP, severe ROP) 4) Treatment for ROP (surgery, cryotherapy)	Assessment at 1 yr of corrected age Not further specified

Evidence Table 5B. Studies Evaluating Association of LBW to Audiology Outcomes
Part II

Author, Year UI#	Predictors	Predictor Measures	Outcomes	Outcome Measures
Gerdes 1995 95264241	Cardiovascular or Pulmonary: Surfactant use	ND	**CNS:** Cerebral palsy Cognitive delay Mental retardation **Ophthalmology:** Visual impairment, Blindness **Audiology:** Hearing Disorder, Deafness **Pulmonary:** 1) Asthma 2)e/o CLD 3) respiratory support @ 1yr **Growth:** Height, Weight, HC **Other:** hospital re-admissions, h/o surgery	Mental retardation Bayley Scales MDI<69

Evidence Table 5B. Studies Evaluating Association of LBW to Audiology Outcomes
Part II

Author, Year UI#	Predictors	Predictor Measures	Outcomes	Outcome Measures
Marlow 2000 20150342	**General:** 1) Birth weight 2) Apgar score 3) CRIB scores **CNS:** 1) Maximum bilirubin level 2) Abnormal cerebral US scan **Audiology:** 1) Sensorineural hearing loss **Cardiovascular/Pulomonary:** 1) Duration of intubation, respiratory support, oxygen, pH<7.2, base excess 2) Dopamine 3) Furosemide 4) Indomethacin use **Other:** 5) Netilmicin 6) Vancomycin 7) Positive blood cultures 8) Bilirubin >200 [mol/l 9) Bilirubin>GA x 10 10) Creatinine >60 mmol/l 11) Netilmicin 12) Vancomycin Combination of the above: 1) Bili.200 + acidosis 2) Bili> 200 + sepsis 3) Bili >200+ netilmicin 4) Bili> 200+ vancomycin 5) Bili>200+ furosemide 6) Peak bili+ acidosis 7) Peak bili+ sepsis 8) Peak bili+ netilmicin 9) Peak bili+ furosemide 10) Creatinine>60+ netilmicin or vancomycin or furosemide 11) Netilmicin+furosemide 12) Vancomycin+ furosemide	Not further specified	In case control component: **Audiology:** 1) Sensorineural hearing loss (SNHL) of 50 dB within 9 months from birth In Longitudinal component: **CNS:** 1) Cerebral palsy at 12 months of age in the 2 groups (SNHL and control group)	Cases of SNHL were identified if the hearing loss had been identified within 3 months of discharge home, (within 9 mo from birth); after excluding cases with conductive hearing loss, possible congenital cause, or had neonatal bacterial meningitis

Evidence Table 5B. Studies Evaluating Association of LBW to Audiology Outcomes
Part II

Author, Year UI#	Predictors	Predictor Measures	Outcomes	Outcome Measures
Lee 1998 98842293	**General:** 1) Candidemia and/or Candidal meningitis	Diagnosis of Candidemia: by at least one positive Blood Culture Diagnosis of Candidal meningitis: by isolation of Candida in the CSF or >45x10^6 WBCs in the CSF and candidemia.	**CNS:** 1) Neurodevelopmental disabilities (NDDs) 2) Cognitive delay 3) Cerebral palsy **Ophthalmology:** 1) Legal blindness **Audiology:** 1) Hearing loss **Growth:** 1) Growth retardation	1) Bayley Scales of Infant development; MDI, PDI for ages < 24 mo. 2) Stanford-Binet Intelligence Scale and Peabody Development Motor Scales for ages > 24 mo. 3) Scores obtained by psychologists, psychometricians, pediatricians specialized. Neurodevelopmental Disabilities: 1) Cerebral palsy (all types and severity) 2) Legal blindness (corrected VA of the better eye<20/200) 3) Hearing loss (neurosensory hearing loss in the better ear > 30 dB) (done by certified audiologist 4) And/or cognitive delay (MDI>3 SDs below the mean) Growth retardation: Weight, Height, HC > 2 SDs below the mean
DeRegnier 1997 98041177	Cardiovascular/ Pulmonary: Chronic lung disease	Classification based on the duration of supplemental oxygen requirements. "No CLD" – breathing room air at 28 days "Mild CLD" – requiring supplemental oxygen at 28 days but not at 36 weeks PMA Sever CLD" – reqiring oxygen at 28 days and 36 weeks PMA	**General:** Motor and cognitive delay Cerebral palsy **Opthalmology:** Visual impairment Blindness **Audiology:** Hearing loss Deafness **Growth:** Weight Z score Length Z score Head circumference Z score **Other:** any adverse outcome	(Between 3-6 yrs CA) Bayley PDI & MDI

252

Evidence Table 5B. Studies Evaluating Association of LBW to Audiology Outcomes

Part II

Author, Year UI#	Predictors	Predictor Measures	Outcomes	Outcome Measures
Kurkinen-Raty 1998 98387235 *sample from the same big population as 20284814	General : PROM	Diagnose was through clinical assessment or with the use of a PROM-test, which detects insulin growth factor binding protein-1 in the cervico-vaginal secretions, or with the use of a nitrazine test.	**CNS:** Motor delay Cerebral delay **Ophthalmology:** Visual Blindness **Audiology:** Hearing disorders Pulmonary: Chronic lung disease **Growth:** weight percent **Other:** Days of re-hospitalization Steroid therapy at followed up	Neurologic exams Diagnosis of CLD was made if infants required oxygen, continuous bronchodilator, or steroid tx because of respiratory signs and symptoms. Diagnoses of RDS were made based on need for respiratory support, radiologic findings, and clinical assessments
Kurkinen-Raty, 2000 20284814 *sample from the same big population as 98197235	General predictors: Birth weight GA Antenatal steroids Cord pH Bronchopulmonary dysphasia (BPD) Other predictors: Indicated preterm delivery Spontaneous perterm delivery	BPD diagnoses were based on radiologic finding	**CNS:** Motor delay Cerebral palsy **Ophthalmology** Visual impairment **Audiology** Hearing disorder **Pulmonary** Chronic lung disease (CLD) at 1 year **Growth:** Wt, Ht, HC	Motor delay = abnormalities of tone or reflexes but functionally normal or borderline CP = spastic diplegia or hemiplegia or spastictetraplegia Diagnosis of CLD was made if infants required oxygen, continuous bronchodilator, or steroid tx because of respiratory signs and symptoms.

253

Evidence Table 5B. Studies Evaluating Association of LBW to Audiology Outcomes
Part III

Author, Year	Associations found	Potential Biases
Northern Neonatal Nursing Initiative Trial Group 1996 96304894	No significant differences by Griffith's Developmental quotients, incidence of CP, seizures, hearing disorders. Initial demographics available in an earlier study.	Study was government and private funded
Hack 1996 97066007 Pediatrics		No data on funding source

Hack 1996 associations:

	MR (MDI<84)	CP	Blind	Deaf	Major Neurosensory abnormal +MDI<80
1982-1988	52%	10%	10%	-	49%
1990-1992	34%	10%	2%	6%	35%

20-month Neurodevelopmental outcomes did not change appreciably between the 2 eras. 20% of infants had subnormal cognitive function (MDI<70) and 10% had CP during 1990-1992 period. One third of infants with BW 500-750 gram had major neurosensory abnormalities and / or MDI<80.

Hack 2000 20358826:

MDI Score < 70:
CLD: 55% (49/89); 2.18 (1.20-3.94)
MDI Score<70 (multi stepwise logistic regression)
Male sex: 2.73 (1.52-4.92)
Social risk: 1.48 (1.09-2.00)
CLD: 2.18 (1.20-3.94)
OR adjusted for sex, social risk & BW:

Gr III-IV IVH:
50% (16/32);   8.55 (3.52-20.76)
50% (8/16);   4.45 (1.54-12.84)
50% (17/34);   5.48 (2.41-12.47)
CLD: 30% (27/89); 3.09 (1.51-6.35)
Sepsis: 14% (13/93); 3.47 (1.16-10.36)
Jaundice: 26% (6/23); 5.15 (1.63-16.22)
Mult. Stepwise Logistic regression:
Male sex: 2.79 (1.02-7.62)
Sepsis: 3.15 (1.05-9.48)
Jaundice: 4.80 (1.46-15.73)
Predictors of neurologic abnormality were a severely abnormal finding on cerebral ultrasound (OR, 8,09; 95% CI 3.69-17.71) and chronic lung disease (OR 2.46; 95% CI 1.12-5.40); predictors of deafness were male sex (OR 2.79 95% CI 1.02-7.62), sepsis (OR 3.15 95 % CI 1.05-9.48), and jaundice (maximal bilirubin level >171)

Hack 2000 Potential Biases: The authors concluded that there is an urgent need for research into the etiology and prevention of neonatal morbidity.

254

Evidence Table 5B. Studies Evaluating Association of LBW to Audiology Outcomes
Part III

Author, Year	Associations found	Potential Biases

Wood 2000 20373840	Infants 22-25 weeks GA developmentally assessed at median 30 months
	• 138/283 had disability 49%(64 met criteria for severe disability)
	• 49% no disability
	• 53/283 severely delayed 19%(Bayley below 3 SD)
	• 32/283 2-3 below SD 11%
	• 28 severe neuromotor disability 10%
	• 7 blind or perceived light only 2%
	• 8 hearing loss that was uncorrectable or required hearing aids 3%
	Survived without overall disability
	  22 wks---------0.7 %
	  23 wks---------5%
	  24 wks---------12%
	  25 wks---------23%
	Severe disability at 30 months
	  22 ---------------0.7%
	  23 --------------3%
	  24 --------------6%
	  25 --------------9%
	• no relation between morbidity pattern and either gestational age &multiple birth
	• boys were likely to be disabled than girls
		Severe disability common; children born extremely premature

255

Evidence Table 5B. Studies Evaluating Association of LBW to Audiology Outcomes
Part III

Author, Year	Associations found	Potential Biases
Singer 1997 98049057	Evaluation at 36 months corrected age. VLBW, VLBW with BPD, full term (FT).	Single region, but at least it is a region Unclear if examiners were blinded to groups status Study was government funded

Bayley MDI
% with MDI below 70

		% with MDI below 70
VLBW	90 ± 16 (38-126)	11%
VLBW w/ BPD	84 ± 24 (10-116)	21%
FT	96 ± 12 (57-127)	4%

P = 0.001 for VLBW vs. VLBW w/ BPD

Singer 2001
21163669

Bayley PDI
% with PDI below 70

		% with PDI below 70
VLBW	98 ± 20 (33-122)	9%
VLBW w/ BPD	84 ± 29 (8-127)	9%
FT	103 ± 15 (58-128)	1%

P = 0.001 for VLBW vs. VLBW w/ BPD

At 3 years BPD predicted poorer motor outcome but not poorer mental outcome.

Receptive DQ: BPD < VLBW < Term, p < 05

Receptive DQ < 85: BPD 49%, VLBW 34%, Term 30%, BPD < VLBW + Term p < .05

Expressive DQ: BPD < VLBW + Term, p < .05

Expressive DQ<85: BPD 44%, VLBW 25%, Term 25% BPD < VLBW + Term p < .05

Communication DQ: BPD < VLBW + Term, p < .05

Communication DQ < 85: BPD 43%, VLBW 31%, Term 28%, NS

Rank order listing of risk factors in order of magnitude of effect and the number of communication DQ lowered by the risk factor: PDA lowered DQ by 13 points, Minority race by 6 points, lower socioeconomic status by 5 points, and higher neurologic risk by 5 points. p .001

Bayley Scales MDI:
BPD 83.7 ± 24, VLBW 90 ±16, Term 96.4 ± 12, BPD < VLBW < Term, p< 0.05

Bayley Scales PDI:
BPD 84.1 28, VLBW 97.4 19, Term 102.8 14
BPD < VLBW + Term, p< .05

ROP: BPD 43%, VLBW 4%, p= .001

Seizures: BPD 7%,

Neurologic score: BPD 1.3 ± 2, VLBW 58 ± 1, p < .001

256

Evidence Table 5B. Studies Evaluating Association of LBW to Audiology Outcomes
Part III

Author, Year	Associations found	Potential Biases
Schmidt 2001 21298249	1) There was no difference in primary outcomes between the 2 groups at 18 months of age. 2) Among the 574 infants who were assigned to prophylaxis with indomethacin, 271 (47%) died or survived with impairment as compared with 261 of 569 infants (46%) assigned to placebo (OR: 1.1; 95% Confidence intervals; 0.8-1.4) 3) In VLBW infants, prophylaxis with indomethacine does not improve the rate of survival without neurosensory impairments at 18 months of age 4) There was no difference in any of the secondary outcomes between the 2 groups, at 18 months of age. **Primary: Composite / CNS Outcomes:** **Indomethacin vs. Placebo** • Death or impairment 271/574(47%) vs. 261/569 (46%) • Death before 18 mo 121/595 (21%) vs 111/594 (19%) • Cerebral palsy 58/467 (12%) vs 55/477 (12%) • Cognitive delay (MDI<70 by Bayley scale 118 /444 (27%) vs 117/457 (26%) **Audiology outcome:** • Hearing loss requiring amplification 10/456 (2%) vs 10/466 (2%) **Ophthalmology outcome:** • Bilateral blindness 9/456 (2%) vs 7/472 (1%) (Odds ratios adjusted for BW stratum and Center) **Secondary CNS outcomes** were not affected by indomethacin administration: • Hydrocephalus requiring shunt 15/470 (3%) vs 9/480 (2%) • Seizure disorder 8/470 (2%) vs 7/483 (1%) • Microcephaly 49/461 (11%) vs 54/475 (11%) Kaplan Meier estimates of survival in the 2 groups: • 0 months n=601 vs 601 • 6 months n=479 (80%) vs 490 (82%) • 12 months n=473 (79%) vs 487 (81%) • 18 months n=470 (78%) vs 483 (80%)	1) By using the Bayley test at 18 mo the authors found that more than one quarter of all surviving infants had moderate to severe cognitive delays, defined by MDIs< 70. The validity of the MDI score at this age as a predictor of later intellectual functioning remains to be determined. 2) At a post hoc calculation the study had a 90% power to detect a 20% reduction in risk, had it existed 3) Authors report that the outcome assessments were done blindly by investigators unaware of treatment groups assignments 4) Authors report that they had almost complete ascertainment for the primary outcome at 2 yrs of age.

Evidence Table 5B. Studies Evaluating Association of LBW to Audiology Outcomes
Part III

Author, Year	Associations found	Potential Biases
Battin 1998 99002694	**CNS outcomes:** Major impairment was present in 36% of infants born at 23-25 wks GA, during 1991-1993 (N=44) 1) Cerebral palsy 9/44 (20%) 2) Low MDI 8/44 (18%) **Ophthalmology** outcome: 1) Blind 4/44 (9%) **Audiology** outcome: 1) Deaf 4/44 (9%) **Combined** outcome: 1) Overall impaired 16/44 (36%) 2) Multiple handicaps 6/16 (38%) Analysis of only 24-25 wks GA infants (N=43): Major handicaps: 15/44 (34%) The percentage of infants with major impairments and/ or multiple handicaps, for the 23-25 wks GA group, was the same in 1991-1993 and 1983-1989 periods (However, no data on the number of infants from this cohort that were actually followed up at 18 mo of age)	1) During 1991-93 period there is no concurrent control group for the comparative assessment of neurodevelopmental outcome 2) Group of infants of 23-25 wks GA, born during 1991-1993, was not matched to the historical control group born during 1983-1989. Possibility of confounders cannot be excluded. 3) No data were given on the number of infants in the historical control group that had f/up at 18 mo of age. No data on source of funding
Vohr 2000 20295211	Studied effect of early IVH at 5 to 11 hours of age on IQ distribution and presence of cerebral palsy (CP). Assessed at 36 months CA.	IVH rates seems high No data on funding source

	Early IVH present	Early IVH absent	P value
N	29	249	
Binet IQ	78.7 (25)	87.5 (20)	0.09
Binet IQ < 70	38%	19%	0.03
PPVT-R	76.6 (28)	86.0 (21)	0.15
CP at 36 months	25%	8%	0.01

Later IVH had effect on Binet IQ similar to early IVH.

Evidence Table 5B. Studies Evaluating Association of LBW to Audiology Outcomes
Part III

Author, Year	Associations found	Potential Biases
Piecuch 1997 98012134	Mean age at follow-up was 32 months. Bayley exams were done at 18 months. Neurologic abnormalities and CP did not differ significantly across the gestational ages of 24 to 26 weeks. Between 67% and 89% were normal in each gestational age group. Significant differences (P = 0.036) related to gestational age were found in 18 month Bayley exam scores when group as normal borderline or deficient	All inborn infants No data on funding source

	Normal	Deficient
24 wk	28%	39%
25 wk	47%	30%
26 wk	71%	11%

Significant differences (P = 0.008) related to gestational age were found in the combined end point of CP or an abnormal Bayley exam score:

	Neither	One	Both
24 wk	28%	39%	33%
25 wk	47%	23%	30%
26 wk	63%	34%	3%

Author, Year	Associations found	Potential Biases
Victorian Infant Collaborative study Group, 1997 97466059	All children born outside the level III perinatal centers. Assessment at 2 years corrected age.	Incomplete reporting of demographic data, methods and results. Study was government funded

	1985-1987	1991-1992
n	19	16
Cerebral Palsy	19.1%	12.5%
Cognitive delay	19.1%	18.8%
Blind	5.6%	6.2%
Deaf	0	0
Sensorineural disability		
Mild	15.8%	6.2%
Moderate	0	0
Severe	5.3%	12.5%

259

Evidence Table 5B. Studies Evaluating Association of LBW to Audiology Outcomes
Part III

Author, Year	Associations found						Potential Biases
Victorian Infant Collaborative study Group, 1997 98026322	Birth weight < 1000g; assessed at 2 years corrected age.						Incomplete reporting of demographic data, methods and results. Study was government funded

Cohort	n	DQ < -3 SD	DQ –3 to –2 SD	DQ –2 to –1 SD	DQ> -1 SD
'91-'92	237	5.9%	6.3%	13.9%	73.4%
'85-'87	211	6.2%	4.3%	14.2%	75.4%

Cohort	n	Mild CP	Mod. CP	Severe CP	Any CP	Blindness	Deaf
'91-'92	237	3.8%	1.7%	3.8%	9.3%	2.1%	0.8%
'85-'87	211	NS	NS	NS	6.6%	4.3%	0.5%

Cohort	No disability	Mild Disability	Moderate disability	Severe disability
'91-92 n = 237	71.3%	14.8%	7.2%	6.8%
'85-'87 n = 211	71.6%	15.6%	6.2%	6.6%

Evidence Table 5B. Studies Evaluating Association of LBW to Audiology Outcomes Part III

Author, Year	Associations found	Potential Biases
Ambalavanan 2000 21031370	ELBW: MDI<68 : 12% PDI<68: 20% Major handicap: 28% CP:28% MR 16% Post-hemorrhagic hydrocephalus: 5% Deaf 1.4% Blindness 1% Predictors of major handicap (Low MDI and/or PDI): Grade of IVH, PVL, absence of chorio (in this population, not in most others), NEC≥II; race; multiple gestation, BPD, maternal education For ELBW infants without IVH, the prevalence of major handicap, low MDI, and Low PDI was 25%, 17%, 16%, respectively. For ELBW infants with grade III IVH, the prevalence of major handicap, low MDI, and Low PDI was 33%, 29%, 24% respectively. For ELBW infants with grade IV IVH, the prevalence of major handicap, low MDI, and Low PDI was 69%, 44%, 63% respectively. This study identifies major determinants of adverse neurodevelopmental outcome (i.e. major handicaps, low MDI, low PDI) of ELBW (<1 kg) infants born 1990-1994. Grade of IVH is strong predictor of adverse outcome. But note large % of ELBW without IVH who had major handicap, low MDI, and Low PDI. **BPD** was a significant determinant of low MDI and PDI. Mat education level was significant determinant of neurodevelopmental outcome. NEC, race, multiple gestation, PVL independently contributed to poor outcome in ELBW infant. Lower BW predicted low PDI.	Retrospective, relatively small sample size (218). No data on funding source
Cheung 1999 99146391	Mental score: *Days of ventilation: (N=64) <0.0001* Motor Score: *Days of ventilation: (N=164) <0.004* Mental Score: *Grade of IVH: (N=164) 0.003* Motor Score: *Grade of IVH: (N=164) <0.0001* Mental Score: *Infants <1250g with gr. 3 or 4 IVH: (N=50) <0.001* Motor Score: *Infants <1250g with gr. 3 or 4 IVH: (N=50) <0.001*	No data on funding source

Evidence Table 5B. Studies Evaluating Association of LBW to Audiology Outcomes
Part III

Author, Year	Associations found	Potential Biases
Doyle 2001 21326609 Victorian Infant Collaborative study Group, 1997 97290716 *some subjects were overlapped with 20307288 (stated in text) *possibly overlapped with 98026322	Evaluation at 5 years corrected age: **CP : 23-27 wk survivors (11.3%) 25/221** Blindness : 23-27 wk (1.8%) 4/221 FT controls (0%) FT control 0% **Deafness : 23-27 wk (0.9%) 2/221** FT control 0% **IQ <-2 SD: 23-27 wk (15.4%) 34/221** **Major neurosensory disability** 23 –27 wk (19.6%) 44/225 FT control (4.1%) 10/245 **Major disability among survivors** 23 wk GA: 2/5 (40%) 24 wk GA: 7/21 (33%) 25 wk GA: 13/51 (25%) 26 wk GA: 17/71 (24%) 27 wk GA: 5/79 (6%) Overall 23-27 wk: 19% **OR for survival with major disability at 5 years:** OR each 1 wk increase in GA = 0.59 (95% CI 0.43, 0.8) **Prognostic factors with major disability at 5 years:** IVH, cystic PVL, surgery during primary hospitalization, postnatal steroid treatment. Rates of survival free of major disability for surviving PT infants: None 96/103 =93% One 59/71 =83 % Two 23/43 =53 % Three 3/9 =33% Four 0/1 = 0 Evaluation at 2 years corrected age. Data shown are for births in 1991-1992. Gestational age Sensorineural disability (% of survivors) |	n	Severe	Moderate	Mild	None
---	---	---	---	---	---
23 weeks	5	29%	20%	40%	20%
24 weeks	21	14.3%	19%	33.3%	33.3%
25 weeks	51	5.9%	21.6%	25%	47%
26 weeks	68	8.8%	11.8%	20.6%	58.8%
27 weeks	74	1.4%	10.8%	23%	64.9%

Overall	219	6.4%	14.6%	24.2%	54.8% |
					
					Decrease in disability with increase in gestational age was significant, p = 0.014.
					Also showed significant fall in severe disability with increase in gestational age, Odds ratio = 0.58 (0.36-0.94)
					Comparison of cohorts born in 1985-1987 vs. 1991: 1992 did not demonstrate any difference between cohorts.
						Perinatal data lacking on some infants,
						Especially outborn (in level II or I)
						Different methods of testing IQ
						Different times of assessing
						Neurodevelopmental outcome
						Some children not evaluated at 5 years
						(evaluated at 2 years)
						210/401 preterm infants were assessed
						    at both 2 and 5 years
						The classification of disability or no
						    disability was the same at both 2 and
						    5 years (90.5% agreement; k=0.691)
						Inadequate discussion of study
						    population demographics
						Also various surrogate data
						Study was government funded

262

Evidence Table 5B. Studies Evaluating Association of LBW to Audiology Outcomes

Part III

Author, Year	Associations found	Potential Biases
Corbet 1995 95264244	**Growth AT 1 YR:** Mean measurements of Height (74 cm), weight (9.1 kg) and HC (46 cm) and growth percentiles were equivalent in the 2 groups.	The incidence of severe impairment in the 19% of infants who did not return for evaluation at the age of 1 yr may be higher than in those who were evaluated.
	Health Status AT 1 YR: No difference in parameters between 2 groups	
	1) Surgeries (33% vs 34%) 2) Readmission to hospital (45% vs 39%)	Source of funding not reported.
	2) CLD (11% vs 10%) 4) Medications for CLD (14% vs 14%)	The neurodevelopmental evaluation of
	3) Respiratory support (4% vs 2%)	infants at 1 yr may not be absolutely reliable for the estimation of later
	4) Med. for chronic neurologic problems (1% vs 2%)	outcome.
	5) Asthma (this only was s/s : 9% vs 3%) 8) Eczema (2% vs 1%)	
	Neurodevelopmental Outcome: No difference in the outcomes between the 2 groups in these parameters.	The estimated mental retardation is likely to be low, and the estimated CP
	1) Mean MDI (values <50= 49): 2) Mean MDI (only children with MDI>69)	is likely to be high, compared to estimates at 2 and 3 yrs.
	2) Number of children with MDI<69: 4) Number of children with PDI<69	
	3) Mean PDI (values<50=49) 6) Mean PDI (only children with PDI>69)	
	CNS Impairment: No difference in any impairments between 2 groups	
	1) Present: 43% vs 37% 2) Absent: 57% vs 63%	
	2) Mild/moderate: 20% vs 14% 4) Severe:23% vs 23%	
	3) MDI<69: 17% vs 16% 6) MDI: 69-84: 18% vs 14%	
	4) CP mild: 8% vs 7% 8) CP moderate/severe: 7% vs 7%	
	Audiology:	
	1) B/L sensorineural hearing deafness: 0% vs 1%	
	2) Deafness not needing amplification: 0% vs 1%	
	Ophthalmology:	
	1) B/L blindness: 3% vs 2% 2) Visual defect: 8% vs 8%	
	Worst examination	
	2) No ROP: 30% vs 33% 2) Mild/moderate ROP: 53% vs 52%	
	3) Severe ROP: 17% vs 15% 4) Surgical treatment for ROP:10% vs 12%	
	4) Cryotherapy for ROP: 5% vs 6%	
	Last examination	
	5) No ROP: 69% vs 72% 2) Mild/moderate ROP: 26% vs 22%	
	6) Severe ROP: 5% vs 6% 4) Surgical treatment for ROP: 4% vs 4%	
	7) Cryotherapy for ROP: 2% vs 3%	
	Infants who survived after treatment at birth with single dose synthetic surfactant fare as well in terms of growth, development and late morbidities as infants who survive without treatment. No difference in medical history during first year of life, growth, incidence of visual or auditory defects, CP, neurodevelopmental delay at 1 yr adjusted age.	

Evidence Table 5B. Studies Evaluating Association of LBW to Audiology Outcomes
Part III

Author, Year	Associations found		Potential Biases
Gerdes 1995 9526424	Severe ROP: 1 dose: 47(16)	3 dose: 35(11)	25% loss to follow up, equal in both groups; 1 year follow-up does not predict long-term outcome from all infants
	Physical evidence of CLD: 1 dose: 43(18)	3 dose: 40(15)	No data on funding source
	Medication for CLD: 1 dose: 35(14)	3 dose: 30(11)	
	Medication for chronic neurologic disease: 1 dose: 12(5)	3 dose: 3(1)	"Prenatal and postantal exclusion criteria were identical to those used in an
	Index<2 SD (%): 1 dose: 29(15)	3 dose: 30(13)	earlier prophylactic trial of this synthetic surfactant"
	Impairment present: 1 dose: 106(44)	3 dose: 92(35)	Died by 1-year adjusted age
	No impairment: 1 dose: 123(51)	3 dose: 155(59)	Lost to follow-up
	Severity of impairment: Mild/moderate: 1 dose: 40(17)	3 dose: 39(15)	
	Serious: 1 dose: 66(27)	3 dose: 53(20)	
	Types of impairments: MDI<69: 1 dose: 40(16)	3 dose: 38(14)	
	Moderate/severe CP: 1 dose: 22(9)	3 dose: 16(6)	
	Bilateral sensorineural deafness: 1 dose: 5(2)	3 dose: 10(2)	
	Deafness not requiring amplification: 1 dose: 5(2)	3 dose: 2(1)	
	Bilateral blindness: 1 dose: 10(4)	3 dose: 4(2)	
	Visual defect: 1 dose: 24(10)	3 dose: 22(8)	

Evidence Table 5B. Studies Evaluating Association of LBW to Audiology Outcomes
Part III

Author, Year	Associations found	Potential Biases
Marlow 2000 20150342	Pulmonary and Other predictors evaluation for **Audiology outcome.** Children with sensorineural hearing loss [15] as compared to control group[30] had longer periods of: 1) Intubation, (14 ds vs 2 ds) 2) Ventilation (34 ds vs 6 ds) 3) Oxygen therapy (57 ds vs 10 ds) 4) Acidosis (12 ds vs 0.5 ds), and 5) More treatments with dopamine (33% vs 7%)or 6) Furosemide (87% vs 53%) 7) Neither P/T of aminoglycosides 8) nor duration of jaundice 9) or level of bilirubin varied between the 2 groups. SNHL was more likely when : 1) netilmicin use coexisted with the peak of bilirubin (87% vs 14%)_ 2) when acidosis occurred when bilirubin was over 200 [lmol/l, (31% vs 4%) 3) when furosemide was used in the face of high creatinine levels (64% vs 27%) 4) when furosemide was used with netilmicin (67% vs 37%) **CNS outcome at 12 mo:** At 12 months of age evidence of cerebral palsy was present in 7/15 (47%) of children with SNHL vs 2/30 (7%) of children without SNHL.(p=0.022)	1) Very small sample size (cases with SNHL only 15) 2) Analyzed too many predictors and combination thereof, for very few outcomes. Very wide confidence intervals; and even those predictors found to be associated with the SNHL this may have been due to chance. 3) The association found between SNHL and cerebral palsy was <u>not</u> based on an adjusted analyses for possible confounders; 4) The 2 groups were different in many factors that were associated with both SNHL and CP Not reported source of funding

Evidence Table 5B. Studies Evaluating Association of LBW to Audiology Outcomes
Part III

Author, Year	Associations found	Cases	Controls	Potential Biases
Lee 1998 98442293	**Growth, CNS and Audiology, and ophthalmology outcomes for** prematures<1250 g with candidemia/candida meningitis **Growth:** 1) No difference in Growth retardation: **CNS:** 1) No difference in MDIs of survivors 2) Lower PDIs in survivors 3) No difference in overall Neurodevelopmental disabilities (NDDs) 4) Cerebral palsy **Ophthalmology:** 1) Vision loss **Audiology:** 1) Hearing loss (All the children with NDDs had Cerebral palsy with or without visual or hearing deficit) Prematures<1250 g with candidemia/candida meningitis had: Higher Combined mortality and NDDs	7/14 survivors(50%) 83 ±20 71 ±21 4/14 (29%) 4/14 (29%) 2/14 (14%) 2/14 (14%) 60% (OR=3.9; 1.2-12.6)	11/21 survivors (50%) 90 ±20 (p>0.05) 87±18 (p<0.05) 3/21 (14%) (p>0.05) 3/21 (14%) 1/21 (5%) 1/21 (5%) 28% (p< 0.05)	Cannot exclude missed association due to the small number of patients analyzed n both groups

Evidence Table 5B. Studies Evaluating Association of LBW to Audiology Outcomes
Part III

Author, Year	Associations found	Potential Biases
DeRegnier 1997 98041177	**Chronic lung disease** *Any adverse outcome:* 2/54 12/54 P<0.001 18/56 *Sensorineural hearing loss:* 0/54 0/54 P<0.05 3/56 *Low MDI<2 SD from mean:* 0/54 4/54 P<0.05 5/56 *Low PDI<2 SD from mean:* 1/54 4/54 P<0.05 7/56 *Weight Z-score:* *No numbers given* <0.05 *Chronic lung disease and cerebral palsy, unilateral blindness, length Z-score, head circumference Z-score are not significant.*	Matching scheme used is likely to be ineffective Large proportion of study population excluded by their matching strategy: subjects excluded were: 329/387=85% with no chronic lung disease; 53/111=47.7% with mild chronic lung disease; 122/180=68% with severe chronic lung disease No data on funding source
Kurkinen-Raty 1998 98387235 ***sample from the same big population as 20284814**	Retrospective controlled cohort study of early PROM between 17 and 30 weeks of gestation. Assesments at one year corrected age. N = 55 for early PROM and 56 for control. Outcome <u>Early PROM</u> <u>Control</u> <u>OR (CI)</u> Cerebral palsy 18% 16% 1.2 (0.4, 3.1) Delayed motor Development 9% 16% 0.5 (0.2, 1.7) Visual disability 4% 4% 1.0 (0.1, 7.5) Hearing loss 7% 9% 0.8 (0.2, 3.2) Good nuerosensory development 67% 61% 1.2 (0.6, 2.2) Early PROM seems to be a major obstetric and neonatal problem with pulmonary ramifications extending beyond the neonatal period. However, most of these infants can be saved.	No data on funding source

Evidence Table 5B. Studies Evaluating Association of LBW to Audiology Outcomes
Part III

Author, Year	Associations found	Potential Biases
Kurkinen-Raty, 2000 20284814 ***sample from the same big population as 98197235**	**CLD at 1 year age:** Indicated PT delivery: (81) 12/81 (15%) Spontaneous PT delivery: (94) 3/94 (3%) RR 4.6 (1.4, 1.6) **Growth:** Indicated PT delivery: (81) Spontaneous PT delivery: (94) Weight RR =0.03 (-5.3, 0.3) L RR = 0.002 HC RR = 0.03 **CP:** Indicated PT delivery: (81) 5/81 (6%) Spontaneous PT delivery: (94) 10/94 (11%) RR=0.6 (0.25-1.6) **Delayed motor:** Indicated PT delivery: (81) 8/81 (6%) Spontaneous PT delivery: (94) 8/94 (9%) RR 1.2 (0.5-3.0) **Visual disability:** Indicated PT delivery: (81) Spontaneous PT delivery: (94) RR =1.9 (0.5, 7.8) **Hearing loss:** Indicated PT delivery: (81) Spontaneous PT delivery: (94) RR =1.9 (0.5, 7.8) This study demonstrated that premature infants who were born due to 'indicated maternal/fetal reasons' vs. spontaneous preterm delivered infants had worse pulmonary outcome a 1 yr age. More infants in 'indicated' group were SGA and were significantly smaller than control group at 1 yr in Wt, HT, and HC. There was no difference between groups in neurosensory outcomes.	Outcome not well defined Difficult to know if lack of difference between groups is due to sample size or event rate. No data on funding source

268

Evidence Table 6A. Studies Evaluating Association of LBW to Behavioral Disorders

Part I

Author, Year UI#	Demographics	Inclusion Criteria	Exclusion Criteria	Disease/Condition Type (N)	Study Design (Duration)

Nadeau 2001 21163667	Location: Canada
	Years of Birth: 1987-1990
	Median GA (range), wk:
	  Cases: 27.4±1.1
	  Control: 39.8±1.6
	Median BW (range), g:
	  Cases: 1024.3±204.2
	  Control: 3453.4±497.8
	Male:
	  Cases: 51%
	  Control: 50%
	Race: ND
	Enrolled: 129
	Evaluated: 86 → 61 (50 controls)
	Number of sites: 1
		Cases: GA<29 weeks, BW<1500 g
		Controls: Normal BW children, born at the same hospital during the same time period
			Cases:
			Lost to follow-up at 5 years 9 months: families had moved away (33), parents' refusal (10)
			Lost to follow-up at age 7: families had moved away (10), parents' or school's refusal (13)
				Cases: EP/VLBW infants (86→61)	Prospective cohort (at 18 months, 5 years 9 months, and age 7)

Robson 1997 9055145	Location: Canada Years of Birth: ND Mean GA (range), wk: 32.6±3.4 Mean BW (range), g: 1758.7±521.7 Male: 36% Race: ND Enrolled: 132 Evaluated: 85 Number of sites: 2	LBW cohort: ≤ 2500 g Admitted to neonatal intensive care units at 2 hospitals in a mid-sized Canadian city. English-speaking mothers. Families lived within 100 km of either hospital. Assessments at 7 mos and 12 mos of age.	Significant visual or motor impairments or any other gross neurological or physical anomalies.	Cases: 85 LBW infants No control group	Prospective single-arm cohort study

Evidence Table 6A. Studies Evaluating Association of LBW to Behavioral Disorders
Part I

Author, Year UI#	Demographics	Inclusion Criteria	Exclusion Criteria	Disease/Condition Type (N)	Study Design (Duration)
Breslau 1996 8836807	Location: US Years of Birth: 1983-1985 Mean GA (range), wk: ND Mean BW (range), g: Urban LBW: 14.7%<1500 g, 21.4% 1501-2000 g, 63.9% 2001-2500 g. Suburban LBW: 17.4%<1500 g, 17.9% 1501-2000 g, 64.7% 2001-2500 g. Urban NBW: ND Suburban NBW: ND Male: Urban LBW: 42% Suburban LBW: 52% Urban NBW: 48% Suburban NBW: 54% Race (% African-American): Urban LBW: 80% Suburban LBW: 11% Urban NBW: 48% Suburban NBW: 3% Enrolled: 1095 Evaluated: 823 Urban LBW: 238 Suburban LBW: 235 Urban NBW: 176 Suburban NBW: 174 Number of sites: 2	LBW cohort: ≤ 2500 g NBW cohort: > 2500 g Born between 1983-85, 6- 7 yrs old during 1990-92 when the fieldwork took place. From 2 major hospitals in southeast Michigan: one urban and one suburban. (In each hospital, random samples of LBW and NBW children were drawn).	From the target sample: Children with severe neurologic impairment: severe mental retardation, severe cerebral palsy, blindness.	At 6 yrs (823): Cases: LBW 473: Urban LBW (238) Suburban LBW (235) Controls: NBW 350: Urban NBW (176) Suburban NBW (174)	Nonrandomized comparison study (6 years)

Evidence Table 6A. Studies Evaluating Association of LBW to Behavioral Disorders

Part I

Author, Year UI#	Demographics	Inclusion Criteria	Exclusion Criteria	Disease/Condition Type (N)	Study Design (Duration)
Breslau 2000 20298367	Location: US Years of Birth: 1983-1985 Mean GA (range), wk: ND Mean BW (range), g: ND Male: ND Race (% African-American): Urban LBW: 80% Suburban LBW: 11% Urban NBW: 74% Suburban NBW: 3% Enrolled: 1095 Evaluated: 823→717 Number of sites: ND	LBW cohort: ≤ 2500 g NBW cohort: > 2500 g Born between 1983-85, 6- 7 yrs old during 1990-92; when the initial assessment took place. Follow-up assessment at age 11 (1995-1997). From 2 major hospitals in southeast Michigan: one urban and one suburban. (in each hospital, random samples of LBW and NBW children were drawn).	From the target sample: Children with severe neurologic impairment: severe mental retardation, severe cerebral palsy, blindness.	At 11 yrs (717): Cases: LBW 411: Urban LBW (217) Suburban LBW (194) Controls: NBW 306: Urban NBW (164) Suburban NBW (142)	Nonrandomized comparison study (11 years)

Evidence Table 6A. Studies Evaluating Association of LBW to Behavioral Disorders
Part I

Author, Year UI#	Demographics	Inclusion Criteria	Exclusion Criteria	Disease/Condition Type (N)	Study Design (Duration)
Hille 2001 21319264	Location: US, Canada, Germany, Netherlands Years of Birth: US: 1984-1987 Canada: 1977-1982 Germany: 1985-1986 Netherlands: 1983 Mean GA (range), wk: US: 27±2.3 Canada: 27±2.3 Germany: 29±2.0 Netherlands: 29±2.3 Mean BW (range), g: US: 853±114 Canada: 834±126 Germany: 888±101 Netherlands: 882±105 Male: US: 40% Canada: 45% Germany: 45% Netherlands: 42% Race: White 93% Enrolled: 523 Evaluated: 408 Number of sites: 1	Survivors from 4 population based cohorts of ELBW infants in 4 countries: US – the neonatal brain-hemorrhage cohort (NBH): BW<2000 g Canada – McMaster ELBW cohort (McM): BW<1000 g Germany – Bavarian longitudinal study of children at biological risk (BLS): BW<1500 g and GA<32 weeks Netherlands – the project on preterm and small for gestational age infants (POPS): BW<1500 g and GA<32 weeks	No assessments of CBCL at age 8-19	Cases: ELBW infants from 4 population based cohorts in 4 countries (108): USA (80) Canada (150) Germany (78) Netherlands (100) Controls/Normative Samples: USA had 1200 4 – 11 year old normative controls. Netherlands had 1172 11 year old normative controls. Canada had 145 full-term controls Germany had 335 full-term controls.	Prospective single-arm cohort study

Evidence Table 6A. Studies Evaluating Association of LBW to Behavioral Disorders
Part I

Author, Year UI#	Demographics	Inclusion Criteria	Exclusion Criteria	Disease/Condition Type (N)	Study Design (Duration)
Katz 1996 97145056	Location: UK Years of Birth: 5/83- 4/85 Median GA (range), wk: 29.2±2.5 (26-34) Mean BW (range), g: 1227.5±341.4 (740-2240) Male: Cases: 52% Controls: 55% Race: Cases: 75% White, 19% Black, 6% Asian Controls: 75% White, 12.5% Black, 12.5% Asian Enrolled: 212 Evaluated: 64 (40 controls) Number of sites: 2	≤34 weeks, no major congenital anomaly, 3 cranial u/s in first week of life	Lost to follow-up Too impair due to multiple cognitive, sensory, or motor disabilities, to complete testing	Cases: Preterm infants (64) Controls: Full-term comparison sample (40)	Prospective cohort (6-8 years)
Sajaniemi 1998 99041674	Location: Finland Years of Birth: 1989-1991 Mean GA: Sample 1: 28.9 (23-35) Sample 2: 39.4 (36-43) Mean BW: Sample 1: 1205 (560-2360) Sample 2: 3461 (2510-5360) Male: ND Race: ND Enrolled: ND Evaluated : 160 Number of sites: 1	For Preterm Group (sample 1): GA: 23-34 wks Mother referred to University Central Hospital of Helsinki for threatened preterm delivery Born between 1989-1991 For Full term group (Sample 2): Born in Metropolitan Helsinki Visiting pediatric services in Helsinki for acute infectious diseases	For Preterm group If mothers had chorioamnionitis If mother had insulin dependent diabetes Children with congenital anomalies, by U/S For Full term group Chronic diseases Developmental delay	Sample 1: Preterm infants (80) Sample 2 Full term enrolled at: 20-28 mo of age (80)	Retrospective comparative study (24 mo CA)

273

Evidence Table 6A. Studies Evaluating Association of LBW to Behavioral Disorders
Part II

Author, Year UI#	Predictors	Predictor Measures	Outcomes	Outcome Measures
Nadeau 2001 21163667	General: GA Other: Family adversity Index	Evaluated at 5 years 9 months, was developed using SES data such as the family status (two-parent, single-parent, blended), age of each parent, their respective levels of education, and professional occupations. 0=low ~ 7=high	**CNS:** Neurodevelopmental: Motor function Cognitive delay Behavioral disorders	Neuromotor development index: Huttenlocher neurological task test McCarthy Scales of Children's Abilities Behaviors wre assessed by peers, teachers, and parents: RCP, TRF, parent's CBCL
Robson 1997 9055145	Developmental status Quality of home environment Early Medical risk Infant temperament	Development measured by The Bayley Scales of Infant Development Quality of Home environment at 7 and 12 mos of age: The HOME Inventory, paternal education, The Blishen Index, preschool version of the HOME Inventory in early childhood Early Medial Risk measured by the Morbidity Scale Infant Temperament and Development: The Carey Infant Temperament Questionnaire when the infants are 7 months of age corrected for prematurity.	**Behavior** Behavior at 5.5 years of age: Inattention Impulsivity	McCarthy Scales of Children's Abilities by the examiner Parental report from the Child Behavior Checklist Task performance test, vigilance tasks Matching Familiar Figures Test
Breslau 1996 8836807	General: 1) LBW (vs Normal BW= NBW) 2) Urban (vs suburban setting) 3) Maternal smoking during pregnancy	BW <2500g Racial composition, whether mothers completed high school, marital status, maternal smoking during pregnancy, maternal substance abuse/dependence during pregnancy.	ADHD (attention deficit hyperactivity disorder) Separation anxiety disorder Simple phobia Overanxious disorder Oppositional defiant disorder	The National Institute of Mental Health Diagnostic Interview Schedule for Children-Parent Teacher Report Form

274

Evidence Table 6A. Studies Evaluating Association of LBW to Behavioral Disorders
Part II

Author, Year UI#	Predictors	Predictor Measures	Outcomes	Outcome Measures
Breslau 2000 20298367	General: 4) LBW (vs Normal BW= NBW) 5) Urban (vs suburban setting) 6) Maternal smoking during pregnancy	BW <2500g Racial composition, whether mothers completed high school, marital status, maternal smoking during pregnancy, maternal substance abuse/dependence during pregnancy.	Behavior assessment at 11 yrs of age. (Assessment at 6 yrs: reported in 1996 publication) 1) Behavioral problems in 3 domains: Attention, Externalizing behaviors, Internalizing behaviors 2) Severe attention problems (above a cutoff point of 67)	Mother's rating was done with: Child Behavior Checklist (CBCL) Teacher's rating was done with Teacher Report Form (TRF) (teachers were blind to the BW information of the child) Assessments at 11 yrs were conducted blindly to the results of assessments at 6 yrs (reported in another publication) 1) Attention problem subscale; 20 items 2) Externalization problem subscale: 2 subclasses 3) Internalization problem subscale: 3 subclasses
Hille 2001 21319264	Birth weight	ND	Behavior Attention	CBCL – Parents: Total problem score Internalizing behavior (anxious, Socratic), Externalizing behavior (aggressive and delinquent), Social, thought, attention problems
Katz 1996 97145056	General: GA CNS: 1) Intracranial/ Intraventricular hemorrhage 2) Periventricular leukomalacia (cystic PVD) 3) PVD (if unilateral or bilateral periventricular echogenic lesions present on at least 3 scans)	IA IVH: no lesion= consistently NC scans. Mild lesion = germinal hem or small IVH or PVD or mild vent dilation without hem. Severe lesion: blood distends the vents or in parenchyma, or multicystic PVC.	CNS: Neurodevelopmental: Attention IQ	Measured by CPT test (Continuous Performance Test), measuring errors of omission or commission. Is also measured by CBCC (Child Behavior Check List): parents check off behavior related to attention and hyperactivity. Measured by British Abilities Scale

Evidence Table 6A. Studies Evaluating Association of LBW to Behavioral Disorders
Part II

Author, Year UI#	Predictors	Predictor Measures	Outcomes	Outcome Measures
Sajaniemi 1998 99041674	**General:** 1) Prematurity per se 2) Premature with BW< 1000 g vs premature with BW > 1000 g 3) Preeclampsia 4) SGA 5) Duration of NICU stay **CNS:** 1) PVL 2) IVH **Pulmonary:** 1) Duration of ventilation	Not further specified	**CNS:** Neurologic outcome Developmental outcome Temperament profile Behavioral profile	Neurologic outcome: 1) Cerebral palsy 2) Free of major disabilities Developmental outcome: 1) Bayley Scales of Infant Development 2) Mental Development Index (MDI) Temperament: Toddler Temperament questionnaire (TTQ) (contains 97 statements) 9 temperament dimensions: 1) Activity 2) Rhythmicity 3) Approach 4) Adaptability 5) Intensity 6) Mood Persistence 7) Distractability 8) Threshold Behavior: Infant Behavior Record: 1) Social responsiveness 2) Attention 3) Affect 4) Energy level 5) Goal directedness during the test (24 mo CA)

Evidence Table 6A. Studies Evaluating Association of LBW to Behavioral Disorders
Part III

Author, Year	Associations found			Potential Biases
Nadeau 2001 21163667	EP/VLBW, n = 61 and controls, n = 44.			No data on funding source
		EP/VLBW	Control	Significance	Data on neuromotor and intellectual functioning only collected once
	Normal neuromotor function	67%	97%	NS	Data on behavior collected once
	Abnormal neuromotor function	33%	3%		
	McCarthy IQ [mean (SD)]	100.3 (19.1)	112.8 (16.2)	P < 0.01	
	Behavioral ratings at 7 years age:				
	Peers rated EP/VLBW's as significantly more sensitive/ isolated than controls				
	Teachers rated EP/VLBW's as significantly more inattentive than controls				
	Parents rated EP/VLBW's as more hyperactive than controls				
	Significantly = P < 0.01				
Robson 1997 9055145	• Developmental status and the quality of the home environment correlate with hyperactivity.			Internal validity B
	• Medical risk, infant temperament, quality of home environment and developmental status correlate with attention.			
	• A nurturing home environment fosters development of self-regulating behaviors in LBW.			
Breslau 1996 8836807	• LBW was significantly associated with ADHD but not with separation anxiety disorder, simple phobia, overanxious disorder, or oppositional defiant disorder.			Internal validity B Parent ratings, questionnaire results are biased but corroborated by teachers who are blinded to BW of children helps to corroborate.
	• Both the mothers' and teachers' ratings significantly correlated with increased ADHD in LBW infants and this relationship is stronger in urban than in suburban communities.			
	• LBW children with the lowest IQ have highest incidence of ADHD.			
	• The urban group was primarily black, more mothers had not completed high school and more were single. However, maternal marital status, history of substance abuse/dependence and smoking during pregnancy were not associated with ADHD.			

277

Evidence Table 6A. Studies Evaluating Association of LBW to Behavioral Disorders

Part III

Author, Year	Associations found				Potential Biases
Breslau 2000 20298367	1) Information from mothers and teachers on children's **behavior problems** at age 11 revealed that the effect of LBW on attention problems differed between urban and suburban settings. 2) LBW children had an excess of **attention problems** in the urban disadvantaged communities and not in the suburban middle class communities. 3) LBW infants in the urban setting had twice as high incidence of attention problems than in urban NBW. 4) In suburban setting there was no difference in severe attention problems between LBW and NBW children. 5) LBW children had externalizing problems both in the urban and suburban settings (however this effect was mainly accounted for by maternal smoking in pregnancy). 6) No LBW effect was observed with respect to internalizing problems 7) Regardless of LBW status, maternal smoking during pregnancy was associated with an increase in externalizing problems 8) No association found between maternal smoking during pregnancy and internalizing or attention problems				1) Recollection bias: The Hx of maternal smoking during pregnancy was elicited when the child was 6 yrs old. This bias would have resulted in underestimation of the confounding effect of smoking during pregnancy. 2) Diagnosis bias: Although there was correspondence of the findings of teachers reports (who were blind to the LBW status of children) and the mothers reports, mothers report could have definitely been biased (worse scores from mothers of LBW infants)
	OVERALL SCORES	Attention scores	Internalizing	Externalizing	
	MOTHER'S SCORES				
	Urban				
	• LBW (n=217)	58.8	52.7	52.2	
	• NBW (n=164)	55.8	51.5	50.4	
	Suburban				
	• LBW (n=194)	55.1	50.4	48.4	
	• NBW (n=142)	53.8	48.6	46.3	
	TEACHER'S SCORES				
	Urban				
	• LBW (n=186)	56.9	50.3	53.9	
	• NBW (n=151)	54.7	48.8	48.5	
	Suburban				
	• LBW (n=180)	53.7	49.0	48.5	
	• NBW (n=135)	54.0	48.7	48.3	

Hille 2001 21319264	ELBW vs. Controls
	    Total problem score:
	    Boys: 3.3-9.8 points higher in ELBW vs. norm/ control
	    Girls: 3.7-5.9 points higher in ELBW vs. norm/ control
	
	Social, thought, and attention difficulty scales were 0.5-1.2 SD higher in ELBW children vs. norm/control children (statistical significance in European countries). Study identified similar types of behavioral problems in all 4 countries in ELBW infants. This suggests that problems with attention, social, and thought problems are a function of experiences of children who were born ELBW, and not to cultural differences.
	
	Internalizing and externalizing behavior scores: no difference for all 4 groups (except for one cohort for internalizing scores)
	
	ELBW children had higher total problem scores than normative/control children
					(None)
					Study was privately funded

Katz	Attention deficit is measured by the CPT test (error of omission). Hyperactivity and impulsivity is measured by the				Exactly how FT No data on

Evidence Table 6A. Studies Evaluating Association of LBW to Behavioral Disorders

Part III

Author, Year	Associations found	Potential Biases
1996 97145056	CPT test (error of commission). There were no differences among the preterm infants with mild, moderate and severe intracranial lesions. However, there was a significant increase in both errors of commission and omission in preterm with mild lesions compared to full term infants as well as in preterm with severe lesions compared to full term infants. With increasing severity of lesions in preterm infants, increasing percentage in each group commit errors of commission. Even in the absence of detectable intracranial lesions, preterm infants are still at higher risk for developing attention deficits than full term infants.	controls were selected in an unbiased way is not described. This study does not explore relationship of attention deficits identified with CPT test with actual school performance and achievement in this group of preterm infants. This study includes older preterm 26-34 weeks and does not include the extremely preterm 24-25 wk infants.

Evidence Table 6A. Studies Evaluating Association of LBW to Behavioral Disorders
Part III

Author, Year	Associations found	Potential Biases
Sajaniemi 1998 99041674	The neurological outcome of preterm infants was: For Cerebral palsy: Free from major disabilities MDI 1) All prematures: 17.5% 82.5% 103 2) Prematures < 1000 gs: 23.5% 23.5% 98 3) Prematures > 1000 gs: 13.5% 85.6% 107 The developmental outcome: Preterm infants had significantly lower MDI scores when compared to full terms (Full terms 124) When temperament was considered: the premature children were significantly less active; more adaptive; less intensive; more positive in mood and had lower sensory threshold than the healthy control term children. When behavior was assessed (Infant's Behavior Records): the preterms were significantly less goal directed; less attentive, and had lower endurance than the controls. When Bayley neurodevelomental was assessed: 1) the preterms performed significantly less well than the controls. 2) Low Bayley scores correlated with temperament scores of high rhythmicity, positive mood, low persistence and high threshold 3) Low Bayley scores correlated with IBR scores 4) No strong relationship between temperament characteristics and cognitive performance. Preterm infants had significantly lower MDI compared to full terms: • Preterm infants were different in 5/9 items of temperament profile compared to full terms: less active (p<0.008), more adaptive (p<0.02), less intense (p<0.01), more positive in mood (p<0.0004), lower in threshold to respond (p<0.0003) • Preterm infants were different in 3/5 items in IBR profile when compared to full terms: less goal directed, less attentive, lower in endurance Predictors evaluation: • From the perinatal risk factors: preeclampsia, SGA, PVL and IVH were not associated with developmental outcome or temperament profiles. • PVL, IVH were associated with shorter attention span (1/5 items in IBR profile); when preterms compared to full terms. • Duration of NICU stay was not associated with Bayley score • Duration of ventilation was not associated with Bayley score • Duration of ventilation and days in NICU were associated with the 5 items of IBR profile; Duration of ventilation was associated with 1/9 items of temperament profile	• Post hoc multiple comparisons were done between preterms and full terms for the multiple individual items of the tests used. • Cannot exclude selection bias • No matching between groups cannot exclude the presence of confounders. • Interactions between • Predictor may have masked some real associations; Possible interactions were not formally tested • Cannot exclude Diagnosis bias, as no information is given on the blinding of the personnel doing the outcome evaluation, of the child's PMHx.

Evidence Table 6B. Studies Evaluating Association of LBW to School Performance and Learning Disabilities Part I

Author, Year UI#	Demographics	Inclusion Criteria	Exclusion Criteria	Disease/Condition Type (N)	Study Design (Duration)
Hille 1994 8071753	Location: Netherlands Year of birth:1983 Description of group: VLBW Mean GA (range), wk: <32 weeks Mean BW (range), g: <1500 g Male: ND Race: ND Enrolled: 1338 Evaluated: 813 Number of sites: 1	Cases: Participants of the Project on Preterm and Small for Gestational Age Infants, a nationwide collaborative study 2) Perinatal data collection and follow-up until 2 years of age and assessments at 5 and 9 years 3) VLBW (very preterm) GA< 32 weeks at birth BW<1500 g.	ND	Cases: VLBW (or very preterm): 813 No control group	Prospective (single arm) cohort
Stathis 1999 99325758	Location: Australia Years of Birth: :1977-1986 Median GA (range), wk: 27.7(27.3-28.1) Mean BW (range), g: 860 (837-833) Male: 36% Race: ND Enrolled: 124 Evaluated: 87 Number of sites: 1	BW 500-999g survived to discharge Cared for in study NICU Enrolled in follow-up programs	ND	ELBW survived infants (87)	Prospective cohort (followed at 4, 8, 12, months)

Cherkes-Julkowski 1998 98262696	Location: ND
	Years of Birth: ND
	Mean GA (range), wk: ND
	Mean BW (range):
	  Cases: 4.14±1.87 lbs
	  Controls: 7.30±1.87 lbs
	Male:
	  Cases: 61%
	  Controls: 50%
	Race: ND
	SES: "middle class"
	Enrolled: 48
	Evaluated: 28 (20 controls)
	Number of sites: 1
		Preterm:
		<38 wks, BW<5 lbs, no congenital disorders, no retrolenteal fibroplasia, discharge from hospital prior to 42 wks conceptional age, mother willing to participate
		Controls: participats were enrolled in a longitudinal sudy before their second month of age
			ND	Preterms (28)
				
				Controls: full term infants (20)
					Retrospective cohort

Evidence Table 6B. Studies Evaluating Association of LBW to School Performance and Learning Disabilities

Part I

Author, Year UI#	Demographics	Inclusion Criteria	Exclusion Criteria	Disease/Condition Type (N)	Study Design (Duration)
Marlow 1993 8466264	Location: UK Years of birth:1980-1981 Description of group: VLBW Mean GA (range), wk: ND Mean BW (range), g: ≤1250 g Male: ND Race: ND Enrolled: 72 Evaluated: 51 Controls: 59 Number of sites: 1	Cases: VLBW ≤1250g at birth and without cerebral palsy at 6 years. Controls: 1) Control group (full term) matched for age, race, and sex, and school-matched.	Major disabilities (CP or major sensory impairment)	Cases: VLBW: 51 Controls: Full term/ controls: 59	Nonrandomized comparison trial

282

Evidence Table 6B. Studies Evaluating Association of LBW to School Performance and Learning Disabilities
Part II

Author, Year	Predictors	Predictor Measures	Outcomes	Outcome Measures
Hille 1994 8071753	General predictors: 1. BW 2. GA 3. Gender 4. Perinatal factors: congenital malformations, Apgar scores, intracranial hemorrhage, septicemia, assisted ventilation >7 days, serum bilirubin, thyroxine levels. 5. Socioeconomics 6. Performance at 5 years of age: Development, neuromotor function, speech/language, hyperactivity and school performance.	Assessment at 5 years of age: 1. Neurologic examination according to Touwen 2. Dutch test of speech and language development 3. Visual fields, acuity 4. Audiometry 5. Groningen Neurobehavioral concentration test 6. Child Behavior Checklist 7. Handedness 8. Kind of school 9. School results	At 9 years of age : School performance Special education	Questionnaire: kind of school (mainstream or special education), grade and need for extra help from teachers, remedial teaching, or speech therapy.
Stathis 1999 99325758	CNS Predictors 1) Other: head circumference category 2) Head growth velocity	Self-explanatory	**CNS:** Neurodevelopmental: Cognitive delay Behavioral disorders-ADHD School problems Learning disabilities	Academic problems--Answer questionnaires given to teacher ADHD--Dr. Paul rating scale McCarthy's scales
Cherkes-Julkowski 1998 98262696	General: GA Other: Mother perception of child competence	ND	**CNS:** Cognitive delay Neurodevelopmental School problem Neurological Impairment (NI) Attention Deficit Disorder (ADD) **Audiology:** Language	Cognitive delay, measured by Stanford-Binet School programs (school concerns = SC) Learning disabilities (LD) Neurological Impairment (NI) Attention deficit Disorder (ADD) Language impairment = LI – dx made by speech and language clinician

283

Evidence Table 6B. Studies Evaluating Association of LBW to School Performance and Learning Disabilities
Part II

Author, Year	Predictors	Predictor Measures	Outcomes	Outcome Measures
Marlow 1993 8466264	General predictors: VLBW	BW ≤ 1250g	At 8 years of age: School performance Behavior disorder	School performance: mathematics test (NFER Nelson), Schonell S1 graded word spelling test, Suffolk reading test, handwriting, fine motor skills. Behavior Measurements: parental questionnaire Rutter A(2), and teacher questionnaire using Rutter B(2) and Connors hyperactivity scale.

Evidence Table 6B. Studies Evaluating Association of LBW to School Performance and Learning Disabilities

Part III

Author, Year	Associations found	Potential Biases	Comments
Hille 1994 8071753	• School performance at 9 years of age is best predicted by performance at 5 years of age. • At 9 year of age, 19% were in special education and 81% in mainstream education. • At 9 years of age, only 44% of the nondisabled prematurely born children were in mainstream education at an age-appropriate level without special assistance. • GA <28 wks, BW < 1250 g, male gender and socioeconomics were significantly related to education outcome. Neonatal illnesses were not associated with school outcome at 9 years of age. • Majority of children having difficulty in school at 5 years of age had difficulty in school at 9 years of age.	Children labeled as having difficulty in school early in education (i.e. at 5 years of age) may continue to be treated as such within the system. Therefore independent evaluation of these children's performance at 9 years of age may reveal more useful information.	Internal validity A According to this study, early school problems are not transient.
Stathis 1999 99325758	Head circumference category at 8 months corrected age related to learning delay greater than one year when assessed at 6 years: HC Category n % with delay < 3rd percentile 23 61% (39, 80) 3rd to 10th 13 77% (46, 95) P = 0.004 > 10th 40 30% (17, 47) Head circumference category at 12 months CA did predict McCarthy General Cognitive index at six years, but head circumference category at 24 months CA did not significantly predict McCarthy CGI at 6 years. Head circumference and head growth velocity was not shown to have a relationship with attention deficit hyperactivity disorder. *Head circumference category < 10th vs. greater than 10th percentile at four and* *8 months corrected age were significantly associated with McCarthy CGI at* *6 years age*	One nursery High rate of patients lost to follow-up (30%) Small numbers: limited ability to detect small differences; high chances of type 2 error	Study was privately funded
Marlow 1993 8466264	• Even in the presence of normal IQ, premature children are more likely to underachieve in school compared to full-term peers. • Forty-eight percent in preterm group had difficulty in one or more subjects compared with 19% in full term group. • Both teachers and parents report behavior problems of restlessness, hyperactivity, inattention, unresponsive/apathetic, fearful/afraid of new situations. • Motor difficulties and mathematics test best correlate with later school performance problems.		Internal validity B

285

Evidence Table 7. Studies Evaluating Association of LBW to Ophthalmologic Outcomes

Part I

Author, Year UI#	Demographics	Inclusion Criteria	Exclusion Criteria	Disease/Condition Type (N)	Study Design (Duration)
Page 1993 94051493	Location: Canada Years of Birth: 1986-1987 Mean GA (range), wk: 27±1.8 (23-32) Mean BW (range), g: 942±197 (400-1250) Male: 38% Race: White 100% Enrolled: 138 Evaluated: 110 → 50 Number of sites: 1	BW<1250 g admitted to Toronto's Hospital for sick children Survived the neonatal periods and had at least one eye examination between 28 and 42 of life that documented the severity of ROP	No 12-month follow-up reports	VLBW infants at 12-month follow-up (110) VLBW infants at 24-months follow-up (50)	Retrospective cohort (12, 24 months)
Cryo-ROP 1994 94304375 *The original large population of CRYO-ROP	Location: US Years of Birth: 1/1986 to 11/1987 Mean GA (range), wk: 26.0±1.9 to 29.6±2.1 Mean BW (range), g: 781±156 to 1061±144 Male: 48% Race: White 56%, Black 35%, Hispanic 6%, Other 3% Enrolled: 4099 Evaluated: 2759 Number of sites: 23	BW < 1251 g Survived at least 28 days No serious ocular anomaly, such as cataract, glaucoma, or chorioretinitis, and no major systemic malformations Parental consent Initial eye examination by a study-certified ophthalmologist by 49 days after birth	Death <28 days; serious ocular anomaly or systemic malformations, lack of consent; first eyes exam with 4 qd Death (264) Lost to follow-up (1076)	Zone and Stage of ROP (2759): Zone I (46) Zone II, stage 3+, 9-12 sectors (139) Zone II, stage 3+, 5-8 sectors (64) Zone II, stage 3+, 1-4 sectors (47) Zone II, stage 3 (241) Zone II, stage 2 (484) Zone II, stage 1 (500) Zone III (319) Other ROP (22) No ROP (896)	Prospective cohort (1 year)

286

Evidence Table 7. Studies Evaluating Association of LBW to Ophthalmologic Outcomes

Part I

Author, Year UI#	Demographics	Inclusion Criteria	Exclusion Criteria	Disease/Condition Type (N)	Study Design (Duration)

Keith 1995 95288128	Location: UK
	Years of Birth: 1977-1992
	Mean GA (range), wk:
	  Sample 1: 26.0±2.3
	  Sample 2: 26.1±2.2
	Mean BW (range), g:
	  Sample 1: 783±136
	  Sample 2: 786±133
	Male: ND
	Race: ND
	Enrolled: 457
	Evaluated: 434
	Number of sites: 1
		ELBW infants, BW < 1000g
		Survival to hospital discharge
		Eye exams done
			ND
			
			Not seen by the ophthalmologist: transferred to another level-3 center for ongoing care (17); unknown reasons (6)
				Sample 1: ELBW survivors born 1977-1984 (145)
				Sample 2: ELBW survivors born 1985-1992 (312)
					Prospective cohort (16 years)

Foreman 1997 97271716	Location: UK
	Years of Birth: 4/1994-4/1996
	Mean GA (range), wk:
	  Cases: 29.38
	  Controls: 39.88
	Mean BW (range), g:
	  Cases: 1413±302
	  Controls: 3437±625
	Male: 63%
	Race: ND
	Enrolled: 114
	Evaluated: 16 (16 controls)
	Number of sites: 1
		Healthy preterm infants
		GA 27 –32 weeks; weight within the normal range for GA
		Normal on all criteria of Standard child health surveillance program from 7.5 to 48 months
		Each could be matched with FT control on gender, post-natal age at testing, and on SEC.
		Healthy controls from School population
		Controls: children drawn from a school population who were known to have been full-term, normal delivered and whose uneventful medical and developmental histories were confirmed by parents, general practitioners, and teachers
			ND	Healthy preterm infants (16)
				Controls: Matched full term controls (16)
					Prospective cohort (6.1 years)

Evidence Table 7. Studies Evaluating Association of LBW to Ophthalmologic Outcomes
Part I

Author, Year UI#	Demographics	Inclusion Criteria	Exclusion Criteria	Disease/Condition Type (N)	Study Design (Duration)
Tin 1998 99046171 *also in CNS table	Location: North of England Years of Birth: 1983, 1990-1991 Median GA (range), wk: ND Mean BW (range), g: ND Male: ND Race: ND Enrolled: 1983 (230); 1990-1 (566) Evaluated: 1983 (230); 1990-1 (566) Number of sites: 5	GA 23-31 weeks	ND	1983 cohort (230): Child reviewed without difficulty (204) Child traced with difficulty (14) Child seen with difficulty after child was traced (12) 1990 to 1991 (566): Child reviewed without difficulty (505) Child traced with difficulty (26) Child seen with difficulty after child was traced (35)	Prospective cohort *2 Cohorts of different time periods
Dogru 1999 99168711	Location: Japan Years of Birth: 4/1994-4/1996 Mean GA (range), wk: Sample 1: 27.6±2.9 Sample 2: 26.9±1.4 Sample 3: 26.3±3.1 Controls: 29.6±2.6 Mean BW (range), g: Sample 1: 1016±207 Sample 2: 836±178 Sample 3: 874±218 Controls: 1193±241 Male: 49% Race: ND Enrolled: 144 Evaluated: 78 (66 controls) Number of sites: 1	Premature infants (BW < 1500 g, GA < 37 weeks) with ROP Controls: randomly selected premature subjects with no ROP	Physical and mental disabilities or any CNS and ocular disorder	Premature infants: (Sample 1, 2, and 3): Premature infants with ROP (78) Sample 1: ROP stage 1 (53) Sample 2: ROP stage 2 (11) Sample 3: ROP stage 3 (14) Controls: Premature infants without ROP (66)	Prospective cohort (18-24 months)

Evidence Table 7. Studies Evaluating Association of LBW to Ophthalmologic Outcomes

Part I

Author, Year UI#	Demographics	Inclusion Criteria	Exclusion Criteria	Disease/Condition Type (N)	Study Design (Duration)
Pennefather 1999 20002011	Location: UK Years of Birth: 1/1/90-12/31/91 Mean GA (range), wk: ND Mean BW (range), g: ND	All surviving children <32wk GA born in geographically deprived region in Northern UK Survived to 2 years old	No examined at age 2 years old	Preterm infants (558)	Prospective cohort and retrospective review of patient records (2-3 years)
Pennefather 2000 20217908	Male: ND Race: ND Enrolled: 566 Evaluated: 558				
* This study also should be mentioned in multiple outcome and CNS table	Number of sites: ND				
Tin 2001 21143595	Location: North of England Years of Birth: 1990-1994 Median GA (range), wk: 23-27 Mean BW (range), g: ND	GA < 28 weeks Surviving (born 1990-1991) when 2 years old Surviving (born 1992-1994) when 18 months	ND	Sample 1: Preterm infants, SpO$_2$ 88-98% (123) Sample 2: Preterm infants, SpO$_2$ 70-90% (126)	Prospective cohort
*1990-1991 sample is same as 99046171	Male: ND Race: ND Enrolled: 1990-1 (781); 1992-1994 (ND) Evaluated: 249 (for current review) Number of sites: ND	Assessed for CP and ophthalmic For current review, only SpO$_2$ 88-98% and SpO$_2$ 70-90% groups were included			

Evidence Table 7. Studies Evaluating Association of LBW to Ophthalmologic Outcomes
Part II

Author, Year	Predictors	Predictor Measures	Outcomes	Outcome Measures

Page 1993 94051493	*General predictors:*
	1) Birth weight
	2) GA
	
	CNS predictors:
	1) Intracranial/ Intraventricular hemorrhage
	2) Periventricular leukomalacia
	
	Ophthalmology predictors:
	1) Retinopathy of prematurity
	2) Myopic at 12 months post-term
	
	Cardiovascular or pulmonary predictors:
	1) PDA
	2) Days ventilated
	3) Days in O$_2$
		ROP - ICROP
		Others not defined
		Myopic - >0.25 D
			Ophthalmology outcomes:
			Visual impairment
			Strabismus
			Refractive error
			  Myopia
			  Astigmatism
				Myopia - spherical equivalent of 0.25 diopters
				
				High Myopia - spherical equivalent of 4.0 diopters
				
				Astigmatism - > 1 diopter in any meridian or cycloplegic refraction
				
				Anisometropia - spherical equivalent >2 D between eyes (both refracted)

Cryo-ROP 1994 94304375
 	
*The original large population of CRYO-ROP
	Ophthalmology predictors:
	Retinopathy of prematurity
		ROP defined by examination according to the ICROP	**Ophthalmology:**
			Visual impairment
			Structural outcome
				ROP outcomes (structural):
				  I. Only peripheral changes, no mascular distortion
				  II. Mascular displacement
				  III. Retinal fold involving macula
				  IV. Retrolental opacity entotal retinal detachment and/or total pupillary occlusion to retinal detachment
				
				Functional outcome:
				  a. Normal fixation
				  b. Presence/absence of nystagmus
				  c. Strabismus
				  d. Refractive error (spherical equivalence)

Evidence Table 7. Studies Evaluating Association of LBW to Ophthalmologic Outcomes

Part II

Author, Year	Predictors	Predictor Measures	Outcomes	Outcome Measures
Keith 1995 95288128	General predictors: Birth cohort: 1977-1984 vs. 1985-1999	ND	Ophthalmology outcomes: 1) blindness 2) severe ROP	Eye exam with ICROP classification. Sheridan-Gardner test - visual outcome. Snellen's eye chart - visual outcome.
Foreman 1997 97271716	GA	28-32 week prematurity vs. full term controls	CNS Attention skill Ophthalmology Visual-perceptual skills Visual-motor skills	Point-to-Target test Complex visual search test Cartoon comparison test Overlapping figures Goillin incomplete figures
Tin 1998 99046171 *also in CNS table	General: GA (23-31 wks)	ND	CNS: CP Neurodevelopmental: Mental retardation (IQ < 75) Other: disability (severe, sever sensorimotor) Other: development - assessed by Griffith's mental and developmental scales Ophthalmology Visual impairment Blindness Other: Severe ROP with Cryotherapy	Definition of "severe disability" and "severe sensorimotor disability" were not given in this article. They referred to the wrong reference for these definitions, therefore, I am unable to find the definitions. Reference population for Griffith's scales were "preterm babies in the study S serious sensorimotor disability"
Dogru 1999 99168711	ROP	Staging of retinopathy was based on International Classification of Retinopathy of Prematurity (The Committee for the Classification of Retinopathy of Prematurity, 1984)	Ophthalmology: Visual acuity	Preferential looking method

Evidence Table 7. Studies Evaluating Association of LBW to Ophthalmologic Outcomes
Part II

Author, Year	Predictors	Predictor Measures	Outcomes	Outcome Measures
Pennefather 1999 20002011	*General Predictor:* GA **CNS:** 1) IVH 2) Periventricular leukomalacia 3) Ventriculomegaly/Ventricular Dilation **Ophthalmology:** 1) ROP 2) Refractive error	ND	**CNS:** Cerebral palsy	Retrospective review of patient records
Pennefather 2000 20217908 *** This study also should be mentioned in multiple outcome and CNS table**	Other: Family Hxg strabismus, Developmental disability, CP		**Ophthalmology:** Visual impairment (cortical)(CVI) Cicatricial ROP Strabismus	Visual acuity, visual fields
Tin 2001 21143595 ***1990-1991 sample is same as 99046171**	*General predictors:* GA *Other predictors:* SpO₂ policies (88-98% vs.70-90%)	SpO₂ policies were obtained retrospectively	**CNS:** Cerebral palsy **Ophthalmology:** Blindness Severe ROP Rx with cryotherapy	Threshold ROP: (Cryo-ROP definition) stage 3 plus acute ROP extensive permanent cicatricial retinal scanning

Evidence Table 7. Studies Evaluating Association of LBW to Ophthalmologic Outcomes

Part III

Author, Year	Associations found	Potential Biases	Comments
Page 1993 94051493	Outcome: Incidence of myopia at 12 mo postterm age: Overall incidence of myopia in cohort (BW<1251 g) was 15% (4.5% severe myopia) At 12 months age: Increased severity of ROP predicted increased severity of myopia (p=0.001) Overall, 16% of infants had myopia, and 4.5% had severe myopia at 12 months age. To show incidence of myopia according to severity of ROP: 10% of infants with No or Stage 1 ROP had myopia 54% of infants with Stage 3 ROP had myopia 23% of infants with Stage 3 ROP had severe myopia The likelihood of myopia at 12 months age doubled with each increment in ROP stage. - At 24 months age: 80% of 50 children showed deteriorating vision. - 13 of 16 (81%) showed worsening of their myopia after 12 months age. Overall, the incidence of myopia and severe myopia increased among 50 infants followed to 2 years: 38% had myopia 0.25-4 Diopters; 24% had myopia >4 Diopters. BW was negatively associated with incidence of myopia (p=0.002). BW<750 g 3.2 fold odds of myopia vs. 751-1000 g. - BW <750 g 10 fold odds of myopia vs. 1001-1250 g. - Incidence of strabismus was positively associated with severity of ROP (e.g. no ROP 6% vs. Strabismus at 12 mo in infants who had Stage 3 ROP 38%). There was further increased diagnosis of strabismus at 24 months age. Months of age in infants who had had Stage 3 ROP (38% to 62%). 100% of infants who had Grade III or IV IVH had strabismus	Retrospective NB and ophthalmic chart review 36% eye reports available at 24 months. Also 24 month sample was biased toward children at greatest risk of myopia. Children with normal eye results at 12 months age were discharged from further follow-up at 18 months post-term age. This may have led to underdiagnosis of myopia due to lack of detection of progressive myopia. Infants born 1986-1987 (not a bias, but a limitation) Used other pop reference figures for norms	No data on funding source This study demonstrates the importance of low birth weight, ROP severity, and IVH in the development of myopia and strabismus.

293

Evidence Table 7. Studies Evaluating Association of LBW to Ophthalmologic Outcomes
Part III

Author, Year	Associations found	Potential Biases	Comments
Cryo-ROP 1994 94304375	The more posterior the zone of ROP and /or the greater the extent of Stage 3+ ROP, the worse the structural and functional ophthalmic outcomes. Zone II without plus disease, Zone III, or no ROP was associated with low rate of unfavorable outcome. CNS injury may affect ophthalmic function (e.g. nystagmus and strabismus).	(None)	Study was government and privately funded Biweekly or weekly eye exams until fully vascularized or until threshold ROP (>5 contiguous or 8 cumulative clock hours) stage 3 with plus disease. Only data from eyes that served as controls (untreated) are included in this segment.

*The original large population of CRYO-ROP	Visual function by ROP Classification
	ICROP Abnl.Fixation %Nystagmus %Strabismus
	Zone I............................44%...............6%...........25%
	Zone II
	   Stage 3, 9-12 sectors 57%...........39%...........33%
	Zone II,
	   Stage 1...................2%...............1%............10%
	No ROP..................1%...............1%............6%
	
	% of Eyes with refractive error (≥2 diopters myopia) by ROP severity
	No or Stage 1 ROP (<5%)
	Zone II, Stage3+, 9-12 sectors (62%)
	Zone I (40%)		

Keith 1995 95288128	**Any ROP:** Birth Cohort 1977 –1984 (141) 68/141 48.2 % 1985-1992 (293) 105/293 35.6% OR=0.60 (0.40-0.90) P<0.02 **Severe ROP:** 1977 –1984 (141) 36/141 25.4 % 1985-1992 (293) 52/293 17.4% OR=0.62 (0.38-1.02) NS **Blindness:** 1977 –1984 (141) 2/141 1.4 % 1985-1992 (293) 2/293 0.6% OR=0.43 (0.05-3.5) NS	Data are from care center No outborn infants in either cohort so data are not generalizable to outborn ELBW infants Twenty-three surviving ELBW's could not be located to determine ROP status.	No data on funding source 16 year study; 1001 ELBW infants; 457 survived to discharge; 434 seen by same ophthalmologist. Twenty children not seen by ophthalmologist.

294

Evidence Table 7. Studies Evaluating Association of LBW to Ophthalmologic Outcomes
Part III

Author, Year	Associations found	Potential Biases	Comments
Foreman 1997 97271716	*Visual-motor coordination:* PT v. FT NS diff **Visual-spatial attention skill**: Significant difference between Preterm and Full term in complex visual search scores (failure to find figure and latency to find) and cartoon comparisons PT 2.94 FT 0.81 P<0.05 *Visual-form perception*: NS difference between Preterm and full term in latency to respond to overlapping figure and Gollin incomplete figure tests. PT 22.2% FT 21.9% NS diff Compared to matched, FT controls, the PT school age group performed poorly on 2 measures visual-motor tests. Thus in the absence of detectable disability, prematurity is associated with visual-motor and attentional impairments that persist through 16 years age.	Small sample size Incomplete data analysis	No data on funding source
Tin 1998 99046171 ***also in CNS table**	*Result of 1983 cohort at 6 years:* **Severe disability:** Sample 1: 4.4%, Sample 2 : 2.1%, Sample 3: 50% *IQ < 75 without sensorimotor disability:* Sample 1 : 4.9%, Sample 2: 0, Sample 3 : 25% *Severe sensorimotor disability:* Sample 1: 5.9%, Sample 2 : 21.4%, Sample 3 : 41.7% *Severe sensorimotor or cognitive disability:* Sample 1 : 8.4% (5 - 13.1%, 95% CI) Sample 2 : 21.4% (4.7-50.8%) Sample 3: 41.7% (15.2-72.3%) **Result of 1990 cohort at 2 years:** *Severe disability:* Sample 1: 7.9%, Sample 2: 15.4%, Sample 3: 57.1% **High f/u rate is critical because it may underestimate incidence of the outcome.**	No definitions of outcome, incomplete methods description, wrong reference	Study was privately funded
Dogru 1999 9168711	Stage 3 ROP had significantly lower visual acuity scores compared to stage 1- 2 or no ROP at 18-24 months (P<0.0001)	(None)	No data on funding source

295

Evidence Table 7. Studies Evaluating Association of LBW to Ophthalmologic Outcomes
Part III

Author, Year	Associations found	Potential Biases	Comments
Pennefather 1999 20002011	Strabismus in 70/558 (12.5%) infants GA<32 week. **The incidence of strabismus increased with decreasing GA (p=0.0004),** increasing severity of ROP (p=0.0001), and decreasing general developmental quotient (GMDS) (p<0.0001).	Prospective evaluation but retrospective collection of neonatal data; therefore, probable incomplete collection of variable reason for present and absent data	No data on funding source
Pennefather 2000 20217908 *** This study also should be mentioned in multiple outcome and CNS table**	Stabismus present in 28 (52%) of patients with CP (P< 0.001) **OR (95% CI) of Strabismus if following predictor was present:** Cicatricial ROP: 4.94 (1.1-22.12), p0.037 Fam Hx of Strabismus: 4.15 (2.19-7.88), p<0.00005 Refractive Error: 2.71 (1.3-5.66), p=0.008 GMDS 78-100: 3.34 (1.46-7.64), p =0.004 GMDS <77: 46.2 (17.1-125), p<0.00005 This study confirms findings of other studies that strabismus is increased in premature infants with decreasing GA and is increased with increasing severity of ROP and CP. Independent factors related to strabismus are cicatricial ROP, refractive error, family hx of strabismus, and developmental delay (especially delayed hand-eye coordination)	No demographic data was report (the cohort was described elsewhere)	
Tin 2001 21143595 ***1990-1991 sample is same as 99046171**	Premature infants who had oxygen saturation range (SpO2) between 88-98% for at least first 8 weeks of life developed severe ROP requiring treatment with cryotherapy four times greater than infants who had SpO2 range between 70-90. Incidence of severe ROP with Cryotherapy (SpO2 range 88-98%)=28% Incidence of severe ROP with Cryotherapy (SpO2 range 70-80%)= 6% Incidence of Blindness in the two study groups: Premature infants with SpO2 range 88-98%: 4 / 65 Premature infants with SpO2 range 70-80%: 0 / 65 Incidence of CP in the two study groups: Premature infants with SpO2 range 88-98%: 17% Premature infants with SpO2 range 70-80% 15% The lower SpO2 range was not associated with difference in CP. Differences in SpO2 policies (70-90% vs. 88-98%) did have a major impact on the proportion who developed severe ROP, but had no effect on survival or on incidence of CP among premature survivors.	Different pulse oximeters No attempt to document real SpO2 or how often SpO2 fell outside recommended ranges (or vice versa). Narrow limits broached often > wider limits.	ROP screening conformed to national guidelines

Evidence Table 8. Studies of Treatment Effects for LBW Infants with Retinopathy of Prematurity (ROP)

Part I

Author, Year UI#	Demographics	Inclusion Criteria	Exclusion Criteria	Disease/Condition Type (N)	Study Design (Duration)
Cryo-ROP, 1990, 1996, and 2001 (x3) 91024693, 96180078, 21375786, 21375787, 21375788 Repka 1998 98426775 *sample from the large population of 94304375 (CRYO-ROP)	Location: US Years of Birth: from 1/1986 to 11/1987 Mean GA (range), wk: 1 yr follow-up: 26.3±1.8 5.5 yr follow-up: 26.3±1.7 (bilateral threshold ROP; 26.3±1.8 (asymmetric threshold ROP) 10 yr follow-up: 26.3±1.8 Mean BW (range), g: 1 yr follow-up: 800±165 5 yr follow-up: 801±165 (bilateral threshold ROP, 800±165 (asymmetric threshold ROP) 10 yr follow-up: 800±165 Male: ND Race: ND Enrolled: 291 Evaluated: 246 (at 1-year exam), 234 (at 5.5-year exam), 247 (at 10-year exam) Number of sites: 23	BW < 1251 g Survived at least 28 days Diagnosis of threshold ROP	ND {(At 1-year follow-up: Died before the 1-year follow-up (36) Unable to follow-up for the 1-year exam (14) At 5.5-year & 10-year follow-up: Died before the 5.5-year & 10-year exam (36)} Lost to follow-up for the 10-year exam (8)	At 1-year exam: VLBW infants with ROP (241) At 5.5-year exam: VLBW infants with ROP (234) – bilateral threshold ROP (191); asymmetric threshold ROP (43) At 10-year exam: VLBW infants with ROP (234)	Randomized controlled trial (1, 5.5, 10 years)
Cryotherapy for Retinopathy of Prematurity Group 1993 93191597	Location: US Years of Birth: 1986-1987 Mean GA (range), wk: 26.3±1.8 Mean BW (range), g: 800±165 Male: ND Race: ND Enrolled: 236 Evaluated: 236 Number of sites: 23	All infants <1251g, who participated in CRYO-ROP Multicenter trial and had threshold (severe) ROP.	See original study	Infants with threshold ROP (236)	3.5 years

Evidence Table 8. Studies of Treatment Effects for LBW Infants with Retinopathy of Prematurity (ROP)
Part I

Author, Year UI#	Demographics	Inclusion Criteria	Exclusion Criteria	Disease/Condition Type (N)	Study Design (Duration)

Algawi 1994 95001766	Location: UK
	Years of Birth:
	  Sample 1: 2/1992-11/1992
	  Sample 2: 1/1987-2/1992
	Mean GA (range), wk:
	  Sample 1: 24-32
	  Sample 2: 25-30
	Mean BW (range), g:
	  Sample 1:700-1200
	  Sample 2: 620-1500
	Male: 53%
	Race: ND
	Enrolled: 32
	Evaluated: 32
	Number of sites: 1
		Premature infants with threshold ROP (stage 3+ disease of 5 or more contiguous clock hours [30° sector] or 8 cumulative clock hours) or more	ND	Sample 1: Laser Treatment (12)
				Sample 2: Cryotherapy Treatment (20)
					Prospective cohort

Ling 1995 95391616	Location: UK Years of Birth: 1992-1993 Median GA (range), wk: 25.5 (24-27) Median BW (range), g: 725 (589-887) Male: 38% Race: White 100% Enrolled: 13 Evaluated: 13 Number of sites: 1	All premature infants in 1 unit who developed threshold ROP and treated with diode laser therapy	ND	Infants with ROP treated with Diode laser (13)	Before and after trial (6, 12, and 18 months)

Evidence Table 8. Studies of Treatment Effects for LBW Infants with Retinopathy of Prematurity (ROP)
Part I

Author, Year UI#	Demographics	Inclusion Criteria	Exclusion Criteria	Disease/Condition Type (N)	Study Design (Duration)
Connolly 1998 984267776	Location: US Years of Birth: 11/1989-5/1992 Mean GA (range), wk: 25.4 (23-32) Mean BW (range), g: 731 (440-1318) Male: 44% Race: ND Enrolled: 52 Evaluated: 25 Number of sites: 1	Premature infants with symmetric threshold ROP underwent bilateral treatment	ND (Stage 4 or 5 ROP in one or both eyes Refused to cooperate with monocular occlusion during Snellen testing Limited cognitive ability that precluded Snellen or illiterate e-chart acuity testing)	Sample 1: Laser Treatment (21 eyes) Sample 2: Cryotherapy Treatment (21 eyes)	RCT and follow-up (5.8 [4.3-7.6] years)
Shalev 2001 21331013	Location: US Years of Birth: 1991-1992 Mean GA (range), wk: 24.8 (23.4-27.0) Mean BW (range), g: 631 (540-846) Male: 60% Race: 30% Enrolled: 19 Evaluated: 10 Number of sites: 1	Threshold ROP treated with laser or cryotherapy	ND Lost to follow-up (2) Died at 4 months of age (2) Refusal (3)	Infants with threshold ROP (10)	RCT with prospective follow-up (7 years and 6 months)
O'Connor 2002 21635822	Location: UK Years of birth: 1985-1987 Mean GA (range), wk: 31.06±3.09 Mean BW (range), g: 1400 (iqr 1150, 1562) Male: ND Race: ND Enrolled: 505 Evaluated: 505 Number of sites: 5	All infants <1701g, who survived 3 weeks. Born to mothers who were residents in the study areas, admitted to one of 5 NICUs.	ND	Premature infants (254) Control (169)	10-12 years

299

Evidence Table 8. Studies of Treatment Effects for LBW Infants with Retinopathy of Prematurity (ROP)
Part II

Author, Year	Predictors	Predictor Measures	Outcomes	Outcome Measures
Cryo-ROP, 1990, 1996, and 2001 (x3) 91024693, 96180078, 21375786, 21375787, 21375788 Repka 1998 98426775 *sample from the large population of 94304375 (CRYO-ROP)	*Ophthalmology predictors:* Threshold retinopathy of prematurity At 5.5-year & 10-year follow-up: Cryotherapy vs. No Cryotherapy	At least 5 contiguous clock hours or 8 cumulative clock hours of stage 3 ROP in zone 1 or 2 in the presence of "plus disease" (dilation and tortuosity of the posterior retinal vessels) Monocular visual acuity (using log of minimal angle of resolution visual acuity chart)	**Ophthalmology:** Visual impairment (visual acuity) Structural outcome Blindness Distance snellen acuity Near snellen acuity Visual field Medical and surgical ophthalmologic interventions Cerebrospinal fluid shunting surgery	Visual acuity - • "normal": ≥1.6 cycles per degree • "below normal": 8.0 to <1.6 cycles per degree • "poor": <0.8 cycles per degree • "blind": eyes judged to have no light perception, eyes for which the tester was unable to estimate acuity, which were judged by a physician to have total retinal detachment Structural outcome - • Posterior retinal fold • Retinal detachment involving zone 1 of the posterior pole • Retrolental tissue or "mass" obscuring the view of the posterior pole Favorable Functional outcome: Favorable visual acuity: better than 20/200 Unfavorable visual acuity: worse than 20/200 or blind Goldmann perimetry to measure visual field extent along 8 meridian using V4e and III 4 e stimuli
Cryotherapy for Retinopathy of Prematurity Group 1993 93191597	Retinopathy of Prematurity (ROP) (Specifically threshold ROP treated with cryotherapy or no cryotherapy)	Threshold ROP as per CRYO-ROP definition.	**Visual impairment** Blindness	Visual acuity (HOTV, Grating) Unfavorable outcome (HOTV 20/200 or worse, Grating <6.4 cycles per degree; blind): this outcome is combination of poor + blind Myopia:≥2 <6 diopters; ≥6 diopters

Evidence Table 8. Studies of Treatment Effects for LBW Infants with Retinopathy of Prematurity (ROP)

Part II

Author, Year	Predictors	Predictor Measures	Outcomes	Outcome Measures
Algawi 1994 95001766	Ophthalmology Retinopathy	ND	**Ophthalmology:** Visual impairment: Refractive error Visual fixation Preferential looking	Visual functions were assessed by either fixation pattern or preferential looking technique
Ling 1995 95391616	ROP	Threshold as for Cryo-ROP trial	**Ophthalmology** Visual function	Favorable outcome (anatomical) defined as a normal posterior funus on BIO exam performed by observer who had not done Rx. Functional outcomes assessed using Keeler preferential looking cords acuity greater or equal to 0.8 cycles per degger defined 1 yr. Age
Connolly 1998 984267776	ROP	Threshold as for Cryorop trial - 5 or more contiguous or 8 cumulative clock-hours of stage 3 ROP in zone I or II in the presence of "plus" disease	**Ophthalmology Outcomes:** Visual impairment Refractive error Visual acuity	Visual acuity 20/50 or better =good Visual acuity 20/60 or worse = poor
Shalev 2001 21331013	ROP	Threshold as for Cryorop trial	**Ophthalmology** Visual function outcome Structural outcome	Favorable outcome = normal posterior fundus. Refraction by retinoscopy Functional outcomes: Keeper preferential looking cards . Favorable function was grating acuity greater than or equal to 0.8 cycles/degree (as per CRYO ROP study at 1 year)

301

Evidence Table 8. Studies of Treatment Effects for LBW Infants with Retinopathy of Prematurity (ROP)
Part II

Author, Year	Predictors	Predictor Measures	Outcomes	Outcome Measures
O'Connor 2002 21635822	Birth weight ROP	BW self-explanatory (grams) ROP not stated, but c/w ICROP	**Visual impairment** Blindness	Visual acuity: Normal (20/20); ≥Moderately reduced = worse than 20/40. Contrast sensitivity (Pelli Robson chart) Steroacuity (TNO plates) Perimetry (visual fields) (Damato campimeter) Color vision (desaturated D15 test) Strabismus (cover test and prism test) Refractive error (cycloplegic refraction) Eye size and dimensions of its components (N.D.)

Evidence Table 8. Studies of Treatment Effects for LBW Infants with Retinopathy of Prematurity (ROP)

Part III

Author, Year	Associations found	Potential Biases	Comments
Cryo-ROP, 1990, 1996, and 2001 (x3) 91024693, 96180078, 21375786, 21375787, 21375788	**At 1-year follow-up:** Fundus photography: Unfavorable posterior pole outcome at 1 yr Cryotherapy Rx 191 eyes 25.7% Control 194 eyes 47.4% P<0.001 Unfavorable structural outcome (retinal detachment, macular fold, etc) at 1 yr Cryotherapy Rx 208 eyes 49% Control 203 eyes 66% Unfavorable functional (Teller Visual Acuity) outcome at 1 yr Cryotherapy Rx 160 35% Control 158 56.3%	(None)	Study was government and private funded 5 ½ year follow-up of preterm infants with BW <1251 g with Threshold ROP randomized to cryotherapy vs. no cryotherapy groups. Both had high incidence of blindness, impaired visual acuity, and unfavorable outcome. Unfavorable outcomes were significantly less in cryotherapy group vs. control group. Excellent long-term (10 yr) ophthalmic follow-up of PT infants with severe ROP. Cryotherapy assoc with significantly less unfavorable visual function outcome and less unfavorable structural outcome. >44% of cryo Rx eyes have unfavorable visual outcome and 62% have unfavorable structural outcome. Threshold ROP with or without Rx is high for adverse long-term outcome. Infants with BW<1251 g with ROP underwent a large number of ophthalmic interventions through the first 5.5 years of life. Long-term costs of extreme prematurity and ROP include initial ablative therapy for ROP and societal loss due to visual impairment or blindness and ongoing costs for caring for eye problems.
Repka 1998 98426775 **sample from the large population of 94304375 (CRYO-ROP)**	**At 5.5-year follow-up:** Visual acuity Unfavorable outcome: Threshold ROP (control: no cryotherapy) 62% Threshold ROP CRYOtherapy 47% Greater reduction in unfavorable visual acuity outcome in cryo group (P<0.005) **Unfavorable structural outcome** Threshold ROP (control: no cryotherapy) 45% Threshold ROP CRYOtherapy 27% Greater reduction in unfavorable structural outcome in cryotherapy group (P<0.001) **Blindness** Threshold ROP (control: no cryotherapy) 48% Threshold ROP CRYOtherapy 32% Greater reduction in blindness in cryotherapy group (P<0.001) **Visual acuity 20/40 or better** Threshold ROP (control: no cryotherapy) 17% Thresdhold ROP CRYOtherapy 13% No significant difference between groups with respect to proporation of infants with visual acuity 20/40 or better (P=0.19). Among children who had Threshold ROP treated with cryotherapy: 226 / 257 had ocular intervention in addition to cryotherapy (0.9% interventions per child) Vitrectomy 26% (66/257); Scleral buckling 3% (8/257); Lensectomy 18%; Glaucoma medical treatment 4%; Glucoma surgery 2%; amblopia treatment 20%; Strabismus surgery 10%; Cataract surgery 2%; Enucleation 2%; Ventriculoperitoneal shunt (VPS) 11% Among children in the Natural History Cohort with variable ROP: 239 ocular interventions (0.4% interventions per child) Strabismus 6%; Amblyopia Rx 7% (3% if no ROP); VPS 3%		

303

Evidence Table 8. Studies of Treatment Effects for LBW Infants with Retinopathy of Prematurity (ROP)
Part III

Author, Year	Associations found	Potential Biases	Comments
Cryo-ROP, 1990, 1996, and 2001 (x3) 91024693, 96180078, 21375786, 21375787, 21375788	**At 10-year follow-up:** **Unfavorable** Visual outcomes (functional) in Threshold ROP. Comparison of Threshold ROP eyes treated with CRYO vs. Control. Distance Snellen Acuity (≥20/200) CRYO Rx 44% Control 62% Near Snellen Acuity CRYO Rx 43% Control 62%		
Repka 1998 98426775	Blindness CRYO Rx 33% Control 50% Unfavorable Visual Acuity		
Continued	Zone I/Threshold ROP/ CRYO Rx 94% Zone I/Threshold ROP/Control 94% Unfavorable structural outcome Zone I/Threshold ROP/ CRYO Rx 88% Zone I/Threshold ROP/Control 94% Although cryotherapy was beneficial in reducing unfavorable structural and functional outcome vs. no treatment in Threshold ROP eyes, infants with threshold ROP still were at high risk for unfavorable outcome even with cryotherapy, especially infants with Threshold Zone 1 ROP.Vii Visual fields at 10 years age in children enrolled in the CRYO ROP trial who had history of Threshold ROP (cryotherapy vs. control). Visual fields (with or without cryotherapy) were significantly smaller with severe ROP Visual fields in treated eyes were reduced by 30-37% vs. no ROP. Visual fields in control eyes were reduced by 27-33% compared to no ROP. Cryotherapy vs. control preserved sight and visual field in infants with severe ROP. Visual field area was 24 to 26% larger in CRYO Rx eyes vs. Control. Comparison of sighted treated eyes vs. sighted control eyes revealed that cryotherapy reduced visual field by small amount (5%).		

304

Evidence Table 8. Studies of Treatment Effects for LBW Infants with Retinopathy of Prematurity (ROP)
Part III

Author, Year	Predictors/ Conditions	N	Outcome Category	Outcome of Interest/ Instruments used	% with Outcome	Methods of Correlation	Potential Biases	Comments
Cryotherapy for Retinopathy of Prematurity Group 1993 93191597	Cryotherapy	203	vision	Unfavorable outcome HOTV acuity	47%	Cryo group had 19% reduction in unfavorable outcome for HOTV (p<0.01)		
	No Cryotherapy	203	vision	Unfavorable outcome HOTV acuity	58% unfavorable outcome			
	Cryotherapy	193	vision	Unfavorable outcome Grating acuity	52%	Cryo group had 20% reduction in unfavorable outcome for grating (p<0.01)		
	No Cryotherapy	193	vision	Unfavorable outcome Grating acuity	66%			
	Cryotherapy		vision	Myopia ≥2 <6 diopters	20%	More treated eyes had myopia than control eyes. Data not shown is that more control eyes could not be refracted.		
	No Cryotherapy		vision	Myopia ≥2 <6 diopters	15.5%			
	Cryotherapy		vision	Myopia ≥6 diopters	37.7%			
	No Cryotherapy		vision	Myopia ≥6 diopters	27.2%			

Evidence Table 8. Studies of Treatment Effects for LBW Infants with Retinopathy of Prematurity (ROP)
Part III

Author, Year	Associations found	Potential Biases	Comments
Algawi 1994 95001766	Myopia Treat with Laser 6/15 (40%) (Spher Equiv –1.5 to –3.5 D) Treat with Cryotherapy 23/25 (92%) (Spher Equiv –0.5 to –8.0 D) Significantly more myopia in cryotherapy vs. laser group (P=0.0006) Hypermetropia <+3.0 Diopters Treat with Laser 9/15 (60%) Treat with Cryotherapy 2/25 (8%) Clinical significant astigmatism (no significant difference between groups (P=0.4). Treat with Laser 5/15 Treat with Cryotherapy 5/25	Small sample size Cohorts treated at different time, not concurrent and not randomized	No data on funding source There is a high incidence of myopia following treatment for threshold ROP. Myopia occurred less often in the laser treated group vs. cryotherapy treated group.
Ling 1995 95391616	Visual outcome of Threshold ROP treated with diode laser: Structural Outcome (as defined by Cryotherapy Multicenter Trial) at 19.5 months age (range 9.7-25.5. mo) was favorable in all 13 patients (25 eyes). Functional outcome at the same follow-up (n=13): 3 with strabismus; 1 myopic; grating visual acuity (Keeler preferential looking cards) ranged 2.9-14.5 cycles per degree. 7 uniocular and 6 binocular acuity assessments fell within the CRYO-ROP definition of favorable acuity at 1 year of age (≥0.8 cycles per degree uniocular)	(None)	No data on funding source

Evidence Table 8. Studies of Treatment Effects for LBW Infants with Retinopathy of Prematurity (ROP)
Part III

Author, Year	Associations found	Potential Biases	Comments
Connolly 1998 984267776		Excluded large numbers of subjects	No data on funding source

	Laser Treated Threshold ROP	Cryotherapy Treated Threshold ROP	Total
Visual Acuity 20/50 or better	17	8	25
Visual Acuity 20/60 or worse	4	13	17
Total	21	21	42

81% of laser-treated vs. 38 % of cryotherapy treated Threshold ROP had good visual acuity outcome (VA 20/50 or better). The odds that a laser treated eye had a good visual outcome were 6.91 greater than threshold ROP eyes treated with cyrotherapy (95% CI 1.7- 28).

Refractive Error: On average, 23 cryotherapy eyes had a mean spherical equivalent of --5.08 Diopters vs. –3.05 Diopters for 23 laser treated eyes P=0.0072). Thus, cryotherapy eyes had greater amount of myopia than laser treated eyes.

Summary: The odds that eyes treated with laser therapy would have best-corrected visual acuity of 20/50 or better was almost 7 times greater than cryotherapy treated eyes. Also, laser treated eyes had less myopia than cryotherapy treated eyes. Thus, the results suggest that laser photocoagulation for threshold ROP was more likely to result in good visual outcome with less myopia compared to cryotherapy treatment.

Author, Year	Associations found	Potential Biases	Comments
Shalev 2001 21331013	**Associations:** All 10 Laser treated eyes had favorable structural outcome; 2 of 8 cryotherapy eyes had unfavorable structural outcome.	Small numbers for randomized comparison. It is not clear how similar were the groups in terms of original threshold ROP (zone I vs. II)	No data on funding source

Laser-treated vs. cryotherapy treated threshold eyes had more favorable outcome.

	Laser	Cryotherapy	P
Geometric visual acuity	20/33	20/133	0.03
Range	(20/20-20/70)	(20/25 to phthisis)	
Mean refractive error(D)	-6.5	-8.25	0.27

Conclude: Laser therapy for threshold ROP may have long-term visual function advantages over cryotherapy.

Evidence Table 8. Studies of Treatment Effects for LBW Infants with Retinopathy of Prematurity (ROP)
Part III

Author, Year	Associations found						Potential Biases	Comments
	Predictors/Conditions	N	Outcome Category	Outcome of Interest/Instruments used	% with Outcome	Methods of Correlation		
O'Connor 2002 21635822	Full term / Control	169	Visual function	Distance Acuity (Left eye)	-0.08 (-0.1,0.01)			
	BW <1701 all / Premature cohort	254	Visual function	Distance Acuity (Left eye)	0.0 (-0.08,0.1)			
	No ROP / Premature cohort	126	Visual function	Distance Acuity (Left eye)	0.0(-0.08,0.04)			
	Stage 3 or 4 ROP / Premature cohort	7	Visual function	Distance Acuity (Left eye)	0.34(0.21,0.605)			
	Full term / Control	169	Visual function	Binocular Distance Acuity	Normal 93% ≥Moderately reduced 0%	P<0.001 between control vs. premature cohort		
	BW <1701 all / Premature cohort	254	Visual function	Binocular Distance Acuity	Normal 76% ≥Moderately Reduced 3.5%			

Evidence Table 9. Studies Evaluating Association of LBW and Pulmonary Outcome

Author, Year UI#	Demographics	Inclusion Criteria	Exclusion Criteria	Disease/Condition Type (N)	Study Design (Duration)
Als 1994 94358983 (CNS+ Pulmonary)	Location: US Years of Birth: ND Median GA (range), wk: Experiment: 27.1±1.6 Control: 26.5±1.4 Median BW (range), g: Experiment: 827±173 Control: : 862±145 Male: Experiment: 45% Control: 61% Race: Black Experiment: 40% Control: 17% SES I, II/III/IV, and V: Experiment: 45%, 20%, 35% Control: 56%, 17%, 27% Enrolled: 43 Evaluated: 38 Number of sites: 1	BW < 1250 g GA < 30 weeks and more than 24 weeks of estimated GA at birth Mechanical ventilation starting within the first 3 hrs after birth and lasting longer than 24 hrs in the first 48 hrs Alive at 48 hrs Absence of chromosomal or other major genetic anomalies, congenital infections, and known fetal exposure to drugs of addiction Singleton At least one family member with some English-language facility Telephone access Living within the greater Boston area	ND	Experiment: VLBW infants participated in individualized developmental care (20) Controls: VLBW infants received standard care (18)	Randomized controlled trial (2 weeks and 9 months)
Chye 1995 95314864	Location: Australia Years of Birth: 1989 to 1990 Mean GA (range), wk: Cases: 28±1.58 Controls: 28.63±1.26 Mean BW (range), g: Cases: 1055± 234 Controls: 1077±215 Male: 56% Race: ND Enrolled: 80 Evaluated: 78 (78 controls) Number of sites: 1	Cases: 26-33 week GA infants with BPD and discharged home Controls: 26-32 week GA infants without BPD admitted to the hospital within 1 year of the cases, matched for BW with the cases in broad categories (<1000 g, 1000-1499 g and ≥1500 g)	Cases: Trisomy 21 (2)	Cases: Preterm infants with BDP (78) Sample 2: Preterm infants without BPD (78) Subgroups of cases at 12 months corrected age follow-up: Sample 1: BPD no Home O₂ (58) Sample 2: BPD with Home O₂ (20)	Case-control study

Evidence Table 9. Studies Evaluating Association of LBW and Pulmonary Outcome

Author, Year UI#	Demographics	Inclusion Criteria	Exclusion Criteria	Disease/Condition Type (N)	Study Design (Duration)
Kraybill 1995 95264242	Location: USA Years of Birth: 1986-1989 Mean GA: (F/up at 1 year) Sample 1: 28.2 ±1.9 Sample 2: 28.1 ±2.0 Mean BW: Sample 1: 1022 ±177 Sample 2: 1028 ±184 Male: Sample 1: 51% Sample 2: 52% Race: Sample 1: White: 21%, Black: 53%, Hispanic: 23%, Other; 4% Sample 2: White: 34%, Black: 42%, Hispanic: 22%, Other: 2% Enrolled: 323 (survivors at 1 yr) Evaluated: 258 (at 1 yr f/up) Mean GA (F/up at 2 years of age) Sample 1: 28.3 ±1.8 Sample 2: 28.1 ±1.8 Mean BW: Sample 1: 1043 ±165 Sample 2: 1005 ±184 Male: Sample 1: 49% Sample 2: 43% Race: Sample 1: White: 35%, Black: 60%, Other:5% Sample 2: White: 43%, Black: 54%, Other: 3% Enrolled: 136 (survivors at 2 yrs) Evaluated: 118 Number of sites: 2	Premature VLBW: 700-1350 g (Detailed description available in another article)	ND	At 1 yr f/up Sample 1: Synthetic Surfactant at Birth via ET tube: 5 ml/kg (136) Sample 2: Air placebo via ET tube at birth (122) At 2 yr F/up: Sample 1: Synthetic surfactant at birth (57) Sample 2: Air placbo (61)	Randomized placebo-controlled double blind trial (at 1 year and at 2 years CA)

Evidence Table 9. Studies Evaluating Association of LBW and Pulmonary Outcome

Author, Year UI#	Demographics	Inclusion Criteria	Exclusion Criteria	Disease/Condition Type (N)	Study Design (Duration)

Santuz 1995 96023205	Location: Italy
	Years of Birth: 1981-1987
	Mean GA (range), wk:
	  Cases: 30±2 (27-32)
	  Controls: 39±1 (37-40)
	Mean BW (range), g:
	  Cases: 1400±335 (890-1900)
	  Controls: 3335±418 (2800-4100)
	Male:
	  Cases: 75%
	  Controls: 69%
	Race: ND
	Enrolled: 12 (16 controls)
	Evaluated: 12 (16)
	Number of sites: 1
		Cases: Premature, RDS with mechanical vent > 7 days; met criteria for BPD; agreed to cooperate
		
		Control: healthy term school children matched for age, height, weight, habitual level of physical activity
			Cerebral palsy; too young to cooperate	Cases: Preterm infants with BPD (12)
				Controls: Healthy term infants (16)
					Case-control study (6-12 years)

Iles 1997 97280982	Location: UK Years of Birth: ND Mean GA (range), wk: ND Median BW (range), g: 900 (589-1891) Male: ND Race: ND Enrolled: 40 Evaluated: 33 Number of sites: 1	Premature birth Continuous supplemental O2 for 28 days after birth	Refused consent Returned to referring hospital	Premature infants with CLD (33)	Prospective cohort
Cheung 1998 99059896	Location: Canada Years of Birth: 12/93-10/97 Mean GA (range), wk: 25 (24-30) Median BW (range), g: 860 (340-1460) Male: 67% Race: ND Enrolled: 24 Evaluated: 10 Number of sites: 1	VLBW survivors, BW < 1500 g, requiring inhaled nitrous oxide (INO) (continues to be hypoxenic at >90% O$_2$ and MAP 15 ± 2)	Mosaic trisomy 18 Potter's syndrome survived to 1 year of chronological age	VLBW infants treated with INO (10)	Prospective cohort

Evidence Table 9. Studies Evaluating Association of LBW and Pulmonary Outcome

Author, Year UI#	Demographics	Inclusion Criteria	Exclusion Criteria	Disease/Condition Type (N)	Study Design (Duration)
Gross 1998 98375435 (All+Lung) *sample from the same big population as 20284814	Location: US Years of Birth: 1985-1986 Mean GA (range), wk: Sample 1: 28.2±2.1 Sample 2: 28.4±2.0 Controls: 40±1.1 Mean BW (range), g: Sample 1: 1173±345 Sample 2: 1179±354 Controls: 3565±427 Male: Sample 1: 53% Sample 2: 51% Controls: 57% Race: White Sample 1: 86% Sample 2: 85% Controls: 89% Enrolled: 133 (125 controls) Evaluated: 96 (108) Number of sites: 1	All live-born babies 24-31 wk gestation cared for at Crouse Memorial Hospital, survived to discharge Controls: FT AGA, 38-42 wk GA. PT matched to FT for sex, mat. Race, mat. Educa. and marital status (sociodemographic factors).	ND	(Sample 1&2): Preterm infants (96) Sample 1: Preterm infants with BPD (43) Sample 2: Preterm infants without BPD (53) Controls: Full term infants (108)	Prospective cohort (7 years) Cases: 8 died after discharge because of complications of chronic lung disease (2), pneumonia (2), nonrespiratory conditions (4), lost to follow-up (6), and neurodevelopmental delays (23) Controls: lost to follow-up (12), neurodevelopmental delays (5)
Kurkinen-Raty 1998 98387235	Location: Finland Years of Birth: 1990-1996 Mean GA (range), wk: Cases: 28.2 (23.8- 37.2) Controls: 28.4 (22.9-36.9) Mean BW (range), g: Cases: 1138.3±434 Controls: 1272.4±547.2 Male: ND Race: ND Enrolled: 78 (78 controls) Evaluated: 78 (78) Number of sites: 1	Preterm PROM between 17-30 weeks gestation; singleton; delivered > 2 hr after rupture Controls: preterm no PROM; spontaneous preterm delivery matched for GA and year of delivery.	Rupture unconfirmed or transient	Sample 2: Preterm rupture (78) Sample 2: Preterm delivery no rupture (78)	Retrospective cohort

312

Evidence Table 9. Studies Evaluating Association of LBW and Pulmonary Outcome

Author, Year UI#	Demographics	Inclusion Criteria	Exclusion Criteria	Disease/Condition Type (N)	Study Design (Duration)

Subhedar 1999 20257096	Location: UK
	Years of Birth: 6/1995-5/1999
	Mean GA (range), wk:
	  Sample 1: 28 (24-34)
	  Sample 2: 30 (26-34)
	Mean BW (range), g:
	  Sample 1: 1055 (510-2310)
	  Sample 2: 1420 (840-2150)
	Male:
	  Sample 1: 52%
	  Sample 2: 52%
	Race: ND
	Enrolled: 98
	Evaluated: 98
	Number of sites: 1
		Sample 1: Preterm infants with CLD
		Sample 2: Preterm infants without CLD received mechanical ventilation <24 hours + 02< 72 hours
			ND	Sample 1: Preterm infants with CLD (54)
				Sample 2: Healthy preterm infants (44)
					Prospective cohort

Kurkinen-Raty 2000 20284814
 	
*sample from the same big population as 98197235
	Location: Finland
	Years of Birth: 1990-1997
	Mean GA (range), wk:
	  Cases: 30.5±2.1
	  Controls: 30.4±2.1
	Mean BW (range), g:
	  Cases: 1294±469
	  Controls: 1605±427
	Male: ND
	Race: ND
	Enrolled: 103 (103 controls)
	Evaluated: 103 (103)
	Number of sites: 1
		Cesarean delivered singleton, GA 24-33 weeks
		Controls: spontaneously delivered singleton after regular contractions and/or preterm rupture of the membranes no more than 24 hrs before. The mothers were matched one-to-one by gestational age at delivery plu7s or mines 1 week.
			ND	Sample 1: Indicated preterm I.e. preterm birth 'indicated' for maternal/fetal reasons (103)
				Sample 2: Spontaneous preterm delivery due to preterm labor (103)
					Retrospective cohort

Evidence Table 9. Studies Evaluating Association of LBW and Pulmonary Outcome

Author, Year UI#	Demographics	Inclusion Criteria	Exclusion Criteria	Disease/Condition Type (N)	Study Design (Duration)
Brooks 2001 21153125	Location: US Years of Birth: 1988 Mean GA (range), wk: ND Mean BW (range), g: ND Male: ND Race: ND Enrolled: 8071 Evaluated: 8071 Number of sites: 1	< 4 year old selected from randomized, systematic population based sample, weighted to be nationally representative of sampling of African-American and LBW infants who had initial (1988) and follow-up (1991) surveys and asthma reports	ND	VLBW infants (<1500g), MLBW (1500-2499g); NBW (≥2500) infants from NMIHS population (8071)	Prospective cohort Follow-up 3 years 1988-1991

Doyle 2001 21064379
 	
*overlapped sample with Ford, 2000 20380862 in growth table
	Location: Australia
	Years of Birth: 1/1977 to 3/1982
	Mean GA (range), wk:
	  Sample 1: 27.5 ±2.3
	  Sample 2: 29.6 ±1.5
	  Controls: 39.9 ±1.0
	Mean BW (range), g:
	  Sample 1: 859±100
	  Sample 2: 1248±145
	  Controls: 3420±427
	Male:
	  Sample 1: 45%
	  Sample 2: 54%
	  Controls: 62%
	Race: ND
	Enrolled: 210 (60 controls)
	Evaluated: 180 (42 controls)
	Number of sites: 1
		Sample 1: 86 consecutive ELBW survivors (BW 500-999g) born during the 63 months from 1/1/1977
		
		Sample 2: 124 consecutive ELBW survivors (BW 1000-1500g) born during the 18 months from 1/10/1980
		
		Control: 60 randomly selected term infants with BW>2499g born within the Royal Women's Hospital during the last 6 months of the recruitment phase
			ND	Sample 1: Preterm ELBW infants, BW 500-999g (78)
				Sample 2: Preterm ELBW infants, BW 1000-1500g (102)
				Control: Term infants, BW >2499g (42)
					Prospective cohort (14 years)

314

Evidence Table 9. Studies Evaluating Association of LBW and Pulmonary Outcomes
Part II

Author, Year	Predictors	Predictor Measures	Outcomes	Outcome Measures
Als 1994 94358983	Other: Participation in individualized developmental care staffing by specially educated nurses	The psychologist and clinical nurse specialist provided ongoing support for the care teams and parents of the infants in the experimental group in jointly planning and implementing individually supportive care and environments.	**CNS:** Neurodevelopmental: Cognitive delay **Pulmonary:** BPD severity	Baley Scale of Infant Development at 9 months of age Assessed by double-blind review of cranial US scans by a consultant senior radiologist
Chye 1995 95314864	**Bronchopulmonary dysplasia** BPD with Home O_2 BPD without Home O_2	Diagnoses of BPD was based on Bancalari's BPD definition Home oxygen therapy program – infants who were well, feeding satisfactorily and gaining weight, but were unable to maintain adequate oxygenation (93-97% saturation) in room air, and were therefore discharged from hospital under the home oxygen therapy	**Growth** Re-hospitalization	Growth was based on sex-specific National Center of Health Statistics growth chart

315

Evidence Table 9. Studies Evaluating Association of LBW and Pulmonary Outcomes
Part II

Author, Year	Predictors	Predictor Measures	Outcomes	Outcome Measures
Kraybill 1995 95264242	**General:** Surfactant (single dose 5 ml/kg given via ET tube at birth)	As soon as after birth, infants were treated either with 5 ml/kg of surfactant or air placebo, via ET tube.	At 1 yr assessment (NCMH and HCHD cohort): **General:** Overall survival **Pulmonary:** Need for O2 via Nasal canula Need for O2 via CPAP CLD At 2 yr assessment (NCMH cohort) **General:** Overall survival Hospitalization for respiratory illness **Pulmonary:** Bronchodilator regular use Tracheostomy At 1 and 2 yr assessment: **Growth:** Height for age Weight for age HC for age Mean MDI score MDI scores < 2 SDs Mean PSI score PDI scores < 2 SDs Severity of impairments Types of Impairments Any surgery (between 28 ds-1 yr or 1yr to 2 yr) Assessment between 28 ds-12mo: **Ophthalmology:** ROP (No ROP, Mild/moderate, Severe) Tx for ROP(surgery or cryotherapy) ROP presence at latest exam Severe ROP	No further specifications given, except for the followings: Oxygen via Nasal canula : providing alveolar O2 concentrations of : 26%-40%, based on NC flow and NC O2 concentration Bayley Scale of Infant Development: • MDI= Mental Development Index Score • PDI: Psychomotor Development Index Score ROP : (not further definitions) • No ROP, • Mild/moderate • Severe CP (no further definitions) • Mild • Moderate/Severe Severity of impairments: • Severe • Mild/Moderate Types of impairments: • MDI<69 • MDI: 69-84 • Moderate/severe CP • Mild CP • Bilateral sensorineural deafness • Deafness not requiring amplification • Bilateral blindness • Visual defect (1 yr and 2 yr CA)

316

Evidence Table 9. Studies Evaluating Association of LBW and Pulmonary Outcomes

Part II

Author, Year	Predictors	Predictor Measures	Outcomes	Outcome Measures
Santuz 1995 96023205	General Predictor: GA Cardiovascular 1) Chronic Lung Diseases 2) Other: duration of supplemental oxygen	Chronic Lung Disease defined as oxygen dependency for at least 28 days and beyond 36 postmenstrual weeks in association with an abnormal chest radiograph.	Other Outcomes: Cardiovascular: pulmonary hypertension	Measured as AT/RVET ratio = Doppler derived acceleration time to right ventricular ejection time ratio
Iles 1997 97280982	*Cardiovascular or Pulmonary Predictors:* Bronchopulmonary dysplasia *Other Predictors:* ECG with RVH	$DaAO_2$ in 50% O_2 $PaCO_2$ PFT testing to determining V_{max} FRC	**Pulmonary:** Requirement for supplemental O_2 at one year CA; alternately phrased by authors as $SaO_2 < 90\%$ in RA **Other outcomes:** Hospital readmission	ND
Cheung 1998 99059896	Cardiovascular or Pulmonary Predictors: Inhaled nitric oxide (INO)	ND	**Pulmonary:** BPD or CLD (with or without meds) Aspiration pneumonia	PDI + MDI of Bayley Scales of Infant Developmental Index were used. "Neurodevelopmental" outcomes: Disability: one of more of: 1. CP (all types or severity) 2. Legal blindness (corrected visual acuity of the better eye <20/200 3. Hearing loss (sensorineural hearing loss of >30 dB in the better ear) 4. Severe mental retardation (MDI >3 SD below the mean) Delay: does not have disability and either MDI or PDI was >2 SD below the mean. Normal: free of disability or delay and MDI and PDI were within 2 SD of the mean.

317

Evidence Table 9. Studies Evaluating Association of LBW and Pulmonary Outcomes
Part II

Author, Year	Predictors	Predictor Measures	Outcomes	Outcome Measures
Gregoire 1998 95264241	Cardiovascular/Pulmonary: 1) Chronic Lung Disease 2) Bronchopulmonary dysplasia Compared O₂ dependence at 28 days with O₂ dependence at 36 wk	ND	**CNS:** Cerebral palsy Motor and cognitive delay **Audiology:** Hearing Disorders → Free field audiograms **Pulmonary:** Respiratory readmissions PICU admissions **Growth:** Weight, height, head circumference **Other:** Health Outcomes	Giffith's Mental Development Scales Neurologic examinations
Gross 1998 98375435	General: GA Cardiovascular: Bronchopulmonary dysplasia @ 30 wk Other: social data, health data	PT 24-31 wk GA BPD if infants were dependent on supplemental oxygen @ 35 wk PMA	**Pulmonary:** Respiratory symptoms (wheeze, chronic cough, chest congestion) Restriction in activity, Use of respiratory medicines, 7-year pulmonary function studies Bronchodilator responsiveness **Other:** Re-hospitalization Metabolic measures	Lung function testing was performed on SensorMedics 2200 (SensorMedics, Anaheim, Calif) by investigators blinded to children's GA and medical histories
Kurkinen-Raty 1998 98197235	General : PROM	Diagnose was through clinical assessment or with the use of a PROM-test, which detects insulin growth factor binding protein-1 in the cervico-vaginal secretions, or with the use of a nitrazine test.	**CNS:** Motor delay Cerebral delay **Ophthalmology:** Visual Blindness **Audiology:** Hearing disorders **Pulmonary:** Chronic lung disease **Growth:** weight percent **Other:** Days of re-hospitalization Steroid therapy at follow-up	Neurologic exams Diagnosis of CLD was made if infants required oxygen, continuous bronchodilator, or steroid tx because of respiratory signs and symptoms. Diagnoses of RDS were made based on need for respiratory support, radiologic findings, and clinical assessments

318

Evidence Table 9. Studies Evaluating Association of LBW and Pulmonary Outcomes

Part II

Author, Year	Predictors	Predictor Measures	Outcomes	Outcome Measures
Subhedar 1999 20257096	Cardiovascular/Pulmonary: Chronic lung disease	CLD was defined as oxygen dependency for at least 28 days and beyond 36 PMA in association with an abnormal chest radiograph	**Pulmonary:** 1) Pulmonary function-forced vital capacity 2) Minor ventilation forced expiratory volume, forced expiratory flow Other: Heat rate during exercise	Measures OR aerobic power: a) maximum O2 consumption b) max O2 consumption at anaerobic threshold C) running time
Kurkinen-Raty 2000 20284814	General predictors: Birth weight GA Antenatal steroids Cord pH Bronchopulmonary dysphasia (BPD) Other predictors: Indicated preterm delivery Spontaneous preterm delivery	BPD diagnoses were based on radiologic finding	**CNS:** Motor delay Cerebral palsy **Ophthalmology** Visual impairment **Audiology** Hearing disorder **Pulmonary** Chronic lung disease (CLD) at 1 year **Growth:** Wt, Ht, HC	Motor delay = abnormalities of tone or reflexes but functionally normal or borderline CP = spastic diplegia or hemiplegia or spastictetraplegia Diagnosis of CLD was made if infants required oxygen, continuous bronchodilator, or steroid tx because of respiratory signs and symptoms.
Brooks 2001 21153125	General: Birth weight Sex Other: SEC factors (mat age, race, education, SEC status, mat wt gain, mat smoking, poverty status variable) Prenatal history Developmental outcomes	Predictors self-explanatory. Poverty variable based on family income and number of household members, categorized by standard national poverty levels.	**Pulmonary:** M.D. diagnosed asthma in 1st 3 years of life	Diagnosis of asthma based on response of parent to question, "Have you been told by a MD/ RN/other health provider that your child has asthma?"
Doyle 2001 21064379 *overlapped sample with 20380862	General: Birth weight Cardiovascular/Pulmonary: Bronchopulmonary	ND	**Pulmonary:** 1) Asthma 2) Lung function testing 3) readmission to hospital for asthma or pneumonia **Growth:** height **Other:** hospital readmission	Lung function testing, Jaeger Bodyscreen II-Bodybox (Jaeger, Germany), with Masterlab (ML3) software

319

Evidence Table 9. Studies Evaluating Association of LBW and Pulmonary Outcomes
Part III

Author, Year	Associations found			Potential Biases	Comments
Als 1994 94358983	Studied effect of an individualized developmental care plan on Bayley score at 9 months age and occurrence and severity of BPD.			Small number of babies studied Only one NICU Only one neurodevelopmental assessment at 9 months of age Reported timing of IVH different from many other studies High potential for contamination	Study was government funded
		Experimental group	Controls	P value		
	N	20	18			
	Bayley MDI	118.30 (17.35)	94.38 (23.31)	< 0.001		
	Bayley PDI	100.6 (20.19)	83.56 (17.97)	< 0.01		
	No BPD	2/20	3/18			
	Mild BPD	13/20	7/18			
	Moderate BPD	5/20	2/18			
	Severe BPD	0	6/18	0.03		

Evidence Table 9. Studies Evaluating Association of LBW and Pulmonary Outcomes

Part III

Author, Year	Associations found	Potential Biases	Comments
Chye 1995 95314864	Rehospitalization rate (overall) BPD (78) 58% Control (75) 35% RR 1.7 (1.2-2.4) Rehospitalization for respiratory illness BPD (78) 39% Control (75) 20% RR 1.9 (1.1- 3.2) Rehospitalization for poor growth BPD (78) 14% Control (75) 1% RR=1.4 (1.7-82) Rehospitalization for failure to thrive BPD on home O_2 (20) 30% Control no home O_2 (58) 9% RR=3.3 (1.2-8.9) **Growth (wt in kg)** : NS diff between BPD and control BPD M 9.08 F 8.4 Control M 9.37 F 8.82 **Growth (Ht in cm):** NS diff BPD M 73.0 F 72.1 Control M 74.4 F 72.6 **Growth (HC in cm):** NS diff BPD M 46.7 F 46.0 Control M 47.0 F 454. There was a significant increase in **any** rehospitalization in 1st year of life in preterm infants with BPD vs. preterm infants with no BPD. There was a significant increase (2-fold) in rehospitalization for **respiratory illness** in the 1st year of life in preterm infants with BPD vs. preterm infants with no BPD. BPD infants with Home O_2 (N=20) had ~3 fold increased re-hospitalization for failure to thrive. Growth failure was common in both preterm groups (i.e. in infants with no BPD and with BPD <10% in weight at 1 yr age). Re-hospitalization was high in both preterm groups (with and without BPD).	(None)	Study was privately funded

321

Evidence Table 9. Studies Evaluating Association of LBW and Pulmonary Outcomes
Part III

Author, Year	Associations found	Potential Biases	Comments
Kraybill 1995 95264242	Single dose Surfactant tx at birth was not associated with the physical and neurodevelopmental status of VLBW premature infants at 1 yr of corrected age Placebo group vs Surfactant group, at 1 yr of age: 1. Overall survival at 1 yr: 2. Oxygen via NC 3. Oxygen via CPAP: 4. CLD 5. Distribution of pts in both groups across different percentiles: Ht/age, Weight/age and HC/age: were not s/s different across the two groups. 6. Mean MDI score: 7. MDI scores< 2SDs 8. Mean PDI score: 9. PDI scores < 2 SDs: 10. No impairment: 11. Impairment present (total) 12. Severe impairment: 13. Mild/Moderate impairment: 14. Types of impairment: MDI<69: MDI: 69-84: Moderate/severe CP: Mild CP: Bilateral sensorineural deafness: Deafness not requiring amplification Bilateral blindness: Visual defect: Assessment from 28ds-12 mo: • No ROP: • Present ROP overall: • Mild/Moderate ROP: • Severe ROP: • Treatment for ROP overall: Surgery: Cryotherapy: In the NCMH cohort there was no difference in impairments, the severity of impairments and the types of impairments at the 1yr of age assessment		

322

Evidence Table 9. Studies Evaluating Association of LBW and Pulmonary Outcomes
Part III

Author, Year	Associations found	Potential Biases	Comments
Santuz 1995 96023205	Forced vital capacity (FVC): BPD: (N=12) 87±10 Without BPD: (N=16) 96±8 <0.05 Forced expiratory volume(1 sec)(FEV1): BPD: 83±12 Without BPD: 100±8 <0.01 FEF 25-75 (forced expiratory flow between 15-7520 vc): BPD: 77±30 Without BPD: 110±14 <0.01 Oxygen consumption (ml/?/?): BPD: 25.2±10.3 Without BPD: 37.1±10.4 <0.01 Running time (minutes): BPD: 6.1±1.3 Without BPD: 7.9±2.6 <0.05 Minute ventilation: BPD: 20±9.4 Without BPD: 30.7±9 <0.01 Max heat rate during exercise: BPD: 192±7.9 Without BPD: 194±8 Not significant Running time: BPD: 6.1±1.3 Without BPD: 7.9±2.6 P <0.05	Small study Far from comprehensive; likely substantial section bias Compares prematures with BPD to term infants without BPO; unclear if results are due to BPD or prematurity	No data on funding source

323

Evidence Table 9. Studies Evaluating Association of LBW and Pulmonary Outcomes
Part III

Author, Year	Associations found	Potential Biases	Comments
Iles 1997 97280982	Study of chronic lung disease (CLD) leading to a persistent requirement for supplemental oxygen at one year of age. N % requiring oxygen at one year age Supplemental O2 at discharge 6 50% RVH on ECG 3 100% Alveolar arterial oxygen gradient > 29 kPa in 50% hood oxygen at 35 to 40 weeks PCA predicted need for supplemental oxygen at one year with sensitivity 0.85 and specificity 0.88. PaCO2 greater than 7 kPa at 35 to 40 weeks PCA predicted supplemental oxygen requirement at one year with sensitivity 0.78 and specificity 0.88.	Small number of infants No information regarding early neonatal course No control groups of preterms without CLD	Study was privately funded
Cheung 1998 99059896	Mean MDI 81 ± 21, PDI 64 ± 22 Normal development 31% Neurodevelopmental delay 20% Disabled 50% Severe mental retardation 10% Spastic diplegic CP 30% Hemiplegic CP 10% <3rd %ile for weight 20% <3rd%ile for height 40% <3rd%ile HC 30% BPD 80% Need bronchodilators for CLD 10% Recurrent wheezing but did not need meds 40% Grade 4 IVH 20% Grade 3 IVH 20% VP shunt 30% PVL 10% Sensorineural hearing loss 10%	Very small sample size Descriptive study with no control group for comparison	No data on funding source

324

Evidence Table 9. Studies Evaluating Association of LBW and Pulmonary Outcomes
Part III

Author, Year	Associations found	Potential Biases	Comments
Gross 1998 98375435	Rehospitalization during 1st 2 years: PT with BPD 23/43 (53%) PT without BPD 14/53 (26%) FT 3/108 (3%) Respiratory symptoms in PT with BPD were greater than symptoms in PT without BPD, and both were greater than FT group Pulmonary function Tests: Multiple tests revealed significantly worse PFTs in PT with BPD at rest and after exercise compared to either PT without BPD or FT group. Exercise results: No difference in baseline HR, VO2, RQ, Max VO2, Max RQ, endurance among groups Asthma: PT with BPD 20/43 (47%) PT without BPD 13/53 (25%) FT 23/108 (21%) PT with BPD vs. FT: P<0.001 School age children who were former preterm infants with BPD demonstrated abnormal pulmonary function at 7 years age in contrast to school age children who were preterm infants without BPD or FT AGA control. The children who were preterm infants without BPD had similar pulmonary function as children who were FT AGA controls.	(None)	No data on funding source

325

Evidence Table 9. Studies Evaluating Association of LBW and Pulmonary Outcomes
Part III

Author, Year	Associations found	Potential Biases	Comments
Kurkinen-Raty 1998 98387235	Retrospective controlled cohort study of early PROM between 17 and 30 weeks of gestation. Assements at one year corrected age. N = 55 for early PROM and 56 for control. Outcome — Early PROM — Control — OR (CI) Cerebral palsy — 18% — 16% — 1.2 (0.4, 3.1) Delayed motor Development — 9% — 16% — 0.5 (0.2, 1.7) Visual disability — 4% — 4% — 1.0 (0.1, 7.5) Hearing loss — 7% — 9% — 0.8 (0.2, 3.2) Good nuerosensory development — 67% — 61% — 1.2 (0.6, 2.2) Early PROM seems to be a major obstetric and neonatal problem with pulmonary ramifications extending beyond the neonatal period. However, most of these infants can be saved.	(None)	No data on funding source
Subhedar 1999 20257096	AT/RVET ratio much lower in CLD group p< 0.01. Pulmonary arterial pressure remains persistently elevated in CLD infants until the end of first year of life.	Does not state whether the Doppler evaluators were blinded to the groups	Study was private funded

Evidence Table 9. Studies Evaluating Association of LBW and Pulmonary Outcomes

Part III

Author, Year	Associations found	Potential Biases	Comments
Kurkinen-Raty 2000 20284814	**CLD at 1 year age:** Indicated PT delivery: (81) 12/81 (15%) Spontaneous PT delivery: (94) 3/94 (3%) RR 4.6 (1.4, 1.6) **Growth:** Indicated PT delivery: (81) Spontaneous PT delivery: (94) Weight RR =0.03 (-5.3, 0.3) L RR = 0.002 HC RR = 0.03 **CP:** Indicated PT delivery: (81) 5/81 (6%) Spontaneous PT delivery: (94) 10/94 (11%) RR=0.6 (0.25-1.6) **Delayed motor:** Indicated PT delivery: (81) 8/81 (6%) Spontaneous PT delivery: (94) 8/94 (9%) RR 1.2 (0.5-3.0) **Visual disability:** Indicated PT delivery: (81) Spontaneous PT delivery: (94) RR =1.9 (0.5, 7.8) **Hearing loss:** Indicated PT delivery: (81) Spontaneous PT delivery: (94) RR =1.9 (0.5, 7.8) This study demonstrated that premature infants who were born due to 'indicated maternal/fetal reasons' vs. spontaneous preterm delivered infants had worse pulmonary outcome a 1 yr age. More infants in 'indicated' group were SGA and were significantly smaller than control group at 1 yr in Wt, HT, and HC. There was no difference between groups in neurosensory outcomes.	Outcome not well-defined Difficult to know if lack of difference between groups is due to sample size or event rate.	No data on funding source

327

Evidence Table 9. Studies Evaluating Association of LBW and Pulmonary Outcomes
Part III

Author, Year	Associations found	Potential Biases	Comments
Brooks 2001 21153125	Diagnosis asthma by age 3 years BW ≥ 2500 gm 6.7% BW≥1500-2499gm 10.9% OR=1.4 (1.1-1.8) BW < 1500 (VLBW) 21.9% OR=2.9 (2.3-3.6) African-American 12% OR=1.9 (1.6-2.4) VLBW/African-American OR 2.5 (2.0-3.3) VLBW/white OR=3.1 9 (2.2-4.3) Chronic lung disease (8058) 20.4% OR 3.4 (2.4-4.8) 68% attributable risk for asthma in VLBW children was due to birth weight.	Retrospective classification of BPD may have been limited compared to prospective classification. Potential for selection bias a. identifying asthma children based on parental report of physician-diagnosed asthma. (Evidence of high specificity and PPV) b. defining asthma may vary by physician practice	Study was government funded Objective of study was to estimate the independent contribution of BW to asthma prevalence among children <4 years age. This study found a strong, independent association between low birth weight and asthma.
Doyle 2001 216464379 *overlapped sample with 20380862	Respiratory health and lung function in these preterm children <1501g were mostly normal and comparable with normal control term infants at 14 years	(None)	Study was privately funded

328

Evidence Table 10. Studies Evaluating Association of LBW and Bone and Growth Outcomes
Part I

Author, Year UI#	Demographics	Inclusion Criteria	Exclusion Criteria	Disease/Condition Type (N)	Study Design (Duration)
Forslund 1992 93044002	Location: Sweden Years of Birth: ND Median GA (range), wk: ND Mean BW (range), g: ND Male: ND Race: ND Enrolled: ND Evaluated: 41 (24 controls) Number of sites: ND	ND	ND	Cases: Preterms (41) Controls: Term infants (24)	Unclear (the study design was described in detail in previous papers)

Chye 1995 95314864	Location: Australia
	Years of Birth: 1989 to 1990
	Mean GA (range), wk:
	  Cases: 28±1.58
	  Controls: 28.63±1.26
	Mean BW (range), g:
	  Cases: 1055± 234
	  Controls: 1077±215
	Male: 56%
	Race: ND
	Enrolled: 80
	Evaluated: 78 (78 controls)
	Number of sites: 1
		Cases: 26-33 week GA infants with BPD and discharged home
		Controls: 26-32 week GA infants without BPD admitted to the hospital within 1 year of the cases, matched for BW with the cases in broad categories (<1000 g, 1000-1499 g and ≥1500 g)
			Cases: Trisomy 21 (2)	Cases: Preterm infants with BDP (78)
				Sample 2: Preterm infants without BPD (78)
				
				Subgroups of cases at 12 months corrected age follow-up:
				Sample 1: BPD no Home O_2 (58)
				Sample 2: BPD with Home O_2 (20)
					Case-control study

DeReignier 1997 98041177	Location: Netherlands Years of Birth: 1/1/1987-12/31-1991 Median GA (range), wk: 27.5 Mean BW (range), g: 1015 Male: 48% Race: 38% Black Enrolled: 678 Evaluated: 174 Number of sites: 1	VLBW infants , BW < 1500 g, survived until discharge Matched sever CLD and no CLD infants to mild CLD infants for BW, race, and sex.	Condition independent of CLD known to adversely affect neurosensory status, development, growth; significant congenital anomalies; congenital viral infections; SGA; NEC requiring enterostomy	Matched VLBW infants (89): No CLD (58) Mild CLD (58) Severe CLD (58)	Retrospective cohort (followed until 1 year adjusted age)

Evidence Table 10. Studies Evaluating Association of LBW and Bone and Growth Outcomes
Part I

Author, Year UI#	Demographics	Inclusion Criteria	Exclusion Criteria	Disease/Condition Type (N)	Study Design (Duration)
Gosch 1997 97379896	Location: US Years of Birth: 1989 to 1994 Mean GA (range), wk: Cases: 27.6 (26-29) Controls: 39 (36-40) Mean BW (range), g: Cases: 880 Controls: 3466 Male: 50% Race: ND Enrolled: 5 (5 controls) Evaluated: 5 (5) Number of sites: 1	Participants in a early intervention and family care for blind infants and preschoolers Blind children	ND	Cases: Blind children born preterm (5) Controls: Blind children born full term (5)	Retrospective cohort (24, 36, 48, and 58 months)
Ladd 1998 98357452	Location: US Years of Birth: 1980-1995 Mean GA (range), wk: 30 (23-42) Mean BW (range), g: 1500 (272-4840) Male: 53% Race: ND Enrolled: 249 Evaluated: 249 Number of sites: 1	249 babies with NEC who had their initial surgical care at the James Whitcomb Riley Hospital for Children Indiana University Medical Center campus, with the diagnosis of NEC from 1/1/1908-12/31/1995 were included in the study	Infants with focal, isolated perforations of the ileum were excluded	Infants with NEC (249)	Retrospective cohort (16 years)

330

Evidence Table 10. Studies Evaluating Association of LBW and Bone and Growth Outcomes
Part I

Author, Year UI#	Demographics	Inclusion Criteria	Exclusion Criteria	Disease/Condition Type (N)	Study Design (Duration)
Wang 1998 98244087	Location: Canada Years of Birth: 1/1977 to 5/1992 Mean GA (range), wk: 27.7±2.3 Mean BW (range), g: 954.6±185.9 Male: 48% Race: Caucasian 88.5% SES: low SES category (Blishen index≤40) 47.2% Enrolled: 1007 Evaluated: 514 Number of sites: 1	VLBW infants, BW<1250g, survived to NICU D/C	Missing more than one measurement	VLBW infants (514)	Prospective cohort (36 months)
Connors 1999 99250892	Location: Australia Years of Birth: 1/1987 to 12/1992 Mean GA (range), wk: 27±2.2 Mean BW (range), g: 822.8 ±125 Male: 45% Race: ND Enrolled: 226 Evaluated: 198 Number of sites: 1	ELBW survived infants, BW <1000 g	Died by 2 years corrected age (1) Lost to follow-up (12) Transferred interstate and limited information was available (4)	ELBW infants (198): Sample 1: ELBW with low perinatal risk factors (128) Sample 2: ELBW with high perinatal risk factors (70)	Prospective cohort (2 year CA)

331

Evidence Table 10. Studies Evaluating Association of LBW and Bone and Growth Outcomes
Part I

Author, Year UI#	Demographics	Inclusion Criteria	Exclusion Criteria	Disease/Condition Type (N)	Study Design (Duration)
French 1999 99115141 (CNS + Growth+ All)	Location: Australia Years of Birth: 1990-1992 Median GA (range), wk: Sample 1: 30 (26-32) Sample 2: 29 (27-31) Sample 3: 30 (28.5-31.5) Sample 4: 31 (29-32) Mean BW (range), g: Sample 1: 1435 (905-1810) Sample 2: 1345 (1000-1735) Sample 3: 1517.5 (1210-1660) Sample 4: 1455 (1080-1715) Male: total 57% Race: ND Enrolled: 652 Evaluated: 477 Number of sites: 1	Singleton live-born infants GA <33 weeks	ND	Sample 1: Antenatal steroids x 0 course (311) Sample 2: Antenatal steroids x 1 course (123) Sample 3: Antenatal steroids x 2 courses (20) Sample 4: Antenatal steroids x > 3 courses (23)	Prospective cohort (3 years)
Ford 2000 20380862 *overlapped sample with Doyle, 2001 21064379 in Lung table	Location: Australia Years of Birth: 1/1977 to 3/1982 Mean GA (range), wk: Sample 1: 27.5 ±2.3 Sample 2: 29.6 ±1.5 Controls: 39.9 ±1.0 Mean BW (range), g: Sample 1: 859±100 Sample 2: 1248±145 Controls: 3420±427 Male: 56% Race: ND Enrolled: 206 (60 controls) Evaluated: 179 (42 controls) Number of sites: 1	Cases: Preterm ELBW infants (<1500g) who survived to discharge Control: Full term NBW (BW>2499g) infants group who survived to discharge	Children with CP at age 14 years Lost to follow-up	At 14-year follow-up: Cases (Sample 1&2): Preterm ELBW infants (179) Sample 1: Preterm infants, BW<1000g (79) Sample 2: Preterm infants, BW 1000-1499g (100) Control: Full term NBW infants (42)	Prospective cohort (14 years)

Evidence Table 10. Studies Evaluating Association of LBW and Bone and Growth Outcomes

Part I

Author, Year UI#	Demographics	Inclusion Criteria	Exclusion Criteria	Disease/Condition Type (N)	Study Design (Duration)
Morley 2000 20167446	Location:UK Centers:5 Enrollment period: ND Age at assessement:7.5-8 yrs Trial 1: conducted in 3 centers Total enrolled in trial 1 and 2: N=926 infants with BW< 1850 g Long term f/up at 7.5-8 yrs of age: N=781 of 833 (94%) survivors	Premature BW< 1850 g Survivors of participants in the two RCTs with 2 parallel arms each (assessing effect of different neonatal diets of growth) Age 7.5-8 yrs	ND	GroupA: Prematures/ fed banked breast milk until weight 2000 g or discharge from the NICU N=207 Mean BW: 1397±297 Mean GA:31.1 % of SGA:30% Males: 53% Group B: Prematures/ preterm formula N=213 Mean BW:1387 ±278 Mean GA:31 % of SGAs:35% Males:52% (both groups included 2 parallel arms with or without supplementation with mother's own milk)	Two Randomized clinical trials Trial 1 and 2, with 2 parallel arms in each trial (The results for each trial are presented for the combination of the 2 parallel arms) Trial 1 had : Follow up At 9 mo At 18 mo At 7.5-8 yrs

333

Evidence Table 10. Studies Evaluating Association of LBW and Bone and Growth Outcomes
Part I

Author, Year UI#	Demographics	Inclusion Criteria	Exclusion Criteria	Disease/Condition Type (N)	Study Design (Duration)

Avila-Diaz 2001 21334039	Location: Mexico
	Years of Birth: ND
	Mean GA (range), wk:
	  Sample 1: 39±0.9
	  Sample 2: 30±2.6
	Mean BW (range), g:
	  Sample 1: 3195±323
	  Sample 2: 1294±167
	Male: 51%
	Race: ND
	Enrolled: 82
	Evaluated: 82
	Number of sites: 1
		Informed consent
		48 full-term "healthy" infants and 34 pre-term infants who were predominantly breast-fed
			ND	Sample 1: Full term infants (48)
				Sample 2: Preterm infants (34)
					Prospective cohort (6 months)

Evidence Table 10. Studies Evaluating Association of LBW and Bone and Growth Outcomes

Part II

Author, Year	Predictors	Predictor Measures	Outcomes	Outcome Measures
Forslund 1992 93044002	General: GA	Not given, resulted from previous papers of study with same group	**CNS:** Neurodevelopmental Motor delay **Growth** in height, weight and head circumference	Motor performance was tested by a physiotherapist: used TMI (test of motor impairment) Measurement of height Weight and head circumference by an experienced RN.
Chye 1995 95314864	Bronchopulmonary dysplasia BPD with Home O_2 BPD without Home O_2	Diagnoses of BPD was based on Bancalari' BPD definition Home oxygen therapy program – infants who were well, feeding satisfactorily and gaining weight, but were unable to maintain adequate oxygenation (93-97% saturation) in room air, and were therefore discharged from hospital under the home oxygen therapy	Growth Re-hospitalization	Growth was based on sex-specific National Center of Health Statistics growth chart
DeReignier 1997 98041177	General: GA Cardiovascular/Pulmonary: Chronic lung disease Gastrointestinal: Necrotizing "enterocolitis" Other: Osteomalcia = Socioeconomic status	No CLD- room air at 28 days Mild CLD- requiring O_2 at 28 days but not at 36 wks PCA. Severe CLD- requiring O_2 at 28 days and 36 wks PCA Not included in CLD if O_2 used only for prevention of apnea	**CNS:** Motor delay Cerebral palsy Cognitive delay Mental retardation **Growth:** Weight Height Head circumference **Other** : Hospital readmissions	Motor and cognitive delay: corrected MDI or PDI scores were >2SD below mean (ie correct score <68) Mental retardation Growth: Weight, Length, Head circumference Development: Pediatrician & physical therapist agreed on presence of definitely abnormal position & posture from impaired neuromotor function Hospital readmission in 1st year

335

Evidence Table 10. Studies Evaluating Association of LBW and Bone and Growth Outcomes
Part II

Author, Year	Predictors	Predictor Measures	Outcomes	Outcome Measures
Gosch 1997 97379896	Ophthalmology 1) Other: Blind ELBW 2) Other: blind Term (term control) Other Predictors 1) Nutrition/Growth-lead circumference(cm) 2) Other: days spent in hospital after delivery	Self-explanatory	**CNS:** Other: BDTB (Bielefeld developmental test for blind infants and pre-schoolers at age 18-48 months) **Growth:** Weight Height Head circumference Body mass index	The scales of BDTB including numbers of items and maximum scores listed on table 1
Ladd 1998 98357452	Gastrointestinal: 1) Short gut 2) Necrotizing "enterocolitis" 3) Presence of ileocecal valve 4) Length of bowel reserve	ND	Growth predictors: growth	ND
Wang 1998 98244087	BW	VLBW ≤ 1250 g	Growth Weight Height	At the specified age and reference
Connors 1999 99250892	Birth weight (i.e. ELBW=BW <1 kg) Postnatal Nutrition Growth: <3%tile, 3-9%tile, ≥10%tile)	High perinatal risk: PVH>Grade 2 + ventriculomegaly, NEC, Home O2. Low perinatal risk: none of the above risk factors	CNS: CP Other adverse neurodevelopmental outcome Neurological Exam	Neurodevelopmental outcome assessed by Griffith's Developmental Scales, Motor outcome assessed by Neurosensory Motor Developmental Assessment [NMDA].
French 1999 99115141 (CNS + Growth+ All)	Other: Number of courses of antenatal steroids	ND	**CNS:** Neurodevelopmental CP **Growth:** Weight ratio Height ratio Head circumference ratio Disability	ND Weight, height, or HC compared to national standard "Any disability" = cerebral palsy, IQ< 85, deafness, or visual acuity worse than 6/60

Evidence Table 10. Studies Evaluating Association of LBW and Bone and Growth Outcomes
Part II

Author, Year	Predictors	Predictor Measures	Outcomes	Outcome Measures
Ford 2000 20380862 *overlapped sample with Doyle, 2001 21064379 in Lung table	Birth weight	VLBW < 1500g (<1kg and 1-1.5 kg) vs Normal BW (>2.4 kg)	Growth outcome: Height Weight Head circumference Pubertal development	Growth scores and variables
Morley 2000 20167446	Trial 1: Type of diet in early neonatal period: • Banked donor breast milk vs Preterm formula (with or without supplementation with its mother's milk) Trial 2: • Preterm formula vs term formula (with or without supplementation with mother's milk)	Not further specified	Trial 1: Growth: Assessment at 9 and 18 months post-term: • Weight (kg) • Length (cm) • HC • Subscapular skinfold thickness • Body mass index Assessment at 7.5 –8 yrs: • All of the above • Also weight to hip ratio Trial 2: • Growth at 18 mo • Growth at 7.5-8 yrs	Not further specified
Avila-Diaz 2001 21334039	General predictors: 1) birth weight 2) preterm vs. full-term	ND	Other outcomes: 1) bone mineral contents (BMC) 2) bone area 3) changes in bone mineral content over time	BMC was measured monthly for full-term infants during the first 5 months of extrauterine life and bimonthly for pre-term infants during the first 6 months of extrauterine life

337

Evidence Table 10. Studies Evaluating Association of LBW and Bone and Growth Outcomes
Part III

Author, Year	Associations found	Potential Biases	Comments
Forslund 1992 93044002	Growth and motor performance assessed in preterm children at 8 years of life. • Differences for mean values for weight, height and head circumference not significant • Relationship exists between findings in TMI (test of motor impairment at 4 and 8 years) suggests possibility of identifying motor problems before school age.	A specific population in a certain are that has been studied before Lack of data regarding the population, stated birth weight significant but not listed anywhere	Study was privately funded Cannot generalize, general lack of data The population studied and the study design have been described in detail in previous paper

338

Evidence Table 10. Studies Evaluating Association of LBW and Bone and Growth Outcomes
Part III

Author, Year	Associations found	Potential Biases	Comments
Chye 1995 95314864	Rehospitalization rate (overall) BPD (78) 58% Control (75) 35% RR 1.7 (1.2-2.4) Rehospitalization for respiratory illness BPD (78) 39% Control (75) 20% RR 1.9 (1.1- 3.2) Rehospitalization for poor growth BPD (78) 14% Control (75) 1% RR=1.4 (1.7-82) Rehospitalization for failure to thrive BPD on home O_2 (20) 30% Control no home O_2 (58) 9% RR=3.3 (1.2-8.9) **Growth (wt in kg) :** NS diff between BPD and control BPD M 9.08 F 8.4 Control M 9.37 F 8.82 **Growth (Ht in cm):** NS diff BPD M 73.0 F 72.1 Control M 74.4 F 72.6 **Growth (HC in cm):** NS diff BPD M 46.7 F 46.0 Control M 47.0 F 454. There was a significant increase in **any** rehospitalization in 1st year of life in preterm infants with BPD vs. preterm infants with no BPD. There was a significant increase (2-fold) in rehospitalization for **respiratory illness** in the 1st year of life in preterm infants with BPD vs. preterm infants with no BPD. BPD infants with Home O2 (N=20) had ~3 fold increased re-hospitalization for failure to thrive. Growth failure was common in both preterm groups (i.e. in infants with no BPD and with BPD <10% in weight at 1 yr age). Re-hospitalization was high in both preterm groups (with and without BPD).	(None)	Study was privately funded

Evidence Table 10. Studies Evaluating Association of LBW and Bone and Growth Outcomes

Part III

Author, Year	Associations found	Potential Biases	Comments
DeReignier 1997 98041177	Sensorineural Hearing Loss: 　CLD: No:0 　　Mild:0 　　Severe: 3　　P<0.05 Low MDI (Bayley Scale): 　CLD: No: 0 　　Mild:4 　　Severe:5　　P<0.05 Low PDI (Bayley Scale): 　CLD: No: 1 　　Mild:4 　　Severe:7　　P<0.05 Cerebral Palsy 　No CLD vs Any CLD: 　　Odds ratios: 6.4 　　95% CI: (1.05-139.8) Weight 2-Score: 　CLD: No: 2 score 　　Severe: signify lower weight HC+ Length 2-Score: 　No, Mild, Severe: No significant difference	(None)	No data on funding source
Gosch 1997 97379896	Blind ELBW infants have developmental delay of 1.5 to 2 years that of term blind controls. **At 48 mos, ELBW blind vs Term blind BDTB scores:** Overall score: 169.4±62.4 vs 270.6±50.7, p <0.05 Neuromotor skills: not significant Social maturity: 42± 13.4, 67.4± 10.1, p < 0.05 Cognition: 16.8 ±22.5, 47.5 ±19.7, p< 0.05 Linguistic abilities: 11.2± 11.7, 29.2 ±12.5, p< 0.05 Socioemotional behavior:33±9.6, 44.8±6.3, NS Orientation and mobility: 35.6 ±10.7, 50.8± 5.9, p< 0.05 **ELBW blind infants had significantly lower weight**, height, head circumference and body-mass index than term blind infants.	Extremely small number of subjects only 5, so statistics not reliable Validity of BDTB scale still in question Does not state whether the evaluators were blinded to the groups or whether they were the same throughout the length of study.	No data on funding source

Evidence Table 10. Studies Evaluating Association of LBW and Bone and Growth Outcomes
Part III

Author, Year	Associations found	Potential Biases	Comments
Ladd 1998 98357452	Death rate of children with NEC was 49% 148 subjects with follow-up more than 2 years was evaluated for the impact of the ICV on severe growth retardation (<10 %tile) found that no association between length of bowel resected or status of the ICV, and sever growth retardation.	Extraordinary poor study Populations at follow-up times not described or compared Time of follow-up given only for 1 outcome Massive Bias Results not interpretable	No data on funding source
Wang 1998 98244087	More VLBW infants were classified as "subnormal growth" based on chronologic age vs. adjusted age through 36 months. The % of VLBW children with subnormal growth is therefore affected by adjustment for corrected age through 36 months and varies according to growth references (especially at younger ages 4-8 months). Regardless of adjusted or chronologic age or growth reference, the mean weight and mean height were significantly lower in VLBW (<1250 gm) than term infants at 4 through 36 months age. As infants approach 18 and 36 months age, the deviation from full term infants is less.	Large number of infants were not included in the analyses. They were slightly differed from the study sample in that they had higher BW and GA and less BPD and CP in follow-up	Study was privately funded
Connors 1999 99250892	Weight percentile was strongly associated with lower general growth quotient and lower motor abilities in ELBW infants. Low weight percentile at 2 year was related to adverse developmental outcome in ELBW infants at high perinatal risk or with neurological impairment. There was minimal association between postnatal low weight percentile and adverse neurodevelopmental outcome in ELBW infants who were at low perinatal risk and who had normal neurological exam. This study confirms strong association between low postnatal weight and adverse neurodevelopmental outcome. This association is stronger in infants with high perinatal risk factors and in infants with CNS impairment	(None)	No data on funding source
French 1999 99115141 (CNS + Growth+ All)	No significant association between antenatal corticosteroids and cerebral palsy, weight ratio at 3 years (median, IQR), height ratio median (IQR), head circumference ratio (median, IQR), and any disability (number, %)	Differential loss to follow-up not assessed Small number in severe group	No data on funding source

Evidence Table 10. Studies Evaluating Association of LBW and Bone and Growth Outcomes
Part III

Author, Year	Associations found			Potential Biases	Comments
Ford 2000 20380862 *overlapped sample with Doyle, 2001 21064379 in Lung table	Pubertal development was similar in VLBW and Normal BW infants. At all ages (2,5,8,14 yrs) the children who were VLBW were significantly smaller Wt/ Ht/ HC than normal BW children. Differences in Ht/ Wt/ improved over time, between VLBW and NBW, but VLBW remained smaller than Normal BW.			(None)	No data on funding source
Morley 2000 20167446	Trial 1 There was no association between the neonatal diet (banked donor milk vs preterm formula) and the 6 anthropometrics at any follow up point (9 mo, 18 mo and 7.5-8 yrs) (Growth at 9 mo) (Growth at 18 months) (Growth at 7.5-8 yrs) Trial 2 There was no association between neonatal diet (term vs preterm formula) and the Weight, Height, HC and skinfold thicknesses at any follow up point (18 mo and 7.5 yrs) Except for a significantly lower waist to hip ratio at 7.5 yrs in infants fed preterm vs term formula solely (without supplementation with mother's milk) (0.86 vs 0.89, p<0.001) (Growth at 18 mo) (Growth at 7.5-8 yrs)	Group A: Fed Banked donor milk (with or without supplementation with mother's milk) N=195 N=221 N=206 N= 168 N=181	Group B: Fed preterm formula:(with or without supplementation with mothers' milk) N=174 N=217 N=214 N=166 N=178		

Evidence Table 10. Studies Evaluating Association of LBW and Bone and Growth Outcomes

Part III

Author, Year	Associations found	Potential Biases	Comments
Avila-Diaz 2001 21334039	Study of bone mineral density using DEXA scan. Outcomes at 5 to 6 months; well preterms vs. fullterm. Full term infants (n = 16) had significantly higher (P < 0.05) bone mineral content and bone area in comparison to preterm infants (n = 26). Preterm infants had a significantly higher rate of increase in bone mineral content per day than full term infants suggesting incomplete "catch-up".	Only "healthy" premature infants enrolled Short duration of follow-up - six months Not clear that all preterms were VLBW	Study was government funded A study of bone mineralization in preterm vs. full-terms. Not clear if all preterms were less than 1500 g.

343

Evidence Table 11. Randomized Controlled Trials in LBW Neonates for Growth Outcomes
Part I

Author, Year UI#	Demographics	Inclusion Criteria	Exclusion Criteria	Disease/Condition Type (N)	Study Design (Duration)

Wauben 1998 98387708	Location: Canada
	Years of Birth: ND
	Mean GA (range), wk:
	  Sample 1: 29.9+1.9
	  Sample 2: 30.1+1.5
	  Sample 3: 29.7+1.7
	Mean BW (range), g:
	  Sample 1: 1400±200
	  Sample 2: 1300±200
	  Controls: 1200±200
	Male: ND
	Race: ND
	Enrolled: 37
	Evaluated: 37
	Number of sites: 1
		BWT<1800
		AGA
		>1 week old
		Full feed 5x5d
		Established weight gain
		No GI disease
		No long malformation
			ND	Sample 1: Milk + Fortifier (12)
				Sample 2: Milk + Calcium phosphorus (13)
				Sample 3: Preterm formula-fed (12)
					Randomized controlled trial (3 and 6 months)

344

Evidence Table 11. Randomized Controlled Trials in LBW Neonates for Growth Outcomes
Part I

Author, Year UI#	Demographics	Inclusion Criteria	Exclusion Criteria	Disease/Condition Type (N)	Study Design (Duration)
Morley 2000 20167446	Location: UK Years of Birth: ND Mean GA (range), wk: Trial 1: 　Group A: 31.1 　Group B: 31 Trial 2: 　Group A: 31 　Group B: 31.2 Mean BW (range), g: Trial 1: 　Group A: 1397±297 　Group B: 1387±278 Trial 2: 　Group A: 1399±301 　Group B: 1416±306 Male: Trial 1: 　Group A: 53% 　Group B: 52% Trial 2: 　Group A: 47% 　Group B: 46% Race: ND Enrolled: 833 Evaluated: 781 Number of sites: 5	Premature BW< 1850 g Survivors of participants in the two RCTs with 2 parallel arms each (assessing effect of different neonatal diets of growth) Age 7.5-8 yrs	Lost to follow-up	Trial 1: Group A: Premature infants, breast-fed until weight 2000 g or discharge (207) Group B: Premature infants, preterm formula-fed (213) Trial 2: Group A: Premature infants, standard term formula-fed until weight 2000 g or discharge (181) Group B: Premature infants, premature formula-fed (213)	RCT: Trial 1 and 2, with 2 parallel arms in each trial (at 9 months, 18 months, 7.5-8 years)

345

Evidence Table 11. Randomized Controlled Trials in LBW Neonates for Growth Outcomes
Part II

Author, Year	Predictors	Predictor Measures	Outcomes	Outcome Measures
Wauben 1998 98387708	Other: Feedings: Breast, Milk+ multinutrient fortifier or breast milk + Ca + P supplement only, or preterm formula	ND	Growth: 1) Weight, length, head circumference 2) Body mass + body composition	ND
Morley 2000 20167446	Trial 1: Type of diet in early neonatal period: Banked donor breast milk vs Preterm formula (with or without supplementation with its mother's milk) Trial 2: Preterm formula vs term formula (with or without supplementation with mother's milk)	Not further specified	Trial 1: Growth: Assessment at 9 and 18 months post-term: Weight (kg), Length (cm), HC, Subscapular skinfold thickness, Body mass index Assessment at 7.5 –8 yrs: All of the above, Also weight to hip ratio Trial 2: Growth at 18 mo Growth at 7.5-8 yrs	Not further specified

Evidence Table 11. Randomized Controlled Trials in LBW Neonates for Growth Outcomes
Part III

Author, Year	Associations found			Potential Biases	Comments
	MM+MNF	MM+CaCP	PTF		
Wauben, 1998	*Term:*			Used a "New multinutrient fortifier" design to their specifications. Generalizability?	Study was privately funded
	Weight (kg): 3.3±0.3	3.2±0.4	3.5±0.4	No relation examined between feeding + neurodevelopment. Unclear that their findings have or had any potential for clinical significance.	
	Length (cm): 49.6±1.3	48.4±1.8	49.4±2.3		
	12 months:			Small study- unlikely to find anything other than major differences	
	Weight (kg): 9.0±0.9	9.0±0.9	9.6±1.4	Post-discharge crossover between breast fed→formula fed, further dilutes effect or small #'s	
	Length (cm): 74.9±3.7	75.9±2.5	76.0±2.8		
	Head circumference (cm): 46.9±3.9	46.8±?	6.8±2.0	No correction for multiple comparison, although it is desperately needed	
	Whole body BMC (g): 209.9±27.1	223.0±29.2	243.9±40.6		
	Lean mass (%): 74.0±5.0	73±4.7	73.8±5.6		
	Fat mass (%): 23.6±5.0	24.3±4.7	23.9±5.6		
Morley, 2000	Trial 1: There was no association between the neonatal diet (banked donor milk vs preterm formula) and the 6 anthropometrics at any follow up point (9 mo, 18 mo and 7.5-8 yrs) Trial 2: There was no association between neonatal diet (term vs preterm formula) and the Weight, Height, HC and skinfold thickness at any follow up point (18 mo and 7.5 yrs). Except for a significantly lower waist to hip ratio at 7.5 yrs in infants fed preterm vs term formula solely (without supplementation with mother's milk) (0.86 vs 0.89, p<0.001)			(None)	? Funding

347

Evidence Table 12. Studies evaluating association of LBW and Nutritional Outcomes

Part I

Author, Year UI#	Demographics	Inclusion Criteria	Exclusion Criteria	Disease/Condition Type (N)	Study Design (Duration)
Kennedy 1999 20076945	Location: US Years of Birth: Jan-Dec 1994 Mean GA (range), wk: 31±2.6 (26-34)	Single or twin birth BW less 2000g, follow-up at hospital clinic, completion of 3 screening visits.	ND	Preterm LBW infants (28)	Retrospective cohort (4, 9, 18 months)
Also in growth paper	Mean BW (range), g: 1534±371 (810-2000) Male: ND Race: White 93% Enrolled: 28 Evaluated: 28 Number of sites: 1				

Part II

Author, Year	Predictors	Predictor Measures	Outcomes	Outcome Measures
Kennedy 1999 20076945	General : BW Other: 1) Nutrition/Growth 2) Discharge weight	ND	**Growth:** 1) weight and length 2) Head circumference	1)Denver II Developmental Test 2) "z"-Scroes

Part III

Author, Year	Associations found	Potential Biases	Comments
Kennedy 1999 20076945	**NICU discharge weight:** mean "z" score was-2.97+/- 0.53 below mean BW of term infants **18 months: mean growth in wt, hc&l** :WNL **Denver II:** normal at 18 months	Only 2 infants weighed less than 1kg Lowest GA 26 weeks 26/28 were white	No data on funding source

348

Evidence Table 13. Studies Evaluating Association of LBW and Other Outcomes
Part I

Author, Year UI#	Demographics	Inclusion Criteria	Exclusion Criteria	Disease/Condition Type (N)	Study Design (Duration)
Saarela 1999 99345620	Location: Finland Years of Birth: 1990-1994 Mean GA: Sample 1: 21.2±2.1 Sample 2: 29.3±2.4 Mean BW: Sample 1: 993±242 Sample 2: 1174±238 Male: Sample 1: 62% Sample 2: 54% Race: ND Enrolled: 174 Evaluated: 129 Number of sites: 1	BW<1500 GA<34	Death Multiple congenital anomalies Severe toxoplasmosis Lack of repeat renal n/s	Sample 1: Preterm infants with nephrocalcinosis 26) Sample 2: Preterm infants without Nephrocalcinosis (103)	Prospective cohort (6 years)
Saarela 1999 20069000	Location: Finland Years of Birth: 1990-1994 Mean GA: Sample 1: 26.7 ±2 Sample 2: 27.2 ±2 Mean BW: Sample 1: 905 ±209 Sample 2: 957 ±226 Male: Sample 1: 30% Sample 2: 50% Race: ND Enrolled : ND for total (enrolled cases: 29) Evaluated : 40 Number of sites: 1	Cases with nephrocalcinosis: VLBW treated in the NICU of Oulu University Hospital Born during 1990-1994 Control cases: Matched to the cases VLBW: nearest to the index cases in the hospital records Difference from case's BW less than 250 g Negative renal U/S during neonatal period for nephrocalcinosis Age difference during f/up renal examination less than 8 months from the index cases.	Urinary incontinence	Sample 1: Cases with Neonatal Nephrocalcinosis(20) Sample 2: Controls, matched control cases without neonatal nephrocalcinosis (20)	Prospective comparative longitudinal study [Follow up during early childhood (not specified but the mean age during f/up assessment was 4.6 yrs)

349

Evidence Table 13. Studies Evaluating Association of LBW and Other Outcomes

Part I

Author, Year UI#	Demographics	Inclusion Criteria	Exclusion Criteria	Disease/Condition Type (N)	Study Design (Duration)
Slonim 2000 20214515	Location: USA Years of Birth: 1992-1994 Mean GA: Sample 1: 1704.3 ±52.7 Sample 2: ND Mean BW: Sample 1: 30.9 ±0.2 Sample 2: ND Male: Sample 1: 57% Sample 2: 58% Race: ND Enrolled: 5927 Evaluated: 5750 Number of sites: 16	Patients with prematurity (<37 wks) and either an anatomic defect (congenital heart disease, GI tract anatomic lesion, neurologic complications (e.g., spina bifida, pulmonary lesions e.g., pulmonary agenesis)) or a prematurity related complication (BPD, Hydrocephalus, IVH, Short gut syndrome, trecheostomy, birth asphyxia, cerebral palsy) Admitted in any of the 16 participating in the study PICUs During period 12/1992-12/1994	Patients admitted in PICU in continuous cardiopulmonary resuscitation. Patients not reaching stable vital signs for > 2 hrs	Sample 1 Formerly premature patients admitted in PICU (FPP) (431) Sample 2 Their complement formerly nonpremature admitted in PICU (5.319)	Cross sectional study (FPP were assessed at a mean age of 35 mo and formerly nonprematures were assessed at a mean age of 72 mo in the 2 groups respectively)

350

Evidence Table 13. Studies Evaluating Association of LBW and Other Outcomes
Part II

Author, Year	Predictors	Predictor Measure	Outcomes	Outcome Measures
Saarela 1999 99345620	General : 1) BW 2) GA Audiology: 1) Furosemide Cardiovascular or Pulmonary: 1) Chronic Lung disease Other: 1) Dexamethasone 2) Furosemide use	ND	Other: Nephrocalcinosis	Described natural resolution of nephrocalcinosis

Evidence Table 13. Studies Evaluating Association of LBW and Other Outcomes
Part II

Author, Year	Predictors	Predictor Measure	Outcomes	Outcome Measures
Saarela 1999 20069000	**General:** 1) Neonatal nephrocalcinosis in VLBW infants	Nephrocalcinosis defined by the presence of medullay echogenic densities in the renal tubular pyramids	**General:** Renal function during early childhood (4-5 yrs) 1) Renal tubular function 2) Distal tubular acidification capacity 3) Renal glomerular function ∧ Serum electrolytes ∧ Venous blood pH, pCO2, Base excess, bicarbonates ∧ Urine pH, ∧ Urine β2-microglobulin ∧ Ca/Cr ∧ Ca/Na ∧ Acetazolamide acidification test ∧ Other variables: ∧ Ccr (ml/min/1.73 m2) ∧ FENa (%) ∧ FEK (%) ∧ Tubular reabsorption of Phosphate (TRP) (%) ∧ Maximum tubular reabsorption of phosphate per glomerular filtration rate (TmP/GFR: mmol/l) 4) Kidney growth 5) Systolic blood pressure	Tubular reabsorption of phospate and maximal tubular reabsorption of phosphate per glomerular filtration rate were calculated from the baseline urine and blood sample data. Creatinine clearance were calculated by the method described by Schwartz

Evidence Table 13. Studies Evaluating Association of LBW and Other Outcomes
Part II

Author, Year	Predictors	Predictor Measure	Outcomes	Outcome Measures
Slonim 2000 20214515	**General:** 1) Prematurity with anatomic abnormalities and/or complications of prematurity (prematures vs nonprematures) 2) GA (<26 wks vs 26-32 wks vs >32 wks)	Anatomic abnormalities: Congenital heart disease Anatomical lesions of the GI tract Neurologic abnormalities: such as spina bifida Pulmonary lesions: such as pulmonary agenesis Complications of prematurity: BPD Birth asphyxia Cerebral palsy	**General:** 1) Characteristics of utilization of chronic care resources, PICU resources and characteristics of their PICU admissions: 2) Age of PICU admission 3) PICU readmissions during same hospitalization 4) Chronic care resources utilization 5) At least one chronic care resource used 6) Prior living conditions 7) Discharge location 8) PICU resource use 9) Length of stay in PICU (mean days) 10) PRISM-III score (mean)	Chronic care resources utilization: Ventilator Tracheostomy Gastrostomy Parental nutrition Prior living conditions: Home Institutions Never discharged Chronic hospital Discharge location Home Routine care Intermediate care Another PICU Chronic care PICU resource use: Ventilator Vasopressors Arterial catheter Central venous catheter PRISM-II scores: at first 24 hrs of PICU admission

Evidence Table 13. Studies Evaluating Association of LBW and Other Outcomes
Part III

Author, Year	Associations found			Potential Biases	Comments
Saarela 1999 99345620	Occurrence of nephrocalcinosis (NC) by birth weight.			(None)	Study was privately funded
	BW group	n	% without NC	% with peripheral NC	% with extensive NC		
	<750g	8	50%	25%	25%		
	751-999	36	65%	20%	15%		
	1000-1249	33	85%	5%	10%		
	1250-1499	52	90%	7%	3%		

Association of BW with NC sigificant at P< 0.001.
NC was also significantly associated (p<0.001) with: Gestational age, Presence of RDS, Presence of BPD (O2 at 28 days), Presence of CLD (O2 at 36 weeks), Furosemide use, Dexamethasone use

Evidence Table 13. Studies Evaluating Association of LBW and Other Outcomes
Part III

Author, Year	Associations found	Potential Biases	Comments
Saarela 1999 20069000	Predictors of renal outcome at age 4-5 yr 1) Neonatal nephrocalcinosis in VLBW children seems to lead to some signs of renal tubular dysfunction in early childhood. 2) However, distal tubular acidification, as measured by the actazolamide test 3) and glomerular function appears not to be specifically disturbed by nephrocalcinosis Renal function during early childhood (mean age: 4.6 yrs) Renal tubular function: ⋏ Urinary calcium /Cr and (p<0.004) ⋏ ß2-microglobulin/Cr excretion were higher in the children with nephrocalcinosis (p<0.05) ⋏ There was no difference in the fractional excretion of Na, K, or tubular reabsorption of phospate Distal Tubular Acidification capacity: • There was no difference in the distal tubular acidification capacity, as tested by the acetazolamide test : Abnormal response: Renal glomerular function: ⋏ Creatinine clearance was no different between the 2 groups There was no difference between the 2 groups in the following : ⋏ Serum electrolytes ⋏ Venous blood pH, pCO2, Base excess, bicarbonates ⋏ Urine pH, Kidney growth: ⋏ Kidney growth was impaired by more than 2 SD ⋏ There was no difference in the systolic blood pressure above 97.5 percentile ⋏ None of the children had hematuria		

355

Evidence Table 13. Studies Evaluating Association of LBW and Other Outcomes
Part III

Author, Year	Associations found	Potential Biases	Comments
Slonim 2000 20214515	Utilization of chronic care resources and PICU resources and characteristics of their PICU admissions of former prematures with a prematurity-related complication or an anatomical deformity [431] when compared to nonprematures [5319] was: • PICU survivors: 90% vs 94% (p=0.008) • Age of PICU admission (mean): 35 mo vs 72 mo (p=0.01) • Postoperative care (%): 44% vs 40% (p=0.15) • Prior PICU admissions: 11% vs 5.5% (p=0.01) Chronic care resources utilization: • Ventilator: 7% vs 1% (p=0.001) Tracheostomy: 16% vs 2% (p=0.001) • Gastrostomy: 23% vs 4% (p=0.001) • Parental nutrition: 3% vs 0.6% (p=0.001) At least one chronic care resource used: 30% vs 5.6% , p=0.001 Prior living conditions: • Home: 90% vs 97% (p=0.001) Institutions: 3% vs 1% (p=0.001) • Never discharged: 6.5% vs 2% (p=0.002) • Chronic hospital: 3% vs 1% (p=0.001) Discharge location • Home: 11% vs 6% (p=0.001) Routine care: 63% vs 77% (p=0.001) • Intermediate care: 15% vs 10% (p=0.03) • Another PICU: 1% vs 1.6% (p=0.52) • Chronic care: 1.6% vs 0.7% (p=0.02) PICU resource use: • Ventilator: 45% vs 35% (p=0.007) • Vasopressors: 15% vs 16% (p=0.12) • Arterial catheter: 28% vs 36% (p=0.006) • Central venous catheter: 17% vs 21% (p=0.03) Limits to care (%): 5.5% vs 4% (p=0.11) Length of stay in PICU (mean days): 5.98 ds vs 3.56 ds (p=0.01) PRISM-III score AT 24 HRS (mean): 4.90 vs 4.53 (p=0.80) Those born < 26 wks had a higher utilization of chronic care resources (ventilator, trachesostomy, gastrostomy) and chronic hospital care (p< 0.006) as compared to the other prematures.	There is a strong selection bias in this study as the inclusion criteria used for the selection of the FPPs were strongly correlated with the outcomes studied (the presence of an anatomic abnormality (150/431) or a complication of prematurity (281/483) in FPPs is strongly Correlated with the utilization of chronic care resources)	Funding: Not Reported

356